# CARDIOVASCULAR PHYSIOLOGY CONCEPTS

SECOND EDITION

# CARDIOVASCULAR PHYSIOLOGY CONCEPTS

SECOND EDITION

**Richard E. Klabunde, Ph.D.**

Associate Professor of Physiology

Department of Biomedical Sciences

Ohio University College of Osteopathic Medicine

Athens, Ohio

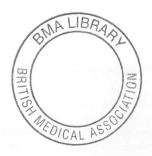

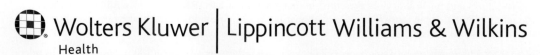

Wolters Kluwer | Lippincott Williams & Wilkins
Health

Philadelphia • Baltimore • New York • London
Buenos Aires • Hong Kong • Sydney • Tokyo

*Acquisitions Editor*: Crystal Taylor
*Product Manager*: Catherine Noonan
*Marketing Manager*: Joy Fisher-Williams
*Vendor Manager*: Bridgett Dougherty
*Manufacturing Manager*: Margie Orzech
*Designer*: Teresa Mallon
*Compositor*: SPi Global

Second Edition

351 West Camden Street
Baltimore, MD 21201

Two Commerce Square
2001 Market Street
Philadelphia, PA 19103

First Edition, 2005

**Library of Congress Cataloging-in-Publication Data**

Klabunde, Richard E.
Cardiovascular physiology concepts / Richard E. Klabunde. — 2nd ed.
p. ; cm.
Includes bibliographical references and index.
ISBN 978-1-4511-1384-6
1. Cardiovascular system—Physiology. I. Title.
[DNLM: 1. Cardiovascular Physiological Phenomena. 2. Heart Diseases—physiopathology. WG 102]
QP101.K553 2012
612.1—dc23

2011014577

To purchase additional copies of this book, call our customer service department at (800) 638-3030 or fax orders to (301) 223-2320. International customers should call (301) 223-2300.

Visit Lippincott Williams & Wilkins on the Internet: http://www.lww.com. Lippincott Williams & Wilkins customer service representatives are available from 8:30 am to 6:00 PM, EST.

9 8 7 6 5 4

CCS0614

# PREFACE

Cardiovascular physiology textbooks have traditionally emphasized biophysical principles such as the behavior of flowing blood, mechanics of muscle contraction, and feedback control systems. In the past two decades, we have gained considerable knowledge about endothelial function, membrane receptors, ion channels, and signal transduction mechanisms that regulate cardiac and vascular function. This new insight into cellular mechanisms has revolutionized not only our understanding of cardiovascular function but also how physicians diagnose and treat patients with cardiovascular disease. *Cardiovascular Physiology Concepts* was written to provide medical, graduate, and allied health science students with a firm foundation in traditional biophysical principles and newer cellular physiology principles.

This textbook incorporates several features to aid the reader in learning: (1) each chapter begins with a list of learning objectives to direct the reader to key concepts, (2) the text is supplemented with problems and clinical cases used to reinforce fundamental physiological concepts, (3) important concepts are summarized at the end of each chapter, (4) relevant reading resources are listed in the chapters, and (5) review questions with explanations are provided as a self-assessment tool for the reader.

Many topics presented in this textbook are placed in a medical context by describing how underlying physiologic concepts relate to disease states, such as arrhythmia, abnormal blood pressure, and heart failure, and to clinical diagnosis and therapeutic intervention. Several of the chapters contain clinical cases to illustrate clinical applications of important physiologic concepts.

The first eight chapters discuss cardiovascular physiology following a traditional organization of topics. The last chapter integrates the material in the preceding chapters by describing how the cardiovascular system responds and adapts to increased demands by the body (e.g., exercise and pregnancy) or to pathophysiologic conditions (e.g., hypotension, hypertension, heart failure, and cardiac valve disease).

Although the basic format of the second edition is similar to the first edition, many chapter sections have been rewritten to enhance clarity and to update our knowledge on specific topics. More than half the figures have been revised or are new in the second edition. Much of the material that was formerly found in an accompanying CD-ROM has now been revised and incorporated into the printed second edition.

Cardiovascular physiology, like all areas of biomedical science, can be overwhelming in the amount of knowledge presented to the reader. For this reason, I have endeavored to present fundamental concepts at a level suitable for medical students in their preclinical years of training. These concepts will be more than sufficient to provide a necessary framework for understanding cardiovascular pharmacology and therapeutics, and cardiovascular pathophysiology. It is my hope that the reader will not only learn how the cardiovascular system functions but will also become awed at the magnificence of the human body.

*Richard E. Klabunde, PhD*
*Athens, Ohio*

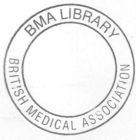

v

# ACKNOWLEDGMENTS

I want to acknowledge the inspiration I received from my graduate advisor, Paul C. Johnson, who taught me by his example to strive for excellence in both teaching and research. I am also grateful to the other physiology faculty at the University of Arizona in the early 1970s for their contagious love and enthusiasm for physiology. Feedback from medical students I have taught for more than 30 years has been invaluable in stimulating me to explore new ways to more effectively teach cardiovascular physiology. I appreciate the helpful suggestions from those who critically reviewed the first edition. These individuals offered many valuable comments that served to enrich the content and format of this second edition. I also want to thank all the talented people at Lippincott Williams & Wilkins who have worked with me on this textbook. Special gratitude is reserved for my loving and patient wife Karen, our four sons, and my parents who always encouraged me to pursue my dreams. Finally, I want to thank God for enabling me to fulfill my dreams.

*Richard E. Klabunde, PhD*
*Athens, Ohio*

# CONTENTS

# INTRODUCTION TO THE CARDIOVASCULAR SYSTEM

Understanding the concepts presented in this chapter will enable the student to:

1. Explain why large organisms require a circulatory system, while single-cell and small multicellular organisms do not.

2. Explain the significance of the series and parallel arrangement of the cardiac chambers, pulmonary circulation, and major organs of the systemic circulation.

3. Describe the pathways for the flow of blood through the heart chambers and large vessels associated with the heart.

4. Explain the importance of negative feedback systems for the control of arterial blood pressure.

## THE NEED FOR A CIRCULATORY SYSTEM

All living cells require metabolic substrates (e.g., oxygen, amino acids, glucose) and a mechanism by which they can remove by-products of metabolism (e.g., carbon dioxide, lactic acid). Single-cell organisms exchange these substances directly with their environment through diffusion and cellular transport systems. In contrast, most cells of large organisms have limited or no exchange capacity with their environment because their cells are not in contact with the outside environment. Nevertheless, exchange with the outside environment must occur for the cells to function. To accomplish this necessary exchange, large organisms have a sophisticated system of blood vessels that facilitates the exchange of substances between cells and blood and between blood and environment. The smallest of these blood vessels, capillaries, are in close proximity to all cells in the body, thereby permitting exchange to occur. For example, each cell in skeletal muscle is surrounded by two or more capillaries. This arrangement of capillaries around cells ensures that exchange can occur between blood and surrounding cells.

Exchange between blood and the outside environment occurs in several different organs: lungs, gastrointestinal tract, kidneys, and skin. As blood passes through the lungs, oxygen and carbon dioxide are exchanged between the blood in the pulmonary capillaries and the gases found within the lung alveoli. Oxygen-enriched blood is then transported to the organs where the oxygen diffuses from the blood into the surrounding cells. At the same time, carbon dioxide, a metabolic waste product, diffuses from the tissue cells into the blood and is transported to the lungs, where exchange occurs between blood and alveolar gases.

Blood passing through the intestine picks up glucose, amino acids, fatty acids, and other ingested substances that have been transported from the intestinal lumen into the blood in the intestinal wall by the cells lining the intestine. The blood then delivers these substances to organs such as the liver for additional metabolic processing and to cells throughout the body as an energy source.

Some of the waste products of these cells are taken up by the blood and transported to other organs for metabolic processing and final elimination into the outside environment through either the gastrointestinal tract or the kidneys.

Cells require a proper balance of water and electrolytes (e.g., sodium, potassium, and calcium) to function. The circulation transports ingested water and electrolytes from the intestine to cells throughout the body, including those of the kidneys, where excessive amounts of water and electrolytes can be eliminated in the urine.

The skin also serves as a site for exchange of water and electrolytes (through sweating), and for exchange of heat, which is a major by-product of cellular metabolism that must be removed from the body. Blood flow through the skin regulates heat loss from the body.

In summary, the ultimate purpose of the cardiovascular system is to facilitate exchange of gases, fluid, electrolytes, large molecules, and heat between cells and the outside environment. The heart and vasculature ensure that adequate blood flow is delivered to organs so that this exchange can take place.

## THE ARRANGEMENT OF THE CARDIOVASCULAR SYSTEM

The cardiovascular system has two primary components: the heart and blood vessels. A third component, the lymphatic system, does not contain blood, but nonetheless serves an important exchange function in conjunction with blood vessels.

The heart can be viewed functionally as two pumps with the pulmonary and systemic circulations situated between the two pumps (Fig. 1.1). The **pulmonary circulation** is the blood flow within the lungs that is involved in the exchange of gases between the blood and alveoli. The **systemic circulation** is comprised of all the blood vessels within and outside of organs excluding the lungs. The right side of the heart comprises the right atrium and the right ventricle. The **right atrium** receives venous blood from the systemic circulation, and the **right ventricle** pumps it into the pulmonary circulation where oxygen and carbon dioxide are exchanged between the blood and alveolar gases. The left side of the heart comprises the left atrium and the left ventricle. The blood leaving the lungs enters

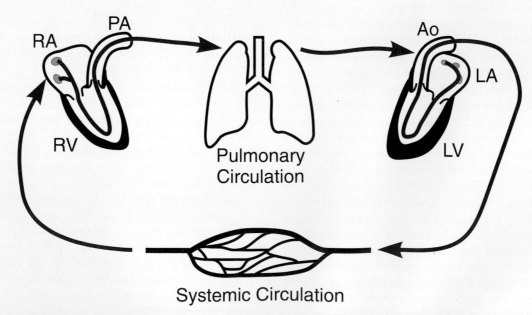

■ **FIGURE 1.1** Overview of the cardiovascular system. The right side of the heart, pulmonary circulation, left side of the heart, and systemic circulation are arranged in series. *RA*, right atrium; *RV*, right ventricle; *PA*, pulmonary artery; *Ao*, aorta; *LA*, left atrium; *LV*, left ventricle.

the **left atrium** by way of the pulmonary veins. Blood then flows from the left atrium into the left ventricle. The **left ventricle** ejects the blood into the **aorta**, which then distributes the blood to all the organs via the arterial system. Within the organs, the vasculature branches into smaller and smaller vessels, eventually forming capillaries, which are the primary site of exchange. Blood flow from the capillaries enters veins, which return blood flow to the right atrium via large systemic veins (the superior and inferior vena cava).

As blood flows through organs, some of the fluid, along with electrolytes and small amounts of protein, leaves the circulation and enters the tissue interstitium (a process termed fluid filtration). The **lymphatic vessels**, which are closely associated with small blood vessels within the tissue, collect the excess fluid from within the tissue interstitium and transport it back into the venous circulation by way of lymphatic ducts that empty into large veins (subclavian veins) above the right atrium.

It is important to note the overall arrangement of the cardiovascular system. First, the right and left sides of the heart, which are separated by the pulmonary and systemic circulations, are **in series** with each other (see Fig. 1.1). Therefore, all of the blood that is pumped from the right ventricle enters into the pulmonary circulation and then into the left side of the heart from where it is pumped into the systemic circulation before returning to the heart. This in-series relationship of the two sides of the heart and the pulmonary and systemic circulations requires that the output (volume of blood ejected per unit time) of each side of the heart closely matches the output of the other so that there are no major blood volume shifts between the pulmonary and systemic circulations. Second, most of the major organ systems of the body receive their blood from the aorta, and the blood leaving these organs enters into the venous system (superior and inferior vena cava) that returns the blood to the heart. Therefore, the circulations of most major organ systems are **in parallel** as shown in Figure 1.2. One major exception is the liver, which receives a large fraction of its blood supply from the venous circulation of the intestinal tract that drains into the

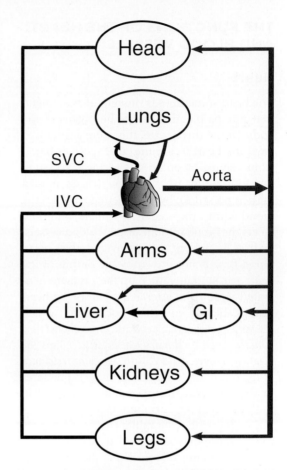

**■ FIGURE 1.2** Parallel arrangement of organs within the body. One major exception is the hepatic (liver) circulation, which receives blood flow from the hepatic portal veins of the gastrointestinal (*GI*) circulation (series) and from the aorta via the hepatic artery (parallel). *SVC,* superior vena cava; *IVC,* inferior vena cava.

hepatic portal system to supply the liver. The liver also receives blood from the aorta via the hepatic artery. Therefore, most of the liver circulation is in series with the intestinal circulation, while some of the liver circulation is in parallel with the intestinal circulation (see Chapter 7).

The parallel arrangement has significant hemodynamic implications as described in Chapter 5. Briefly, *the parallel arrangement of major vascular beds prevents blood flow changes in one organ from significantly affecting blood flow in other organs.* In contrast, when vascular beds are in series, blood flow changes in one vascular bed significantly alter blood flow to the other vascular bed.

## THE FUNCTIONS OF THE HEART AND BLOOD VESSELS

### Heart

The heart sometimes is thought of as an organ that pumps blood through the organs of the body. While this is true, it is more accurate to view the heart as a pump that receives blood from venous blood vessels at a low pressure, imparts energy to the blood (raises it to a higher pressure) by contracting around the blood within the cardiac chambers, and then ejects the blood into the arterial blood vessels.

It is important to understand that organ blood flow is not driven by the output of the heart per se, but rather by the pressure generated within the arterial system as the heart pumps blood into the vasculature, which serves as a resistance network. *Organ blood flow is determined by the arterial pressure minus the venous pressure, divided by the vascular resistance of the organ* (see Chapters 5 and 7). Pressures in the cardiovascular system are expressed in millimeters of mercury (mm Hg) above atmospheric pressure. One millimeter of mercury is the pressure exerted by a 1-mm vertical column of mercury (1 mm Hg is the equivalent of 1.36 cm $H_2O$ hydrostatic pressure). Vascular resistance is determined by the size of blood vessels, the anatomical arrangement of the vascular network, and the viscosity of the blood flowing within the vasculature.

The right atrium receives systemic venous blood (venous return) at very low pressures (near 0 mm Hg) (Fig. 1.3). This venous return then passes through the right atrium and fills the right ventricle; atrial contraction also contributes to the ventricular filling. Right ventricular contraction ejects blood from the right ventricle into the pulmonary artery. This generates a maximal pressure (systolic pressure) that ranges from 20 to 30 mm Hg within the pulmonary artery. As the blood passes through the pulmonary circulation, the blood pressure falls to about 10 mm Hg. The left atrium receives the pulmonary venous blood, which then flows passively into the left ventricle; atrial contraction provides a small amount of additional filling of the left

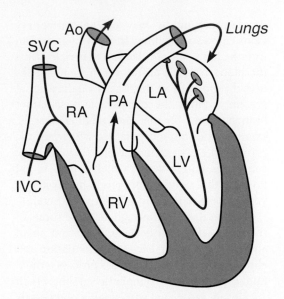

■ **FIGURE 1.3** Blood flow within the heart. Venous blood returns to the right atrium (*RA*) via the superior (*SVC*) and inferior vena cava (*IVC*). Blood passes from the RA into the right ventricle (*RV*), which ejects the blood into the pulmonary artery (*PA*). After passing through the lungs, the blood flows into the left atrium (*LA*) and then fills the left ventricle (*LV*), which ejects the blood into the aorta (*Ao*) for distribution to the different organs of the body.

ventricle. As the left ventricle contracts and ejects blood into the systemic arterial system, a relatively high pressure is generated (100 to 140 mm Hg maximal or systolic pressure). Therefore, *the left ventricle is a high-pressure pump, in contrast to the right ventricle, which is a low-pressure pump*. Details of the pumping action of the heart are found in Chapter 4.

The pumping activity of the heart is usually expressed in terms of its cardiac output, which is the amount of blood ejected with each contraction (i.e., stroke volume) multiplied by the heart rate. Any factor that alters heart rate or stroke volume will alter the cardiac output. The heart rate is determined by specialized cells within the heart that act as electrical pacemakers, and their activity is increased or decreased by autonomic nerves and hormones (see Chapter 2). The action potentials generated by these pacemaker cells are conducted throughout the heart and trigger contraction of cardiac myocytes (see Chapter 3). This results in ventricular contraction and ejection of blood. The force of ventricular contraction, and therefore stroke volume, is regulated by mechanisms intrinsic to the heart, by autonomic nerves and hormones (see Chapters 3, 4, and 6).

The heart has other important functions besides pumping blood. The heart synthesizes several hormones. One of these hormones, atrial natriuretic peptide, plays an important role in the regulation of blood volume and blood pressure (see Chapter 6). Sensory nerve receptors associated with the heart play a role in regulating the release of antidiuretic hormone from the posterior pituitary, which regulates water loss by the kidneys.

## Vascular System

*Blood vessels constrict and dilate to regulate arterial blood pressure, alter blood flow within organs, regulate capillary blood pressure, and distribute blood volume within the body.* Changes in vascular diameters are brought about by activation of vascular smooth muscle within the vascular wall by autonomic nerves, metabolic and biochemical signals from outside of the blood vessel, and vasoactive substances released by endothelial cells that line the blood vessels (see Chapters 3, 5, and 6).

Blood vessels have other functions besides distribution of blood flow and exchange. The endothelium lining blood vessels produces substances that modulate hemostasis (blood clotting) and inflammatory responses (see Chapter 3).

## Interdependence of Circulatory and Organ Function

Cardiovascular function is closely linked to the function of other organs. For example, the brain not only receives blood flow to support its metabolism but also acts as a control center for regulating cardiovascular function. A second example of the interdependence between organ function and the circulation is the kidney. The kidneys excrete varying amounts of sodium, water, and other molecules to maintain fluid and electrolyte homeostasis. Blood passing through the kidneys is filtered, and the kidneys then modify the composition of the filtrate to form urine. Reduced blood flow to the kidneys can have detrimental effects on kidney function and therefore on fluid and electrolyte balance in the body. Furthermore, renal dysfunction can lead to large increases in blood volume, which can precipitate cardiovascular changes that can lead to hypertension or exacerbate heart failure. In summary, organ function is dependent on the circulation of blood, and cardiovascular function is dependent on the function of organs.

## THE REGULATION OF CARDIAC AND VASCULAR FUNCTION

The cardiovascular system must be able to adapt to changing conditions and demands of the body. For example, when a person exercises, increased metabolic activity of contracting skeletal muscle requires large increases in nutrient supply (particularly oxygen) and enhanced removal of metabolic by-products (e.g., carbon dioxide, lactic acid). To meet this demand, blood vessels within the exercising muscle dilate to increase blood flow; however, blood flow can only be increased if the arterial pressure is maintained. Arterial pressure is maintained during exercise by increasing cardiac output and by constricting blood vessels in other organs of the body (see Chapter 9). If these changes were not to occur, arterial blood pressure would fall precipitously during exercise, thereby limiting organ perfusion and exercise capacity. Therefore, a coordinated cardiovascular response is required to permit increased muscle blood flow while a person exercises. Another example of adaptation occurs when a person stands up. Gravitational forces cause blood to pool in the legs when a person assumes an upright body posture (see Chapter 5). In the absence of regulatory mechanisms, this pooling will lead to a fall in cardiac output and arterial pressure, which can cause a person to faint because of reduced blood flow to the brain. To prevent this from happening, coordinated reflex responses increase heart rate and constrict blood vessels to maintain a normal arterial blood pressure when a person stands.

It is important to control arterial blood pressure because it provides the driving

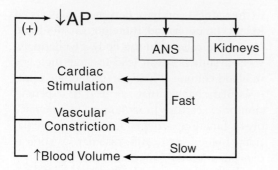

■ **FIGURE 1.4** Feedback control of arterial pressure (*AP*) by the autonomic nervous system (*ANS*) and kidneys. A sudden fall in AP elicits a rapid baroreceptor reflex that activates the ANS to stimulate the heart (increasing cardiac output) and constrict blood vessels to restore AP. The kidneys respond to decreased AP by retaining $Na^+$ and water to increase blood volume, which helps to restore AP. The (+) indicates the restoration of arterial pressure following the initial fall in pressure (i.e., a negative feedback response).

force for organ perfusion. As described in Chapter 6, neural and hormonal (neurohumoral) mechanisms regulating cardiovascular function are under the control of pressure sensors located in arteries and veins (i.e., baroreceptors). These **baroreceptors**, through their afferent neural connections to the brain, provide the central nervous system with information regarding the status of blood pressure in the body. A decrease in arterial pressure from its normal operating point elicits a rapid baroreceptor reflex that stimulates the heart to increase cardiac output and constricts blood vessels to restore arterial pressure (Fig. 1.4). These cardiovascular adjustments occur through rapid changes in **autonomic nerve activity** (particularly through sympathetic nerves) to the heart and vasculature. **Negative feedback** control mechanisms, as this example illustrates, can be defined as a process in which a deviation from some condition (e.g., normal arterial pressure) leads to responses (e.g., cardiac stimulation and vasoconstriction) that diminish the deviation.

In addition to altering autonomic nerve activity, a fall in arterial pressure stimulates the release of **hormones** that help to restore arterial pressure by acting on the heart and blood vessels; they also increase arterial pressure by increasing blood volume through

their actions on renal function. In contrast to the rapidly acting autonomic mechanisms, hormonal mechanisms acting on the kidneys require hours or days to achieve their full effect on blood volume. Hormonal mechanisms include secretion of catecholamines (chiefly epinephrine) by the adrenal glands; release of renin by the kidneys, which triggers the formation of angiotensin II and aldosterone; and release of antidiuretic hormone (vasopressin) by the posterior pituitary. Hormones such as angiotensin II, aldosterone, and vasopressin are particularly important because they act on the kidneys to increase blood volume, which increases cardiac output and arterial pressure.

In summary, arterial pressure is monitored by the body and ordinarily is maintained within narrow limits by negative feedback mechanisms that adjust cardiac function, systemic vascular resistance, and blood volume. This control is accomplished by changes in autonomic nerve activity to the heart and vasculature, as well as by changes in circulating hormones that influence cardiac, vascular, and renal function.

## THE CONTENT OF THE FOLLOWING CHAPTERS

This textbook emphasizes our current knowledge of cellular physiology as well as the classical biophysical concepts that have been used for decades to describe cardiac and vascular function. Chapter 2 describes the electrical activity within the heart, both at the cellular and whole organ level. Chapter 3 builds a foundation of cellular physiology by emphasizing intracellular mechanisms that regulate cardiac and vascular smooth muscle contraction. These cellular concepts are reinforced repeatedly in subsequent chapters. Chapter 4 examines cardiac mechanical function. Chapter 5 summarizes concepts of vascular function and the biophysics of blood flow in the context of regulation of arterial and venous blood pressures. Neurohumoral mechanisms regulating cardiac and vascular function are described in Chapter 6. Chapter 7 describes the flow of blood within different organs, with an emphasis on local regulatory mechanisms. Chapter 8 addresses the ultimate purpose of the cardiovascular system, that is, the exchange of nutrients, gases, and fluid between the blood and tissues. Finally, Chapter 9 integrates concepts described in earlier chapters by examining how the cardiovascular system responds to altered demands and disease states.

## SUMMARY OF IMPORTANT CONCEPTS

- Large organisms require a circulatory system so that metabolic substrates and by-products of cellular metabolism can be efficiently exchanged between cells and the outside environment, as well as transported to distant sites within the body.

- Venous blood returns to the right side of the heart, which pumps the blood into the pulmonary circulation where oxygen and carbon dioxide are exchanged with the gases found within the lung alveoli. Oxygenated blood from the lungs enters the left side of the heart, which pumps the blood at high pressure into the aorta for distribution to various organs via large distributing arteries. Small capillaries within the organs serve as the primary site of nutrient exchange.

- Blood flow within organs is determined primarily by the arterial pressure and by changes in the diameters of blood vessels within the organs brought about by contraction or relaxation of smooth muscle within the walls of the blood vessels.

- Most major organ systems are in parallel with each other so that blood flow in one organ has relatively little influence on blood flow in another organ.

- Negative feedback mechanisms such as the baroreceptor reflex, acting through autonomic nerves and circulating hormones, help to maintain normal arterial pressure.

## REVIEW QUESTIONS

For each question, choose the one best answer:

1. The cardiovascular system
   a. Aids in the transfer of heat energy from organs deep within the body to the outside environment.
   b. Comprises pulmonary and systemic circulations that are in parallel with each other.
   c. Transports carbon dioxide from the lungs to tissues within organs.
   d. Transports oxygen from individual cells to the lungs.

2. Which of the following statements concerning the heart is true?
   a. Cardiac output is the product of ventricular stroke volume and heart rate.
   b. The right and left ventricles are in parallel.

   c. The right ventricle generates higher pressures than the left ventricle during contraction.
   d. The right ventricle receives blood from the pulmonary veins.

3. A patient complains of becoming "light headed" when he is standing upright. Blood pressure measurements reveal a significant fall in arterial pressure upon standing. Which of the following is a likely explanation of this patient's condition?
   a. Excessive activation of baroreceptor negative feedback mechanisms
   b. Excessive fluid retention by the kidneys
   c. Increased heart rate
   d. Reduced cardiac output

## ANSWERS TO REVIEW QUESTIONS

1. The correct answer is "a" because blood flow carries heat from the deep organs within the body to the skin where the heat energy can be given off to the environment. Choice "b" is incorrect because the pulmonary and systemic circulations are in series. Choice "c" is incorrect because carbon dioxide is transported from the tissues to the lungs. Choice "d" is incorrect because blood transports oxygen from the lungs to the tissues.

2. The correct answer is "a" because when the volume per beat (stroke volume) is multiplied by the number of beats per minute (heart rate), the units become volume per minute, which is the flow out of the heart (cardiac output). Choice "b" is incorrect because the right and left ventricles are in series. Choice "c" is incorrect because the left ventricle generates much higher pressures than the right ventricle during contraction. Choice "d" is incorrect because the pulmonary veins empty into the left atrium.

3. The correct answer is "d" because when a person stands up, blood pools in the legs, which reduces the filling of the heart and leads to a fall in cardiac output and arterial pressure, and a decrease in brain blood flow. Choice "a" is incorrect because activation of baroreceptor negative feedback mechanisms ordinarily helps to maintain arterial pressure when standing. Choice "b" is incorrect because increased fluid retention by the kidneys elevates cardiac output and arterial pressure. Choice "c" is incorrect because increased heart rate when standing, which is brought about by the baroreceptor reflex, helps to maintain cardiac output and arterial pressure.

# ELECTRICAL ACTIVITY
# OF THE HEART

# 2

Understanding the concepts presented in this chapter will enable the student to:

1. Describe how changing the concentrations of sodium, potassium, and calcium ions inside and outside the cell affect the resting membrane potential in cardiac cells.

2. Explain why the resting potential is near the equilibrium potential for potassium and the peak of an action potential approaches the equilibrium potential for sodium.

3. Describe the mechanisms that maintain ion concentration gradients across the cardiac cell membrane.

4. Describe the role of voltage-gated $Na^+$, $K^+$, and $Ca^{++}$ channels in the generation of action potentials in pacemaker and nonpacemaker cells of the heart.

5. Describe how autonomic nerves, circulating catecholamines, extracellular potassium concentrations, thyroid hormone, and hypoxia alter pacemaker activity.

6. Describe the role of afterdepolarizations and reentry in the generation of tachycardias.

7. Describe the normal pathways for action potential conduction within the heart and how autonomic nerves, circulating catecholamines, and cellular hypoxia alter conduction velocity within the heart.

8. Describe what each of the waves, intervals, and segments of a normal electrocardiogram (ECG) tracing represents.

9. Recognize the following from an ECG rhythm strip:

   a. Normal sinus rhythm

   b. Sinus bradycardia and tachycardia

   c. Atrial flutter and fibrillation

   d. Atrioventricular (AV) blocks: first, second, and third degree

   e. Premature ventricular complex

   f. Ventricular tachycardia and fibrillation

10. Describe the location for placement of electrodes for each of the following leads: I, II, III, $aV_R$, $aV_L$, and $aV_F$, and precordial $V_1$ to $V_6$.

11. Draw the axial reference system and show the position (in degrees) for the positive electrode for each of the six limb leads.

12. Describe, in terms of vectors, how the QRS complex is generated and why the QRS appears differently when recorded by different electrode leads.

13. Estimate the mean electrical axis for ventricular depolarization from the six limb leads.

## INTRODUCTION

The primary function of cardiac myocytes is to contract. Electrical changes within the myocytes initiate this contraction. This chapter examines (1) the electrical activity of individual myocytes, including resting membrane potentials and action potentials; (2) the way action potentials are conducted throughout the heart to initiate coordinated contraction of the entire heart; and (3) the way electrical activity of the heart is measured using the electrocardiogram (ECG).

## CELL MEMBRANE POTENTIALS

### Resting Membrane Potentials

Cardiac cells, like all living cells in the body, have an electrical potential across the cell membrane. This potential can be measured by inserting a microelectrode into the cell and measuring the electrical potential in millivolts (mV) inside the cell relative to the outside of the cell. By convention, the outside of the cell is considered 0 mV. If measurements are taken with a resting ventricular myocyte, a membrane potential of about −90 mV will be recorded. This **resting membrane potential (Em)** is determined by the concentrations of positively and negatively charged ions across the cell membrane, the relative permeability of the cell membrane to these ions, and the ionic pumps that transport ions across the cell membrane.

#### EQUILIBRIUM POTENTIALS

Of the many different ions present inside and outside of cells, the concentrations of Na⁺, K⁺, and Ca⁺⁺ are most important in determining the membrane potential across the cell membrane. Although chloride ions are found inside and outside the cell, they contribute relatively little to the resting membrane potential. Figure 2.1 shows approximate concentrations of Na⁺, K⁺, and Ca⁺⁺ inside and outside the cell. Of the three ions, K⁺ is the most important in determining the resting membrane potential. In a cardiac cell, the concentration of K⁺ is high inside and low outside the cell. Therefore, a **chemical gradient**

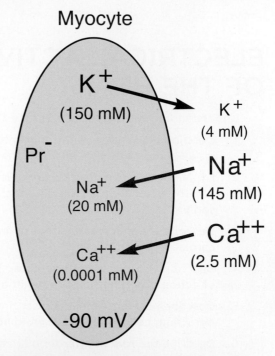

■ **FIGURE 2.1** Concentrations of K⁺, Na⁺, and Ca⁺⁺ inside and outside a cardiac myocyte at a resting membrane potential of −90 mV. *Pr⁻*, negatively charged proteins.

(concentration difference) exists for K⁺ to diffuse out of the cell. The opposite situation is found for Na⁺ and Ca⁺⁺; their chemical gradients favor an inward diffusion. The concentration differences across the cell membrane for these and other ions are determined by the activity of energy-dependent ionic pumps and the presence of impermeable, negatively charged proteins within the cell that affect the passive distribution of cations and anions.

To understand how concentration gradients of ions across a cell membrane affect membrane potential, consider a cell in which K⁺ is the only ion across the membrane other than the large, impermeable, negatively charged proteins on the inside of the cell. In this cell, K⁺ diffuses down its chemical gradient and out of the cell because its concentration is much higher inside than outside the cell (see Fig. 2.1). As K⁺ diffuses out of the cell, it leaves behind negatively charged proteins, thereby creating a separation of charge and a potential difference across the membrane (negative inside the cell relative to outside). The membrane potential that is necessary to oppose the outward movement of K$^+$ down its concentration gradient is termed the **equilibrium potential for K$^+$** (E$_K$; Nernst potential). The **Nernst potential** for K$^+$ at 37°C is as follows:

**Eq. 2-1**    $$E_K = -61 \log \frac{[K^+]_i}{[K^+]_o} = -96 \text{ mV}$$

in which the potassium concentration inside [K$^+$]$_i$ = 150 mM and the potassium concentration outside [K$^+$]$_o$ = 4 mM. The −61 is derived from RT/zF, in which R is the gas constant, z is the number of ion charges (z = 1 for K$^+$; z = 2 for divalent ions such as Ca$^{++}$), F is Faraday constant, and T is temperature (°K). *The equilibrium potential is the potential difference across the membrane required to maintain the concentration gradient across the membrane.* In other words, the equilibrium potential for K$^+$ represents the electrical potential necessary to keep K$^+$ from diffusing down its chemical gradient and out of the cell. If the outside K$^+$ concentration increased from 4 to 10 mM, the chemical gradient for diffusion out of the cell would be reduced; therefore, the membrane potential required to maintain electrochemical equilibrium would be less negative according to the Nernst relationship.

The Em for a ventricular myocyte is about −90 mV, which is near the equilibrium potential for K$^+$. Because the equilibrium potential for K$^+$ is −96 mV and the measured resting membrane potential is −90 mV, a net driving force (**net electrochemical force**) acts on the K$^+$, causing it to diffuse out of the cell. In the case of K$^+$, this net electrochemical driving force is the Em (−90 mV) minus the E$_K$ (−96 mV), resulting in +6 mV. Because the resting cell has a finite permeability to K$^+$ and a small net outward driving force is acting on K$^+$, K$^+$ slowly leaks outward from the cell.

Sodium ions also play a major role in determining the membrane potential. Because the Na$^+$ concentration is higher outside the cell, this ion would diffuse down its chemical gradient into the cell. To prevent this inward flux of Na$^+$, a large positive charge is needed inside the cell (relative to the outside) to balance out the chemical diffusion forces. This potential is

called the **equilibrium potential for Na$^+$ (E$_{Na}$)** and is calculated using the Nernst equation, as follows:

**Eq. 2-2**    $$E_{Na} = -61 \log \frac{[Na^+]_i}{[Na^+]_o} = +52 \text{ mV}$$

in which the sodium concentration inside [Na$^+$]$_i$ = 20 mM and the sodium concentration outside [Na$^+$]$_o$ = 145 mM. The calculated equilibrium potential for sodium indicates that to balance the inward diffusion of Na$^+$ at these intracellular and extracellular concentrations, the cell interior has to be +52 mV to prevent Na$^+$ from diffusing into the cell.

The net driving or electrochemical force acting on sodium (and each ionic species) has two components. First, the sodium concentration gradient is driving sodium into the cell; according to the Nernst calculation, the electrical force necessary to counterbalance this chemical gradient is +52 mV. Second, because the interior of the resting cell is very negative (−90 mV), a large electrical force is trying to "pull" sodium into the cell. We can derive the net electrochemical force acting on sodium from these two component forces by subtracting the Em minus E$_{Na}$: −90 mV − +52 mV equals −142 mV. This large electrochemical force drives sodium into the cell; however, at rest, the permeability of the membrane to Na$^+$ is so low that only a small amount of Na$^+$ leaks into the cell.

The same reasoning can be applied to Ca$^{++}$ as just described for Na$^+$. Its calculated E$_{Ca}$ is +134 mV and net electrochemical force acting on Ca$^{++}$ is −224 mV. Therefore, like Na$^+$, there is a very large net electrochemical force working to drive Ca$^{++}$ into the resting cell; however, in the resting cell, little Ca$^{++}$ leaks into the cell because of low membrane permeability to Ca$^{++}$ at rest.

## IONIC CONDUCTANCES AND MEMBRANE POTENTIAL

As explained, the Em in a resting, nonpacemaker cell is very near E$_K$, and quite distant from E$_{Na}$ and E$_{Ca}$. This occurs because the membrane is much more permeable to K$^+$ in the resting state than to Na$^+$ or Ca$^{++}$. Therefore, Na$^+$ and Ca$^{++}$ have little contribution to the resting Em because Em reflects not only the concentration gradients of individual ions (i.e., the equilibrium potentials) but also the relative permeability of the membrane to those ions. If the membrane has a relatively higher permeability to one ion over the others, that ion will have a greater influence in determining the membrane potential.

Membrane permeability for an ion determines the movement of an ion being driven by a net electrochemical force. Because this ion movement represents an electrical current, it is common to speak in terms of ion conductance (g), which is defined as the ion current divided by the net voltage (net electrochemical force) acting on the ion. Membrane permeability and ion conductance are related in that an increase in membrane permeability for an ion results in an increase in electrical conductance for that ion. Putting these concepts together, it is possible to derive an expression that relates membrane potential (Em) to the relative conductances of all ions and their equilibrium potentials as shown in the following equation:

**Eq. 2-3**   $Em = g'K^+(E_K) + g'Na^+(E_{Na})$
$+ g'Ca^{++}(E_{Ca})$

In Equation 2-3, the Em is the sum of the individual equilibrium potentials for $K^+$, $Na^+$, and $Ca^{++}$, with each multiplied by the membrane conductance for that particular ion relative to the sum of all ion conductances. For example, the relative conductance for $K^+$ ($g'K^+$) = $gK^+/(gK^+ + gNa^+ + gCa^{++})$. If the equilibrium potentials for $K^+$, $Na^+$, and $Ca^{++}$ are calculated using the concentrations shown in Figure 2.1, then Equation 2-3 can be depicted as follows:

**Eq. 2-4**   $Em = g'K^+(-96\ mV)$
$+ g'Na^+\ (+52\ mV)$
$+ g'Ca^{++}(+134\ mV)$

In a cardiac cell, the individual ion concentration gradients change very little, even when $Na^+$ enters and $K^+$ leaves the cell during depolarization. Therefore, *changes in Em primarily result from changes in ionic conductances.* The resting membrane potential (−90 mV) is near the equilibrium potential for $K^+$ (−96 mV) because $g'K^+$ is high in the resting cell, while $g'Na^+$ and

$g'Ca^{++}$ are low. Therefore, the low relative conductances of $Na^+$ and $Ca^{++}$ multiplied by their equilibrium potential values causes those ions to contribute little to the resting membrane potential. When $g'Na^+$ increases and $g'K^+$ decreases (as occurs during an action potential), the membrane potential becomes more positive (depolarized) because the sodium equilibrium potential has more influence on the overall membrane potential. Similarly, a large increase in $g'Ca^+$, particularly when $g'K^+$ is low, will also result in depolarization.

In Equation 2-3, ion concentrations (which determine the equilibrium potential) and ion conductances are separate variables. In reality, the conductance of some ion channels is influenced by the concentration of the ion (e.g., $K^+$-sensitive $K^+$ channels) or by changes in membrane potential (e.g., voltage-dependent $Na^+$, $K^+$, and $Ca^{++}$ ion channels). For example, a decrease in external $K^+$ concentration (e.g., from 4 to 3 mM) can decrease $gK^+$ in some cardiac cells and lead to a small depolarization (less negative potential) instead of the hyperpolarization (more negative potential) predicted by the Nernst relationship or Equation 2-3. In some cells, small increases in external $K^+$ concentration (e.g., from a normal concentration of 4 to 6 mM) can cause a small hyperpolarization owing to activation of $K^+$ channels and an increase in $gK^+$.

---

**PROBLEM 2-1**

High concentrations of potassium are added to cardioplegic solutions used to arrest the heart during surgery. Using the Nernst equation, calculate an estimate for the new resting membrane potential (Em) when external potassium concentration is increased from a normal value of 4 to 40 mM. Assume that the internal concentration remains at 150 mM and that $K^+$ and other ion conductances are not altered.

---

## Maintenance of Ionic Gradients

Membrane potential depends on the maintenance of ionic concentration gradients across the membrane. The maintenance of these concentration gradients requires the expenditure of energy (adenosine triphosphate [ATP] hydrolysis) coupled with ionic pumps. Consider the concentration gradients for Na⁺ and K⁺. Na⁺ constantly leaks into the resting cell, and K⁺ leaks out. Moreover, whenever an action potential is generated, additional Na⁺ enters the cell and additional K⁺ leaves. Although the number of ions moving across the sarcolemmal membrane in a single action potential is small relative to the total number of ions, many action potentials can lead to a significant change in the extracellular and intracellular concentration of these ions. To prevent this change from happening (i.e., to maintain the concentration gradients for Na⁺ and K⁺), an energy (ATP)-dependent pump system (**Na⁺/K⁺-adenosine triphosphatase [ATPase]**), located on the sarcolemma, pumps Na⁺ out and K⁺ into the cell (Fig. 2.2). Normal operation of this pump is essential to maintain Na⁺ and K⁺ concentrations across the membrane. If this pump stops working (such as when ATP is lost under hypoxic conditions), or if the activity of the pump is inhibited by cardiac glycosides such as digoxin, Na⁺ accumulates within the cell and intracellular K⁺ falls. This change

results in a less negative (more depolarized) resting membrane potential primarily because $E_K$ becomes less negative (see Equation 2-1). Besides maintaining the Na⁺ and K⁺ concentration gradients, it is important to note that the Na⁺/K⁺-ATPase pump is **electrogenic** because it extrudes three Na⁺ for every two K⁺ entering the cell. By pumping more positive charges out of the cell than into it, the pump creates a negative potential within the cell. This electrogenic potential may be up to −10 mV, depending on the activity of the pump. Inhibition of this pump, therefore, causes depolarization resulting from changes in Na⁺ and K⁺ concentration gradients and from the loss of an electrogenic component of the membrane potential. In addition, increases in intracellular Na⁺ or extracellular K⁺ stimulate the activity of the electrogenic Na⁺/K⁺-ATPase pump and produce hyperpolarizing currents.

Because Ca⁺⁺ enters the cell, especially during action potentials, it is necessary to have a mechanism to maintain its concentration gradient. Two primary mechanisms remove calcium from cells (Fig. 2.2). The first involves an **ATP-dependent Ca⁺⁺ pump** that actively pumps calcium out of the cell and generates a small negative electrogenic potential.

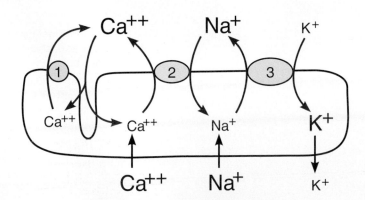

1 = ATP-dependent Ca⁺⁺ pump
2 = Na⁺/Ca⁺⁺ exchanger (3:1)
3 = Na⁺/K⁺-ATPase pump (3:2)

■ **FIGURE 2.2** Sarcolemmal ion pumps and exchangers. These pumps maintain transmembrane ionic gradients for Na⁺, K⁺, and Ca⁺⁺. Na⁺ and Ca⁺⁺ enter the cell down their electrochemical gradient, especially during action potentials, while K⁺ is leaving the cell. Ca⁺⁺ is removed by an ATP-dependent, electrogenic Ca⁺⁺ pump (*1*) and by the electrogenic Na⁺/Ca⁺⁺ exchanger that exchanges three Na⁺ for every one Ca⁺⁺ (*2*). Na⁺ is actively removed from the cell by the electrogenic Na⁺/K⁺-ATPase pump, which brings two K⁺ into the cell for every three Na⁺ that are pumped out.

The second mechanism is the **sodium–calcium exchanger**, through which $Na^+$ and $Ca^{++}$ are transported in opposite directions. The exchanger can operate in either direction across the sarcolemma depending on the Em. In resting cells, the negative Em causes $Na^+$ to enter the cell in exchange for $Ca^{++}$, which leaves the cell. Three sodium ions are exchanged for each calcium ion; therefore, the exchanger generates a small (few millivolts) electrogenic potential that follows the direction of $Na^+$. The opposite occurs in depolarized cells. This exchanger is also strongly influenced by changes in intracellular $Na^+$ concentration. For example, when the activity of the $Na^+/K^+$-ATPase pump is decreased by drugs such as digoxin, the increase in intracellular $Na^+$ concentration reduces the gradient for $Na^+$ movement into the cell through this exchanger, which results in less $Ca^{++}$ efflux, thereby increasing intracellular $Ca^{++}$. As described in Chapter 3, this can lead to an increase in the force of myocyte contraction.

## Ion Channels

Ions move across the sarcolemma through specialized ion channels in the phospholipid bilayer of the cell membrane. These channels are made up of large polypeptide chains that span the membrane and create an opening in the membrane. Conformational changes in the ion channel proteins alter the shape of the channel, thereby permitting ions to transverse the membrane channel or blocking ion movement.

Ion channels are selective for different cations and anions. For example, there are ion channels selective for sodium, potassium, and calcium ions (Table 2-1). Furthermore, a given ion may have several different types

| TABLE 2-1 CARDIAC ION CHANNELS AND CURRENTS | | |
|---|---|---|
| **CHANNELS** | **GATING** | **CHARACTERISTICS** |
| *Sodium* | | |
| Fast $Na^+$ ($I_{Na}$) | Voltage | Phase 0 of myocytes |
| Slow $Na^+$ ($I_f$) | Voltage and receptor | Contributes to phase 4 pacemaker current in SA and AV nodal cells |
| *Calcium* | | |
| L-type ($I_{Ca}$) | Voltage | Slow inward, long-lasting current; phase 2 of myocytes and phases 4 and 0 of SA and AV nodal cells |
| T-type ($I_{Ca}$) | Voltage | Transient current; contributes to phase 4 pacemaker current in SA and AV nodal cells |
| *Potassium* | | |
| Inward rectifier ($I_{K1}$) | Voltage | Maintains negative potential in phase 4; closes with depolarization |
| Transient outward ($I_{to}$) | Voltage | Contributes to phase 1 in myocytes |
| Delayed rectifier ($I_{Kr}$) | Voltage | Phase 3 repolarization |
| ATP-sensitive ($I_{K, ATP}$) | Receptor | Inhibited by ATP; opens when ATP decreases during cellular hypoxia |
| Acetylcholine activated ($I_{K, ACh}$) | Receptor | Activated by acetylcholine and adenosine; Gi-protein coupled; slows SA nodal firing |
| Calcium activated ($I_{K,Ca}$) | Receptor | Activated by high cytosolic calcium; accelerates repolarization |

$I_x$, name of specific current.

of ion channels responsible for its movement across a cell membrane. For example, several different types of potassium channels exist through which potassium ions can move across the cell membrane.

Two general types of ion channels exist: voltage-gated (voltage-operated) and receptor-gated (receptor-operated) channels. **Voltage-gated channels** open and close in response to changes in membrane potential. Examples of voltage-gated channels include several sodium, potassium, and calcium channels that are involved in cardiac action potentials. **Receptor-gated channels** open and close in response to chemical signals operating through membrane receptors. For example, acetylcholine, which is the neurotransmitter released by the vagus nerves innervating the heart, binds to a sarcolemmal receptor that subsequently leads to the opening of special types of potassium channels ($I_{K, ACh}$).

Ion channels have both open and closed states. Ions pass through the channel only while it is in the open state. The open and closed states of voltage-gated channels are regulated by the membrane potential. Fast sodium channels have been the most extensively studied, and a conceptual model has been developed based upon studies by Hodgkin and Huxley in the 1950s using the squid giant axon. In this model, two gates regulate the movement of sodium through the channel (Fig. 2.3). At a normal resting membrane potential (about −90 mV in cardiac myocytes), the sodium channel is in a resting, closed state. In this configuration, the m-gate (activation gate) is closed and the h-gate (inactivation gate) is open. These gates are polypeptides that are part of the transmembrane protein channel, and they undergo conformational changes in response to changes in voltage. The m-gates rapidly become activated and open when the membrane is rapidly depolarized. This permits sodium, driven by its electrochemical gradient, to enter the cell. As the m-gates open, the h-gates begin to close; however, the m-gates open more rapidly than the h-gates close. The difference in the opening and closing rates of the two gates permits sodium to briefly enter the cell. After a few milliseconds, however, the h-gates close and sodium ceases to enter the cell. The closing of the h-gates therefore limits the length of time that sodium can enter the cell. This inactivated, closed state persists throughout the repolarization phase as the membrane potential recovers to its resting level. Near the end of repolarization, the negative membrane potential causes the m-gates to close and the h-gates to open. These changes cause

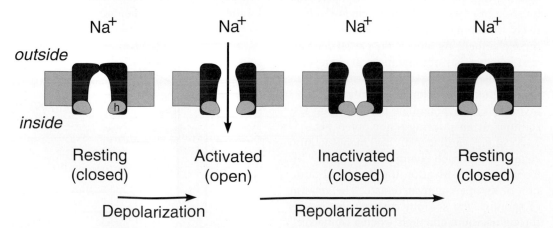

■ **FIGURE 2.3** Open and closed states of fast sodium channels in cardiac myocytes. In the resting (closed) state, the m-gates (activation gates) are closed, although the h-gates (inactivation gates) are open. Rapid depolarization to threshold opens the m-gates (voltage activated), thereby opening the channel and enabling sodium to enter the cell. Shortly thereafter, as the cell begins to repolarize, the h-gates close and the channel becomes inactivated. Toward the end of repolarization, the m-gates again close and the h-gates open. This brings the channel back to its resting state.

the channel to revert back to its initial resting, closed state. Full recovery of the h-gates can take 100 milliseconds or longer after the resting membrane potential has been restored.

The response of the activation and inactivation gates described above occurs when the resting membrane potential is normal (about −90 mV) and a rapid depolarization of the membrane occurs, as happens when a normal depolarization current spreads from one cardiac cell to another during electrical activation of the heart. The response of the fast sodium channel, however, is different when the resting membrane potential is partially depolarized or the cell is slowly depolarized. For example, when myocytes become hypoxic, the cells depolarize to a less negative resting membrane potential. This partially depolarized state inactivates sodium channels by closing the h-gates. The more a cell is depolarized, the greater the number of inactivated sodium channels. At a membrane potential of about −55 mV, virtually all fast sodium channels are inactivated. If a myocyte has a normal resting potential but then undergoes slow depolarization, more time is available for the h-gates to close as the m-gates are opening. This causes the sodium channel to transition directly from the resting (closed) state to the inactivated (closed) state. The result is that there is no activated, open state for sodium to pass through the channel, effectively abolishing fast sodium currents through these channels. As long as the partial depolarized state persists, the channel will not resume its resting, closed state. As described later in this chapter, these changes significantly alter myocyte action potentials by abolishing fast sodium currents during action potentials.

A single cardiac cell has many sodium channels, and each channel has a slightly different voltage activation threshold and duration of its open, activated state. The amount of sodium (the sodium current) that passes through sodium channels when a cardiac cell undergoes depolarization depends upon the number of sodium channels, the duration of time the channels are in the open state, and the electrochemical gradient driving the sodium into the cell.

The open and closed states described for sodium channels are also found in other ion channels. For example, slow calcium channels have activation and inactivation gates (although they have different letter designations than fast sodium channels). Although this conceptual model is useful to help understand how ions transverse the membrane, many of the details of how this actually occurs at the molecular level are still unknown. Nevertheless, recent research is helping to show which regions of ion channel proteins act as voltage sensors and which regions undergo conformational changes analogous to the gates described in the conceptual model.

## Action Potentials

Action potentials occur when the membrane potential suddenly depolarizes and then repolarizes back to its resting state. The two general types of cardiac action potentials include nonpacemaker and pacemaker action potentials. Nonpacemaker action potentials are triggered by depolarizing currents from adjacent cells, whereas pacemaker cells are capable of spontaneous action potential generation. Both types of action potentials in the heart differ considerably from the action potentials found in nerve and skeletal muscle cells (Fig. 2.4). One major difference is the duration of the action potentials. In a typical nerve, the action potential duration is about 1

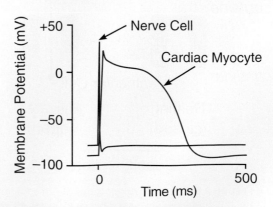

■ **FIGURE 2.4** Comparison of action potentials from a nerve cell and a nonpacemaker cardiac myocyte. Cardiac action potentials are much longer in duration than nerve cell action potentials.

to 2 milliseconds. In skeletal muscle cells, the action potential duration is approximately 2 to 5 milliseconds. In contrast, the duration of ventricular action potentials ranges from 200 to 400 milliseconds. These differences among nerve, skeletal muscle, and cardiac myocyte action potentials relate to differences in the ionic conductances responsible for generating the changes in membrane potential.

## NONPACEMAKER ACTION POTENTIALS

Figure 2.5 shows the ionic mechanisms responsible for the generation of "fast response" nonpacemaker action potentials such as those found in atrial and ventricular myocytes, and Purkinje fibers. By convention, the action potential is divided into five numbered phases. Nonpacemaker cells have a true resting membrane potential (**phase 4**) that remains near

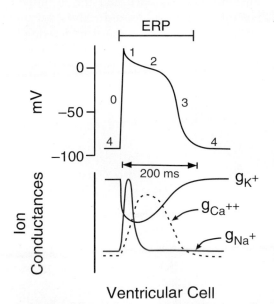

**Ventricular Cell**

■ **FIGURE 2.5** Changes in ion conductances associated with a ventricular myocyte action potential. Phase 0 (depolarization) primarily is due to the rapid increase in sodium conductance ($gNa^+$) accompanied by a fall in potassium conductance ($gK^+$); the initial repolarization of phase 1 is due to opening of special potassium channels ($I_{to}$); phase 2 (plateau) primarily is due to an increase in slow inward calcium conductance ($gCa^{++}$) through L-type $Ca^{++}$ channels; phase 3 (repolarization) results from an increase in $gK^+$ and a decrease in $gCa^{++}$. Phase 4 is a true resting potential that primarily reflects a high $gK^+$. ERP, effective refractory period.

the equilibrium potential for $K^+$ because $gK^+$, through inward rectifying potassium channels (see Table 2-1), is high relative to $gNa^+$ and $gCa^{++}$ in resting cells (see Equation 2-4). When these cells are rapidly depolarized from $-90$ mV to a threshold voltage of about $-70$ mV (owing to, for example, an action potential conducted by an adjacent cell), a rapid **depolarization** (**phase 0**) is initiated by a transient increase in conductance of voltage-gated, fast $Na^+$-channels. At the same time, $gK^+$ falls. These two conductance changes very rapidly move the membrane potential away from the potassium equilibrium potential and closer to the sodium equilibrium potential (see Equation 2-4). **Phase 1** represents an **initial repolarization** caused by the opening of a special type of $K^+$ channels (transient outward) and the inactivation of the $Na^+$ channels. However, because of the large increase in slow inward $gCa^{++}$, the repolarization is delayed and the action potential reaches a **plateau phase** (**phase 2**). This inward calcium movement is through long-lasting (L-type) calcium channels that open when the membrane potential depolarizes to about $-40$ mV. L-type calcium channels are the major calcium channels in cardiac and vascular smooth muscle. They are opened by membrane depolarization (they are voltage-operated) and remain open for a relatively long duration. These channels are blocked by classical L-type calcium channel blockers (e.g., verapamil and diltiazem). **Repolarization** (**phase 3**) occurs when $gK^+$ increases through delayed rectifier potassium channels and $gCa^{++}$ decreases. Therefore, changes in $Na^+$, $Ca^{++}$, and $K^+$ conductances primarily determine the action potential in nonpacemaker cells.

During phases 0, 1, 2, and part of phase 3, the cell is refractory (i.e., unexcitable) to the initiation of new action potentials. This is the **effective (or absolute) refractory period** (ERP, or ARP) (see Fig. 2.5). During the ERP, stimulation of the cell does not produce new, propagated action potentials because the h-gates are still closed. The ERP acts as a protective mechanism in the heart by limiting the frequency of action potentials (and therefore contractions) that the heart can generate. This enables the heart to have adequate time to fill and eject blood. The long ERP also prevents the heart from developing sustained, tetanic contractions like those that occur in skeletal muscle. At the end of the ERP, the cell is in its **relative refractory period.** Early in this period, suprathreshold depolarization stimuli are required to elicit actions potentials. Because not all the sodium channels have recovered to their resting state by this time, action potentials generated during the relative refractory period have a decreased phase 0 slope and lower amplitude. When the sodium channels are fully recovered, the cell becomes fully excitable and normal depolarization stimuli can elicit new, rapid action potentials.

## PACEMAKER ACTION POTENTIALS

Pacemaker cells have no true resting potential, but instead generate regular, spontaneous action potentials. Unlike most other cells that exhibit action potentials (e.g., nerve cells, and muscle cells), the depolarizing current of the action potential is carried primarily by relatively slow, inward Ca$^{++}$ currents (through L-type calcium channels) instead of by fast Na$^+$ currents. The rate of depolarization of pacemaker cells is slow compared to "fast response" nonpacemaker cells, and therefore they are sometimes called "slow response" action potentials.

Cells within the **sinoatrial (SA) node,** located within the posterior wall of the right atrium (RA), constitute the primary pacemaker site within the heart. Other pacemaker cells exist within the AV node and ventricular conduction system, but their firing rates are driven by the higher rate of the SA node because the intrinsic pacemaker activity of the secondary pacemakers is suppressed by a mechanism termed **overdrive suppression.** This mechanism causes the secondary pacemaker to become hyperpolarized when driven at a rate above its intrinsic rate. Hyperpolarization occurs because the increased action potential frequency stimulates the activity of the electrogenic Na$^+$/K$^+$-ATPase pump as a result of enhanced entry of sodium per unit time into these cells. If the SA node becomes depressed, or its action potentials fail to reach secondary pacemakers, overdrive suppression ceases, which permits a secondary

site to take over as the pacemaker for the heart. When this occurs, the new pacemaker outside of the SA node is called an **ectopic focus.**

SA nodal action potentials are divided into three phases: phase 0, upstroke of the action potential; phase 3, the period of repolarization; and phase 4, the period of spontaneous depolarization that leads to subsequent generation of a new action potential (Fig. 2.6).

**Phase 0** depolarization primarily is due to increased gCa$^{++}$ through L-type calcium channels. These voltage-operated channels open when the membrane is depolarized to a threshold voltage of about −40 mV. Because the movement of Ca$^{++}$ through calcium channels is not rapid compared to fast sodium channels (hence, the term "slow calcium channels"), the rate of depolarization (the slope of phase 0) is much slower than that found in other cardiac cells (e.g., in Purkinje cells). As the calcium channels open and the membrane potential moves toward the calcium equilibrium potential, a transient decrease in

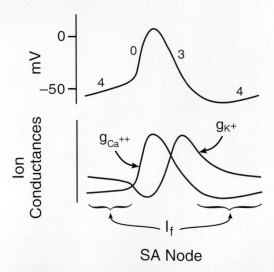

■ **FIGURE 2.6** Changes in ion conductances associated with a sinoatrial (*SA*) nodal pacemaker action potential. Phase 0 (depolarization) primarily is due to an increase in calcium conductance (*gCa$^{++}$*) through L-type Ca$^{++}$ channels accompanied by a fall in potassium conductance (*gK$^+$*); phase 3 (repolarization) results from an increase in gK$^+$ and a decrease in gCa$^{++}$. Phase 4 undergoes a spontaneous depolarization owing to a pacemaker current (*I$_f$*) carried in part by Na$^+$; decreased gK$^+$ and increased gCa$^{++}$ also contribute to the spontaneous depolarization.

gK$^+$ occurs, which contributes to the depolarization as shown in the following equation:

**Eq. 2-5**
**Em = g'K( - 96 mV) + g'Ca( + 134 mV)**

Depolarization causes voltage-operated, delayed rectifier potassium channels to open, and the increased gK$^+$ repolarizes the cell toward the equilibrium potential for K$^+$ (**phase 3**). At the same time, the slow inward Ca$^{++}$ channels that opened during phase 0 become inactivated, thereby decreasing gCa$^{++}$ and contributing to the repolarization. Phase 3 ends when the membrane potential reaches about –65 mV. The phase of repolarization is self-limited because the potassium channels begin to close again as the cell becomes repolarized.

The ionic mechanisms responsible for the spontaneous depolarization of the pacemaker potential (**phase 4**) are not entirely clear, but probably involve multiple ionic currents. First, early in phase 4, gK$^+$ is still declining. This fall in gK$^+$ contributes to depolarization. Second, in the repolarized state, a **pacemaker current (I$_f$)**, or "funny" current, has been identified (see Fig. 2.6). This depolarizing current involves, in part, a slow inward movement of Na$^+$. Third, in the second half of phase 4, there is a small increase in gCa$^{++}$ through T-type calcium channels. T-type ("transient") calcium channels differ from L-type calcium channels in that they open briefly only at very negative voltages (–50 mV) and are not blocked by the classical L-type calcium channel blockers. Fourth, as the depolarization begins to reach threshold, the L-type calcium channels begin to open, causing a further increase in gCa$^{++}$ until threshold is reached and phase 0 is initiated.

To summarize, "slow response" action potentials found in SA nodal cells primarily depend on changes in gCa$^{++}$ and gK$^+$ conductances, with "funny" currents (I$_f$) and changes in gCa$^{++}$ and gK$^+$ conductances playing a role in the spontaneous depolarization.

## REGULATION OF SA NODAL PACEMAKER ACTIVITY

The SA node displays intrinsic automaticity at a rate of 100 to 110 depolarizations per minute. Heart rate, however, can vary between low resting values of 50 to 60 beats/min and over 200 beats/min. These changes in rate primarily are controlled by autonomic nerves acting on the SA node. At low resting heart rates, vagal influences are dominant over sympathetic influences. This is termed **vagal tone**. Autonomic nerves increase SA nodal firing rate by both decreasing vagal tone and increasing sympathetic activity on the SA node in a reciprocal manner. An increase in heart rate is a positive chronotropic response (or **positive chronotropy**), whereas a reduction in heart rate is a negative chronotropic response (or **negative chronotropy**).

Autonomic influences alter the rate of pacemaker firing through the following mechanisms: (1) changing the slope of phase 4; (2) altering the threshold voltage for triggering phase 0; and (3) altering the degree of hyperpolarization at the end of phase 3. Any of these three mechanisms will either increase or decrease the time to reach threshold. Sympathetic activation of the SA node increases the slope of phase 4 (Fig. 2.7) and lowers the threshold, thereby increasing pacemaker frequency (positive chronotropy). In this mechanism, norepinephrine released by sympathetic adrenergic nerves binds to β$_1$-adrenoceptors coupled to a stimulatory G-protein (Gs-protein), which activates adenylyl cyclase and increases cyclic adenosine monophosphate (cAMP; see Chapter 3). This effect leads to an increase in I$_f$ and an earlier opening of L-type calcium channels, both of which increase the rate of depolarization. Repolarization is also accelerated, which shortens overall cycle length and may increase maximal hyperpolarization.

Vagal stimulation releases acetylcholine at the SA node, which decreases the slope of phase 4 (by inhibiting "funny" currents), hyperpolarizes the cell, and increases the threshold voltage required to trigger phase 0. All of these effects cause the pacemaker potential to take longer to reach threshold, thereby slowing the rate (negative chronotropy). The rate of repolarization is reduced, which contributes to increasing overall cycle length. Acetylcholine acts by binding to muscarinic receptors (M$_2$). This decreases cAMP via the inhibitory G-protein (Gi-protein), the opposite effect of sympathetic

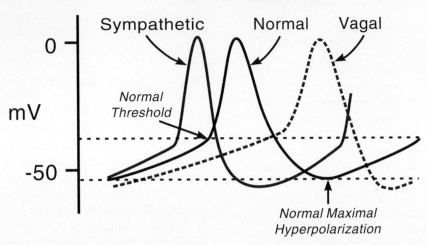

■ **FIGURE 2.7** Effects of sympathetic and parasympathetic (vagal) stimulation on sinoatrial (*SA*) nodal pacemaker activity. Sympathetic stimulation increases the firing rate by increasing the slope of phase 4 and lowering the threshold for the action potential. Vagal stimulation has the opposite effects, and it hyperpolarizes the cell. Horizontal dashed lines represent threshold and maximal hyperpolarization potentials for normal cell.

activation (see Chapter 3). Acetylcholine also activates a special type of potassium channel ($K_{ACh}$ channel) that hyperpolarizes the cell by increasing potassium conductance.

Nonneural mechanisms also alter pacemaker activity (Table 2-2). For example, circulating catecholamines (epinephrine and norepinephrine) cause tachycardia (abnormally high heart rate) by a mechanism similar to norepinephrine

| TABLE 2-2 | FACTORS INCREASING OR DECREASING THE SA NODE FIRING RATE |
|---|---|
| **INCREASING** | **DECREASING** |
| Sympathetic stimulation | Parasympathetic stimulation |
| Muscarinic receptor antagonist | Muscarinic receptor agonists |
| β-Adrenoceptor agonists | β-Blockers |
| Circulating catecholamines | Ischemia/hypoxia |
| Hypokalemia | Hyperkalemia |
| Hyperthyroidism | Sodium and calcium channel blockers |
| Hyperthermia | Hypothermia |

released by sympathetic nerves. Hyperthyroidism induces tachycardia, and hypothyroidism induces bradycardia (abnormally low heart rate). Changes in the serum concentration of ions, particularly potassium, can cause changes in SA node firing rate. Hyperkalemia induces bradycardia or can even stop SA nodal firing, whereas hypokalemia increases the rate of phase 4 depolarization and causes tachycardia, apparently by decreasing potassium conductance during phase 4. Cellular hypoxia depolarizes the membrane potential, causing bradycardia and abolition of pacemaker activity. Increased body temperature (e.g., fever) leads to increased rate of SA nodal firing.

Various drugs used to treat abnormal heart rhythm (i.e., antiarrhythmic drugs) also affect SA nodal rhythm. Calcium channel blockers, for example, cause bradycardia by inhibiting L-type calcium channels, which reduces slow inward $Ca^{++}$ currents during phase 4 and phase 0. Drugs affecting autonomic control or autonomic receptors (e.g., β-blockers and $M_2$ receptor antagonists; β-adrenoceptor agonists) alter pacemaker activity. Digoxin causes bradycardia by increasing parasympathetic activity and inhibiting the sarcolemmal $Na^+/K^+$-ATPase, which leads to depolarization.

## Arrhythmias Caused by Abnormal Action Potential Generation

### ABNORMAL AUTOMATICITY

"Fast response" nonpacemaker action potentials do not ordinarily display automaticity because they are characterized as having a true resting membrane potential that does not undergo spontaneous depolarization. If the fast sodium channels that are responsible for the rapid depolarization during phase 0 are blocked pharmacologically, or inactivated by depolarization caused by cellular hypoxia, the slope and amplitude of phase 0 are significantly depressed, and the action potential appears much like a "slow response" action potential. The depolarization phase of the action potential under these conditions is brought about by slow inward calcium currents carried through L-type calcium channels. Furthermore, like SA nodal pacemakers, these cells may display spontaneous depolarization during phase 4. This **abnormal automaticity** in these transformed "fast response" cells can result in spontaneous action potential generation, thereby producing arrhythmias.

### TRIGGERED ACTIVITY

A second mechanism that can lead to abnormal generation of action potentials is called **triggered activity**. Nonpacemaker cells may undergo spontaneous depolarizations either during phase 3 or early in phase 4, triggering abnormal action potentials. These spontaneous depolarizations (termed **afterdepolarizations**), if of sufficient magnitude, can trigger self-sustaining action potentials resulting in tachycardia (Fig. 2.8). **Early afterdepolarizations** occur during phase 3 and are more likely to occur when action potential durations are prolonged. Because these afterdepolarizations occur at a time when fast $Na^+$ channels are still inactivated, slow inward $Ca^{++}$ carries the depolarizing current. Another type of afterdepolarization, **delayed afterdepolarization**, occurs at the end of phase 3 or early in phase 4. It, too, can lead to self-sustaining action potentials and tachycardia. This form of triggered activity appears to be associated with elevations in intracellular calcium, as occurs

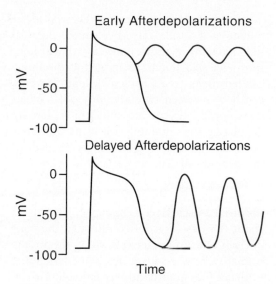

■ **FIGURE 2.8** Early (**top panel**) and delayed (**bottom panel**) afterdepolarizations. If the magnitude of spontaneous depolarization is sufficient, it can trigger self-sustaining action potentials.

during ischemia, digoxin toxicity, and excessive catecholamine stimulation.

## CONDUCTION OF ACTION POTENTIALS WITHIN THE HEART

### Electrical Conduction within the Heart

The action potentials generated by the SA node spread throughout the atria primarily by cell-to-cell conduction (Fig. 2.9). When a single

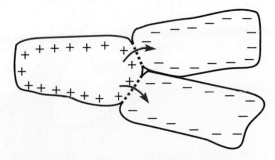

■ **FIGURE 2.9** Cell-to-cell conduction. Cardiac cells are connected together by low-resistance gap junctions between the cells, forming a functional syncytium. When one cell depolarizes, depolarizing currents can pass through the gap junctions (*red arrows*) and depolarize adjacent cells, resulting in a cell-to-cell propagation of action potentials.

myocyte depolarizes, positive charges accumulate just inside the sarcolemma. Because individual myocytes are joined together by low-resistance **gap junctions** located at the **intercalated disks** (see Chapter 3), ionic currents can flow between two adjoining cells. When these ionic currents are sufficient to rapidly depolarize the adjoining cell to its threshold potential, an action potential is elicited in the second cell. This is repeated in every cell, thereby causing action potentials to be propagated throughout the atria. Action potentials in the atrial muscle have a conduction velocity of about 0.5 m/s (Fig. 2.10). Although the conduction of action potentials within the atria is primarily between myocytes, some functional evidence (although controversial) points to the existence of specialized myocytes that serve as conducting pathways within the atria, termed **internodal tracts** (e.g., Bachmann bundle). As action potentials originating from the SA node spread across and depolarize the atrial muscle,

excitation–contraction coupling is initiated (see Chapter 3).

Nonconducting connective tissue separates the atria from the ventricles. Action potentials normally have only one pathway available to enter the ventricles, a specialized region of cells called the **AV node**. The AV node, located in the inferior–posterior region of the interatrial septum separating the left from the right atrium, is a highly specialized conducting tissue (cardiac, not neural in origin) that slows the impulse conduction velocity to about 0.05 m/s. This is one-tenth the velocity found in atrial or ventricular myocytes (see Fig. 2.10).

The delay in conduction between the atria and ventricles at the AV node is physiologically important. First, it allows sufficient time for complete atrial depolarization, contraction, and emptying of atrial blood into the ventricles prior to ventricular depolarization and contraction (see Chapter 4). Second, the low conduction velocity helps to limit the frequency of impulses

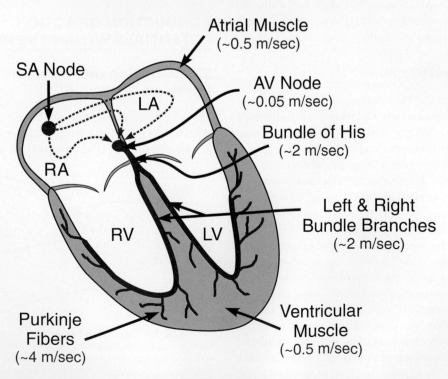

■ **FIGURE 2.10** Conduction system within the heart. Conduction velocities of different regions are noted in parentheses. Note that Purkinje fibers have the highest conduction velocity and the atrioventricular (*AV*) node has the lowest conduction velocity. *SA*, sinoatrial; *RA*, right atrium; *LA*, left atrium; *RV*, right ventricle; *LV*, left ventricle.

traveling through the AV node and activating the ventricle. This is important in atrial flutter and fibrillation, in which excessively high atrial rates, if transmitted to the ventricles, can lead to a very high ventricular rate. This can reduce cardiac output because of inadequate time for ventricular filling (see Chapter 4).

Action potentials leaving the AV node enter the base of the ventricle at the **bundle of His** and then follow the left and right **bundle branches** along the interventricular septum that separates the two ventricles. These specialized bundle branch fibers conduct action potentials at a high velocity (about 2 m/s). The bundle branches divide into an extensive system of **Purkinje fibers** that conduct the impulses at high velocity (about 4 m/s) throughout the ventricles. The Purkinje fiber cells connect with ventricular myocytes, which become the final pathway for cell-to-cell conduction within the ventricles.

The conduction system within the heart is important because it permits rapid, organized, near-synchronous depolarization and contraction of ventricular myocytes, which is essential to generate pressure efficiently during ventricular contraction. If the conduction system becomes damaged or dysfunctional, as can occur during ischemic conditions or myocardial infarction, this can lead to altered pathways of conduction and decreased conduction velocity within the heart. The functional consequence is that it diminishes the ability of the ventricles to generate pressure. Furthermore, damage to the conducting system can precipitate arrhythmias as described later.

## Regulation of Conduction Velocity

The rate of cell-to-cell conduction is determined by several intrinsic and extrinsic factors. Intrinsic factors include the electrical resistance between cells and the nature of the action potential, particularly in the initial rate of depolarization (phase 0). As discussed earlier in this chapter, fast sodium channels are responsible for the rapid upstroke velocity of nonpacemaker action potentials. Increasing the number of activated fast sodium chan-

nels increases the rate of depolarization. The more rapidly one cell depolarizes, the more quickly an adjoining cell depolarizes. Therefore, conditions that decrease the availability of fast sodium channels (e.g., depolarization caused by cellular hypoxia), decrease the rate and magnitude of phase 0, thereby decreasing conduction velocity within the heart. In AV nodal tissue in which slow inward calcium primarily determines phase 0 of the action potential, alterations in calcium conductance alter the rate of depolarization and therefore the rate of conduction between AV nodal cells.

Extrinsic factors can influence conduction velocity, including autonomic nerves, circulating hormones (particularly catecholamines), and various drugs (Table 2-3). Autonomic nerve activity significantly influences the conduction of electrical impulses throughout the heart, particularly in the specialized conduction system. An increase in sympathetic firing (or increased circulating catecholamines) increases conduction velocity via norepinephrine binding to $\beta_1$-adrenoceptors. The activation of parasympathetic (vagal) nerves decreases conduction velocity via the action of acetylcholine on $M_2$ receptors. This is most prominent at the AV node, which has a high degree of vagal innervation. The signal transduction mechanisms coupled to $\beta_1$-adrenoceptors and $M_2$ receptors (Gs- and Gi-proteins) are the same as described in Chapter 3 (see Fig. 3.6) for the regulation of cardiac contraction. A number of drugs can

| TABLE 2-3 | EXTRINSIC FACTORS INCREASING OR DECREASING CONDUCTION VELOCITY WITHIN THE HEART | |
|---|---|
| INCREASING | DECREASING |
| Sympathetic stimulation | Parasympathetic stimulation |
| Muscarinic receptor antagonists | Muscarinic receptor agonists |
| β-Adrenoceptor agonists | β-Blockers |
| Circulating catecholamines | Ischemia/hypoxia |
| Hyperthyroidism | Sodium and calcium channel blockers |

affect conduction velocity by altering autonomic influences or directly altering intercellular conduction. For example, antiarrhythmic drugs that block fast sodium channels decrease conduction velocity in nonnodal tissue; digoxin activates vagal influences on the conduction system, particularly at the AV node; and β-adrenoceptor agonists or antagonists can increase or decrease conduction velocity, respectively.

---

**PROBLEM 2-2**

A drug is found to partially inactivate fast sodium channels. How would this drug alter the action potential in a ventricular myocyte? How would the drug alter conduction velocity within the ventricle?

---

## Abnormal Conduction

When electrical activation of the heart does not follow the normal pathways outlined earlier, the efficiency of ventricular contraction may be reduced, and arrhythmias may be precipitated. For example, if the AV node becomes completely blocked by ischemic damage or excessive vagal stimulation, impulses cannot travel from the atria into the ventricles. Fortunately, latent pacemakers within the ventricular conduction system usually take over to activate the ventricles; however, the lower firing rate of these pacemakers results in ventricular bradycardia and decreased cardiac output. As another example, if one of the bundle branches is blocked, ventricular depolarization still occurs, but the depolarization pathways will be altered, leading to a delay in ventricular activation and reduced contraction efficiency. An ectopic beat originating within the ventricle can cause altered pathways of conduction as well. When this occurs outside of the normal fast conducting system, it alters the pathway of depolarization, and ventricular depolarization has to rely on the relatively slow cell-to-cell conduction between myocytes.

## Tachycardia Caused by Reentry

Reentry is an important mechanism in the generation of tachycardias. Reentry occurs when a conducting pathway is stimulated prematurely by a previously conducted action potential, leading to a rapid, cyclical reactivation as described in Figure 2.11. In this illustration, if a single Purkinje fiber forms two branches (1 and 2), the action potential will divide and travel down each branch (left panel). If these branches then come together into a common branch (3), the action potentials will cancel each other out, and reentry will not occur. An electrode (*) recording from branch 3 would record single, normal action potentials as they are conducted in this branch.

To model what occurs during reentry, suppose that branch 2 (right panel) has a unidirectional block (impulses can travel retrograde but not orthograde) caused by partial depolarization. An action potential traveling down branch 1, after entering the common distal path (branch 3), travels in retrograde fashion through the unidirectional block in branch 2. Within the block, the conduction velocity is reduced because the tissue is depolarized. As the action potential exits the block, if it finds the tissue excitable (i.e., beyond the refractory period), then the action potential will once again be conducted down branch 1 (i.e., reenter branch 1). If the action potential exits the block more rapidly and finds the tissue unexcitable (i.e., within its refractory period), then the action potential will cease to propa-

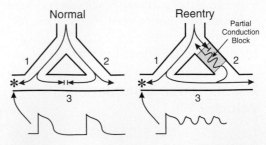

■ **FIGURE 2.11** Mechanism of reentry. With normal conduction of action potentials, impulses traveling down branches 1 and 2 cancel out each other in branch 3. Reentry can occur if branch 2 has impaired conduction and blocks orthograde impulses, but slowly conducts retrograde impulses. If a retrograde impulse emerging from branch 2 reaches excitable tissue (after the ERP, but before the next normal impulse), a premature action potential can be conducted down branch 1. If this occurs with successive action potentials, tachycardia occurs.

gate. Therefore, timing is critical because the action potential exiting the block must find the tissue excitable to continue propagation and thereby establish a reentry circuit.

Because both conduction velocity and refractory state of the tissue are important for reentry to occur, alterations in conduction velocity and tissue refractoriness can either precipitate or abolish reentry circuits. Arrhythmias caused by reentry can be paroxysmal in nature (sudden onset and disappearance) because the conditions necessary to establish and maintain reentry are altered by normal variations in conduction velocity and refractoriness brought about by autonomic and other influences. Changes in autonomic nerve function, therefore, can significantly affect reentry mechanisms, either precipitating in susceptible individuals or terminating reentry circuits. Antiarrhythmic drugs that alter the ERP or conduction velocity can be used to prevent or abolish reentry.

Reentry can occur either globally (e.g., between the atria and ventricles) or locally (e.g., within a small region of the ventricle or atrium) as shown in Figure 2.12. Global reentry between the atria and ventricles often involves accessory conduction pathways such as the bundle of Kent. Accessory pathways allow impulses to be conducted by one or more routes in addition to the normal AV nodal pathway. In the example shown in Figure 2.12, the impulse travels through the accessory pathway, depolarizes the ventricular tissue, and then travels backward (retrograde) through the AV node to reexcite the atrial tissue and thereby establish a counterclockwise global reentry circuit. (The reentry circuit can also occur clockwise in direction.) Global reentry between the atria and ventricles results in supraventricular tachyarrhythmias (e.g., Wolff-Parkinson-White syndrome). Local sites of reentry within a small region of the ventricle or atrium can precipitate ventricular or atrial tachyarrhythmias, respectively.

---

**CASE 2-1**

A patient is diagnosed with a supraventricular tachycardia caused by reentry within the AV node. Explain how using a drug that increases the ERP of the AV nodal tissue can be used to abolish this tachyarrhythmia.

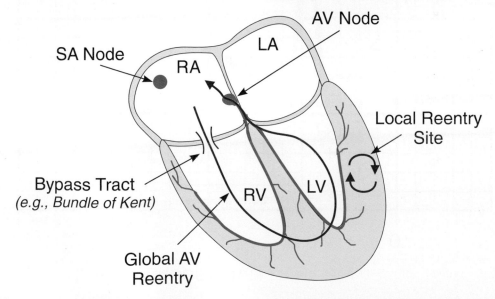

■ **FIGURE 2.12** Global and local reentry. Global reentry can occur between the atria and ventricles utilizing an accessory pathway in addition to the AV node. One such pathway is the Bundle of Kent between the RA and RV, which can lead to retrograde action potential conduction (in this illustration) through the AV node and cause premature excitation of atrial muscle and a supraventricular tachycardia. Local reentry circuits can occur within either the ventricles or atria and produce tachyarrhythmias.

## THE ELECTROCARDIOGRAM

The ECG is a crucial diagnostic tool in clinical practice. It is especially useful in diagnosing rhythm disturbances, changes in electrical conduction, and myocardial ischemia and infarction. The remaining sections of this chapter describe how the ECG is generated and how it can be used to examine changes in cardiac electrical activity.

## ECG Tracing

As cardiac cells depolarize and repolarize, electrical currents spread throughout the body because the tissues surrounding the heart are able to conduct electrical currents generated by the heart. When these electrical currents are measured by an array of electrodes placed at specific locations on the body surface, the recorded tracing is called an ECG

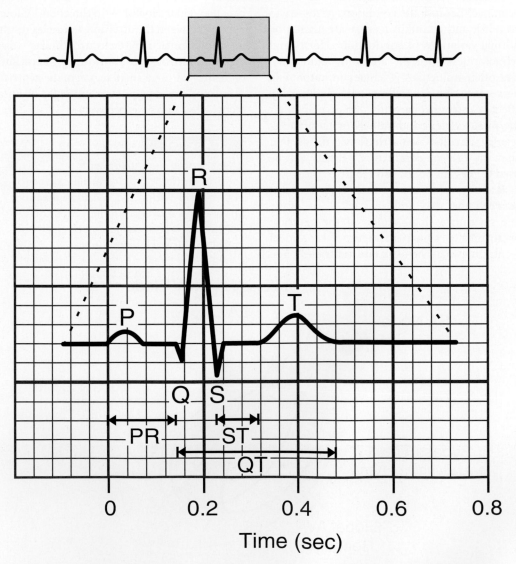

■ **FIGURE 2.13** Components of the ECG trace. An enlargement of one of the repeating waveform units in the rhythm strip shows the P wave, QRS complex, and T wave, which represent atrial depolarization, ventricular depolarization, and ventricular repolarization, respectively. The PR interval represents the time required for the depolarization wave to transverse the atria and the AV node; the QT interval represents the period of ventricular depolarization and repolarization; and the ST segment is the isoelectric period when the entire ventricle is depolarized. Each small square is 1 mm.

(Fig. 2.13). The repeating waves of the ECG represent the sequence of depolarization and repolarization of the atria and ventricles. The ECG does not measure absolute voltages, but voltage changes from a baseline (isoelectric) voltage. ECGs are generally recorded on paper at a speed of 25 mm/s and with a vertical calibration of 1 mV/cm.

By convention, the first wave of the ECG is the **P wave** (Fig. 2.13). It represents the wave of depolarization that spreads from the SA node throughout the atria; it is usually 0.08 to 0.1 seconds in duration (Table 2-4). No distinctly visible wave represents atrial repolarization in the ECG because it is masked by ventricular depolarization and is of relatively small amplitude. The brief isoelectric (zero voltage) period after the P wave represents the time in which the atrial cells are depolarized and the impulse is traveling within the AV node, where conduction velocity is greatly reduced. The period of time from the onset of the P wave to the beginning of the QRS complex, the **PR interval**, normally ranges from 0.12 to 0.20 seconds. This interval represents the time between the onset of atrial depolarization and the onset of ventricular depolarization. If the PR interval is >0.2 seconds, a conduction defect (usually within the AV node) is present (e.g., first-degree AV block).

The **QRS complex** represents ventricular depolarization. The duration of the QRS complex is normally 0.06 to 0.1 seconds, indicating that ventricular depolarization occurs rapidly. If the QRS complex is prolonged (>0.1 seconds), conduction is impaired within the ventricles. Impairment can occur with defects (e.g., bundle branch blocks) or aberrant conduction, or it can occur when an ectopic ventricular pacemaker drives ventricular depolarization. Such ectopic foci nearly always cause impulses to be conducted over slower pathways within the heart, thereby increasing the time for depolarization and the duration of the QRS complex.

The isoelectric period (**ST segment**) following the QRS is the period at which the entire ventricle is depolarized and roughly corresponds to the plateau phase of the ventricular action potential. The ST segment is important in the diagnosis of ventricular ischemia, in which the ST segment can become either depressed or elevated, indicating nonuniform membrane potentials in ventricular cells. The **T wave** represents ventricular repolarization (phase 3 of the action potential) and lasts longer than depolarization.

During the **QT interval**, both ventricular depolarization and repolarization occur. This interval roughly estimates the duration of ventricular action potentials. The QT interval can range from 0.2 to 0.4 seconds depending on heart rate. At high heart rates, ventricular action potentials are shorter, decreasing the QT interval. Because prolonged QT intervals can be diagnostic for susceptibility to certain types of arrhythmias, it is important to determine if a given QT interval is excessively long. In practice, the QT interval is expressed as a corrected QT (QTc) interval by taking the QT interval and dividing it by the square root of the RR interval (the interval between ventricular depolarizations). This calculation allows the QT interval to be assessed independent of heart rate. Normal corrected QTc intervals are <0.44 seconds.

### TABLE 2-4  SUMMARY OF ECG WAVES, INTERVALS, AND SEGMENTS

| ECG COMPONENT | REPRESENTS | NORMAL DURATION (S) |
|---|---|---|
| P wave | Atrial depolarization | 0.08–0.10 |
| QRS complex | Ventricular depolarization | 0.06–0.10 |
| T wave | Ventricular repolarization | [1] |
| PR interval | Atrial depolarization plus AV nodal delay | 0.12–0.20 |
| ST segment | Isoelectric period of depolarized ventricles | [1] |
| QT interval | Length of depolarization plus repolarization—corresponds to action potential duration | 0.20–0.40[2] |

[1]Duration not normally measured.
[2]High heart rates reduce the action potential duration and therefore the QT interval.

## Interpretation of Normal and Abnormal Cardiac Rhythms from the ECG

One important use of the ECG is to enable a physician to evaluate abnormally slow, rapid, or irregular cardiac rhythms. Atrial and ventricular rates of depolarization can be determined from the frequency of P waves and QRS complexes by recording a **rhythm strip**. A rhythm strip is usually generated from a single ECG lead (often lead II). In a normal ECG (Fig. 2.14), a consistent, one-to-one correspondence exists between P waves and the QRS complex; that is, each P wave is followed by a QRS complex. This correspondence indicates that ventricular depolarization is being triggered by atrial depolarization. Under these normal conditions, the heart is said to be in **sinus rhythm**, because the SA node is controlling the cardiac rhythm. Normal sinus rhythm can range from 60 to 100 beats/min. Although the term "beats" is being used here, strictly speaking, the ECG gives information only about the frequency of electrical depolarizations. However, a depolarization usually results in contraction and therefore a "beat."

Abnormal rhythms (arrhythmias) can be caused by abnormal formation of action potentials. A sinus rate <60 beats/min is termed **sinus bradycardia**. The resting sinus rhythm, as previously described, is highly dependent on vagal tone. Some people, especially highly conditioned athletes, may have normal resting heart rates that are significantly <60 beats/min. In other individuals, sinus bradycardia may result from depressed SA nodal function. A sinus rate of 100 to 180 beats/min, **sinus tachycardia**, is an abnormal condition for a person at rest; however, it is a normal response when a person exercises or becomes excited.

In a normal ECG, a QRS complex follows each P wave. Conditions exist, however, when the frequency of P waves and QRS complexes may be different (Fig. 2.14). For example, atrial rate may become so high in **atrial flutter** (250 to 350 beats/min) that not all of the impulses are conducted through the AV node;

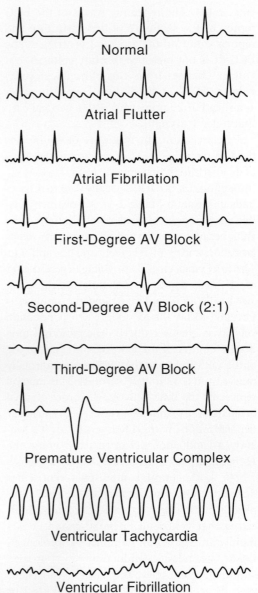

Normal

Atrial Flutter

Atrial Fibrillation

First-Degree AV Block

Second-Degree AV Block (2:1)

Third-Degree AV Block

Premature Ventricular Complex

Ventricular Tachycardia

Ventricular Fibrillation

■ **FIGURE 2.14** ECG examples of abnormal rhythms. *AV,* atrioventricular.

therefore, the ventricular rate (as determined by the frequency of QRS complexes) may be less than half of the atrial rate. In **atrial fibrillation**, the SA node does not trigger the atrial depolarizations. Instead, depolarization currents arise from many sites throughout the atria, leading to uncoordinated, low-voltage, high-frequency depolarizations with no discernable P waves. In this condition, the ventricular rate is irregular and usually rapid. Atrial fibrillation and flutter illustrate an important function of the AV node; it limits the frequency of impulses that it conducts, thereby limiting ventricular rate. This feature is important because when ventricular rates become very high (e.g., >200 beats/min), cardiac output falls owing to inadequate time for ventricular filling between contractions.

Atrial rate is greater than ventricular rate in some forms of **AV block** (see Fig. 2.14). This is an example of an arrhythmia caused by abnormal (depressed) impulse conduction. With AV block, atrial rate is normal, but every atrial depolarization may not be followed by a ventricular depolarization. A **second-degree AV block** may have two or three P waves preceding each QRS complex because the AV node does not successfully conduct every impulse. In a less severe form of AV block, the conduction through the AV node is delayed, but the impulse is still able to pass through the AV node and excite the ventricles. With this condition, termed **first-degree AV block,** a consistent one-to-one correspondence remains between the P waves and QRS complexes; however, the PR interval is found to be >0.2 seconds. In an extreme form of AV nodal blockade, **third-degree AV block,** no atrial depolarizations are conducted through the AV node into the ventricles, and P waves and QRS complexes are completely dissociated. The ventricles still undergo depolarization because of the expression of a secondary, latent pacemaker site (e.g., within the AV junction or from some ectopic foci within the ventricles); however, the ventricular rate is generally slow (<40 beats/min). Ventricular bradycardia occurs because the intrinsic firing rate of secondary, latent pacemakers is much slower than in the SA node. For example, pacemaker cells within the AV node and bundle of His have rates of 50 to 60 beats/min, whereas those in the Purkinje system have rates of only 30 to 40 beats/min. If the ectopic foci are located within the ventricles, the QRS complex will have an abnormal shape and be wider than normal because depolarization does not follow the normal conduction pathways.

---

**CASE 2-2**

A patient is being treated for hypertension with a β-blocker (a drug that blocks β-adrenoceptors in the heart) in addition to a diuretic. A routine ECG reveals that the patient's PR interval is 0.24 seconds (first-degree AV nodal block). Explain how removal of the β-blocker might improve AV nodal conduction.

---

A condition can arise in which ventricular rate is greater than atrial rate; that is, the frequency of QRS complexes is greater than the frequency of P waves (see Fig. 2.14). This condition is termed **ventricular tachycardia** (100 to 200 beats/min) or **ventricular flutter** (>200 beats/min). The most common causes of ventricular tachycardias are reentry circuits caused by abnormal impulse conduction within the ventricles or rapidly firing ectopic pacemaker sites within the ventricles (which may be caused by afterdepolarizations). With ventricular tachycardias, there is a complete dissociation between atrial and ventricular rates because ventricular depolarizations are not being triggered by atrial sites. Both ventricular tachycardia and ventricular flutter are serious clinical conditions because they impair ventricular filling, reduce stroke volume, and can lead to **ventricular fibrillation** (see Fig. 2.14). This latter condition is seen in the ECG as rapid, low-voltage, uncoordinated depolarizations (having no discernable QRS complexes), which results in cardiac output going to zero. This lethal condition can sometimes be reverted to a sinus rhythm by applying strong but brief electrical currents to the heart by placing electrodes on the chest (electrical defibrillation).

The ECG can reveal another type of arrhythmia, **premature depolarizations** (see Fig. 2.14). These depolarizations can occur within either the atria (premature atrial complex) or the ventricles (premature ventricular complex). They are usually caused by ectopic pacemaker sites within these cardiac regions and appear as extra (and early) P waves or QRS complexes. These premature depolarizations are often abnormally shaped, particularly in ventricles, because the impulses generated by the ectopic site are not conducted through normal pathways.

## Volume Conductor Principles and ECG Rules of Interpretation

The previous section defined the components of the ECG trace and what they represent in terms of electrical events within the heart. This section examines in more detail how the appearance of the recorded ECG waveform depends on (1) location of recording electrodes on the body surface; (2) conduction pathways and speed of conduction; and (3) changes in muscle mass. To interpret the significance of changes in the appearance of the ECG, we must first understand the basic principles of how the ECG is generated and recorded.

### VECTORS AND MEAN ELECTRICAL AXIS

The ECG records time-dependent changes in electrical activity within the heart. At a given instant in time, the recording electrodes "see" a summation of all the regions of the heart that are undergoing depolarization or repolarization. To help understand this concept, Figure 2.15 illustrates waves of depolarization originating within the SA node and then spreading into the atrial muscle. When the SA node fires, many separate depolarization waves emerge from the SA node and travel throughout the atria. These separate waves can be depicted as arrows representing individual **electrical**

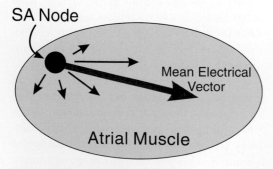

■ **FIGURE 2.15** Electrical vectors. Individual instantaneous vectors of depolarization (*black arrows*) spread across the atria after the sinoatrial (*SA*) node fires. The mean electrical vector (*red arrow*) represents the sum of the individual vectors at a given instant in time.

**vectors**. At any given instant, many individual instantaneous electrical vectors exist; each one represents action potential conduction in a different direction. An instantaneous **mean electrical vector** can be derived by summing the individual instantaneous vectors.

In the heart, the mean electrical vector changes its orientation as different regions of the heart undergo depolarization or repolarization. The direction of the mean electrical vector relative to the axis between positive and negative recording electrodes determines the polarity and influences the magnitude of the recorded voltage as illustrated in Figure 2.16. This illustration depicts the sequence of depolarization within the ventricles by showing four different mean vectors representing different times during depolarization. In this model, the septum and free walls of the left and right ventricles are shown, and each of the four vectors is depicted as originating from the top of the septum where the left and right bundle branches divide. The size of the vector arrow is related to the mass of tissue undergoing depolarization; the larger the arrow (and tissue mass), the greater the measured voltage. The placement of the positive recording electrodes represents leads II and $aV_L$ (described later in this chapter). Before the ventricles undergo depolarization (Panel A), there are no electrical vectors so the voltage recording in either lead will be zero. Early during ventricular activation (Panel B), the first region to depolarize is the interventricular septum, which normally depolarizes from left to right as depicted by the mean electrical vector. The vector is small because the tissue mass is small. Because the vector is heading away from the $aV_L$ positive electrode, this results in a negative voltage in that lead (Q wave of the QRS). The same mean vector, however, when recorded using lead II will not show a change in voltage (no Q wave) because the mean vector is oriented perpendicular to the lead II axis. About 20 milliseconds later (Panel C), the septum is completely depolarized and the apex of the heart begins to depolarize. At this time, the mean electrical vector points downward toward the apex and is heading roughly perpendicular to the $aV_L$ lead axis, thereby generating only a very small positive voltage in $aV_L$.

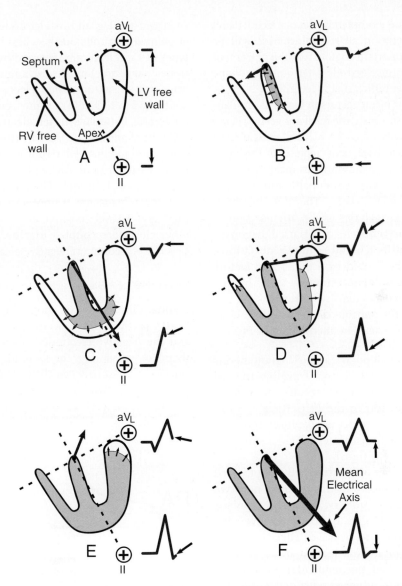

■ **FIGURE 2.16** Generation of QRS complex from two different recording electrodes. **A.** Ventricles prior to depolarization; isoelectric (zero) voltage recorded by electrodes $aV_L$ and II. **B.** Septal depolarization; voltage $aV_L$ < II. **C.** Apical depolarization; voltage $aV_L$ < II. **D.** Left ventricular depolarization (primarily); voltage $aV_L$ > II. **E.** Left ventricular depolarization; voltage in $aV_L$ > II. **F.** Ventricles depolarized; isoelectric voltage in $aV_L$ and II; *red arrow* represents mean electrical axis.

In contrast, the mean vector is heading almost directly towards the lead II positive electrode, which results in a very tall, positive deflection (R wave of the QRS). After another 20 milliseconds (Panel D), the apex and most of the right ventricular free wall are completely depolarized. At this time, the left ventricular free wall depolarizes from the endocardial (inside) to epicardial (outside) surface. The resulting mean vector is mostly heading toward the $aV_L$

electrode and is almost perpendicular to the lead II axis. Therefore, this vector produces a large positive voltage in lead $aV_L$ and a relatively small positive voltage in lead II. The last regions of the left ventricle to depolarize (Panel E) result in a mean vector that is heading somewhat toward lead $aV_L$, and away from lead II. Therefore, $aV_L$ will still record a small positive voltage, whereas lead II will record a small negative voltage (S wave of the QRS). When the ventricles are completely depolarized (Panel F), the voltage in all recording leads will be zero. It is important to note that the placement of the recording electrode determines the shape of the QRS complex that is recorded.

If the four mean vectors in Figure 2.16 (Panels B-E) are summed, the resultant vector (Panel F, large red arrow) is the **mean electrical axis**. The mean electrical axis represents the average of all of the instantaneous mean electrical vectors occurring sequentially during ventricular depolarization. The determination of mean electrical axis is of particular significance for the ventricles and is used diagnostically to identify left and right axis deviations, which can be caused by a number of factors including conduction blocks in a bundle branch and ventricular hypertrophy.

Based on the previous discussion, the following rules can be used in interpreting the ECG:

1. **A wave of depolarization (instantaneous mean electrical vector) traveling toward a positive electrode results in a positive deflection in the ECG trace.** (Corollary: A wave of depolarization traveling away from a positive electrode results in a negative deflection.)
2. **A wave of repolarization traveling toward a positive electrode results in a negative deflection.** (Corollary: A wave of repolarization traveling away from a positive electrode results in a positive deflection.)
3. **A wave of depolarization or repolarization oriented perpendicular to an electrode axis produces no *net* deflection.**
4. **The instantaneous amplitude of the measured potentials depends upon the orientation of the positive electrode relative to the mean electrical vector.**
5. **Voltage amplitude (positive or negative) is directly related to the mass of tissue undergoing depolarization or repolarization.**

## ECG Leads: Placement of Recording Electrodes

The ECG is recorded by placing an array of electrodes at specific locations on the body surface. Conventionally, electrodes are placed on

each arm and leg, and six electrodes are placed at defined locations on the chest. Three basic types of ECG leads are recorded by these electrodes: standard limb leads, augmented limb leads, and chest leads. These electrode leads are connected to a device that measures potential differences between selected electrodes to produce the characteristic ECG tracings. The limb leads are sometimes referred to as **bipolar** leads because each lead uses a single pair of positive and negative electrodes. The augmented leads and chest leads are **unipolar** leads because they have a single positive electrode with the other electrodes coupled together electrically to serve as a common negative electrode.

### ECG LIMB LEADS

**Standard limb leads** are shown in Figure 2.17. **Lead I** has the positive electrode on the left arm and the negative electrode on the right arm, therefore measuring the potential difference across the chest between the two arms. In this and the other two limb leads, an electrode on the right leg is a reference electrode for recording purposes. In the **lead II** configuration, the positive electrode is on the left leg and the

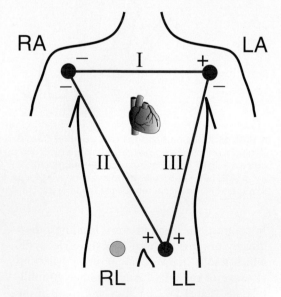

■ **FIGURE 2.17** Placement of the standard ECG limb leads (leads I, II, and III) and the location of the positive and negative recording electrodes for each of the three leads. *RA*, right arm; *LA*, left arm; *RL*, right leg; *LL*, left leg.

negative electrode is on the right arm. **Lead III** has the positive electrode on the left leg and the negative electrode on the left arm. These three limb leads roughly form an equilateral triangle (with the heart at the center), called **Einthoven triangle** in honor of Willem Einthoven who developed the ECG in 1901. Whether the limb leads are attached to the end of the limb (wrists and ankles) or at the origin of the limbs (shoulder and upper thigh) makes virtually no difference in the recording because the limb can be viewed as a wire conductor originating from a point on the trunk of the body.

When using the ECG rules described in the previous section, a wave of depolarization heading toward the left arm gives a positive deflection in lead I because the positive electrode is on the left arm. Maximal positive deflection of the tracing occurs in lead I when a wave of depolarization travels parallel to the axis between the right and left arms. If a wave of depolarization heads away from the left arm, the deflection is negative. In addition, a wave of repolarization moving away from the left arm is seen as a positive deflection.

Similar statements can be made for leads II and III, with which the positive electrode is located on the left leg. For example, a wave of depolarization traveling toward the left leg gives a positive deflection in both leads II and III because the positive electrode for both leads is on the left leg. A maximal positive deflection is obtained in lead II when the depolarization wave travels parallel to the axis between the right arm and left leg. Similarly, a maximal positive deflection is obtained in

lead III when the depolarization wave travels parallel to the axis between the left arm and left leg.

If the three limbs of Einthoven triangle are broken apart, collapsed, and superimposed over the heart (Fig. 2.18), the positive electrode for lead I is defined as being at zero degrees relative to the heart (along the horizontal axis; see Fig. 2.18). Similarly, the positive electrode for lead II is +60° relative to the heart, and the positive electrode for lead III is +120° relative to the heart, as shown in Figure 2.18. This new construction of the electrical axis is called the **axial reference system**. Although the designation of lead I as being 0°, lead II as being +60°, and so forth is arbitrary, it is the accepted convention. With this axial reference system, a wave of depolarization oriented at +60° produces the greatest positive deflection in lead II. A wave of depolarization oriented +90° relative to the heart produces equally positive deflections in both leads II and III. In the latter case, lead I shows no net deflection because the wave of depolarization is heading perpendicular to the 0°, or lead I, axis (see ECG rules).

Three **augmented limb leads** exist in addition to the three bipolar limb leads described. Each of these leads has a single positive electrode that is referenced against a combination of the other limb electrodes. The positive electrodes for these augmented leads are located on the left arm ($aV_L$), the right arm ($aV_R$), and the left leg ($aV_F$; the "F" stands for "foot"). In practice, these are the same positive electrodes used for leads I, II, and III. (The ECG

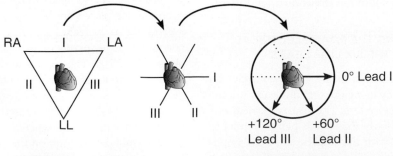

Einthoven's Triangle                    Axial Reference System

■ **FIGURE 2.18** Transformation of leads I, II, and III from Einthoven triangle into the axial reference system. Leads I, II, and III correspond to 0°, +60°, and +120° in the axial reference system. *RA,* right arm; *LA,* left arm; *LL,* left leg.

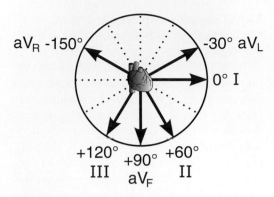

■ **FIGURE 2.19** The axial reference system showing the location within the axis of the positive electrode for each of the six limb leads.

machine does the actual switching and rearranging of the electrode designations.) The axial reference system in Figure 2.19 shows that the $aV_L$ lead is at −30° relative to the lead I axis; $aV_R$ is at −150°, and $aV_F$ is at +90°. It is critical to learn which lead is associated with each axis.

The three augmented leads, coupled with the three standard limb leads, constitute the six limb leads of the ECG. These leads record electrical activity along a single plane, the frontal plane relative to the heart. The direction of an electrical vector can be determined at any given instant using the axial reference system and these six leads. If a wave of depolarization is spreading from right to left along the 0° axis (heading toward 0°), lead I shows the greatest positive amplitude. Likewise, if the direction of the electrical vector for depolarization is directed downward (+90°), $aV_F$ shows the greatest positive deflection.

## DETERMINING THE MEAN ELECTRICAL AXIS FROM THE SIX LIMB LEADS

The mean electrical axis for the ventricle can be *estimated* by using the six limb leads and the axial reference system. The mean electrical axis corresponds to the axis that is perpendicular to the lead axis with the smallest net QRS amplitude (net amplitude = positive minus negative deflection voltages of the QRS complex). If, for example, lead III has the smallest net amplitude (a biphasic QRS with equal positive and negative deflections) and leads I and II are equally positive, the mean electrical axis is perpendicular to lead III, which is 120° − 90°, or +30° (see Fig. 2.19). In this example, lead $aV_R$ has the greatest net negative deflection of the QRS.

It is often important to determine if there is a significant deviation in the mean electrical axis from a normal range, which is between −30° and +90°. Less than −30° is considered a **left axis deviation**, and > +90° is considered a **right axis deviation**. Axis deviations can occur because of the physical position of the heart within the chest or changes in the sequence of ventricular activation (e.g., conduction defects). Axis deviations also can occur if ventricular regions are incapable of being activated (e.g., infarcted tissue). Ventricular hypertrophy can display axis deviation (a left shift for left ventricular hypertrophy and a right shift for right ventricular hypertrophy).

### CASE 2-3

A patient's ECG recording shows that the net QRS voltage is zero (equally positive and negative voltages) in lead I, and that leads II and III are equally positive. What is the mean electrical axis? How would leads $aV_L$ and $aV_R$ appear in terms of net negative or net positive voltages?

## ECG CHEST LEADS

The last ECG leads to consider are the unipolar, precordial **chest leads**. These six positive electrodes are placed on the surface of the chest over the heart to record electrical activity in a horizontal plane perpendicular to the frontal plane (Fig. 2.20). The right arm, left arm, and left leg electrodes are used as a combined negative electrode. The six leads are named $V_1$ to $V_6$. $V_1$ is located to the right of the sternum over the fourth intercostal space, whereas $V_6$ is located laterally (midaxillary line) on the chest over the fifth intercostal space. With this electrode placement, $V_1$ overlies the right ventricular free wall,

## ELECTROPHYSIOLOGICAL CHANGES DURING CARDIAC ISCHEMIA

The ECG is a key tool for diagnosing myocardial ischemia and infarction. A 12-lead ECG can identify the extent, location, and progress of damage to the heart following ischemic injury. For example, altered conduction can result in exaggerated Q waves in specific leads following some types of myocardial infarction. Ischemia can also damage conduction pathways, leading to arrhythmias or changes in the shape of the QRS complex. Furthermore, ischemia can produce injury currents flowing from the depolarized ischemic regions to normal regions that can shift the isoelectric portions of the ECG, resulting in upward or downward shifts in the ST segment recorded by overlying electrodes.

The mechanisms by which ischemia and infarction alter the ECG are complex and not fully understood. We do know, however, that tissue hypoxia caused by ischemia results in membrane depolarization. As ATP levels decline during hypoxia, there is a net loss of $K^+$ as it leaks out of cells through $K_{ATP}$ channels (normally inhibited by ATP) and as a result of decreased activity of the $Na^+/K^+$-ATPase pump. Increased extracellular $K^+$, coupled with decreased intracellular $K^+$, causes membrane depolarization. This depolarization inactivates fast sodium channels as previously described, thereby decreasing action potential upstroke velocity. One result is decreased conduction velocity. Changes in refractory period and conduction velocity can lead to reentry currents and tachycardia. Membrane depolarization also alters pacemaker activity and can cause latent pacemakers to become active, leading to changes in rhythm and ectopic beats. Finally, cellular hypoxia results in the accumulation of intracellular calcium, which can lead to afterdepolarizations and tachycardia.

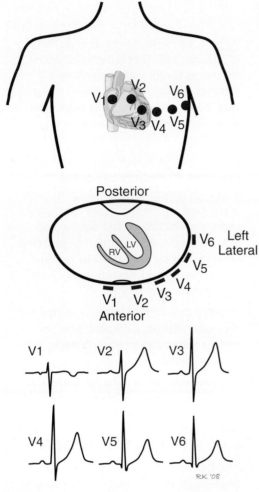

■ **FIGURE 2.20** Placement of the six precordial chest leads and the normal appearance of the ECG recording for leads $V_1 - V_6$. These electrodes record electrical activity in the horizontal plane, which is perpendicular to the frontal plane of the limb leads.

and $V_6$ overlies the left ventricular lateral wall. The rules of interpretation are the same as for the limb leads. For example, a wave of depolarization traveling toward a particular electrode on the chest surface elicits a positive deflection. Normal electrical activation of the ventricles results in a net negative deflection in $V_1$ and a net positive deflection in $V_6$ as shown in Figure 2.20.

## SUMMARY OF IMPORTANT CONCEPTS

- The membrane potential is determined primarily by the concentration of sodium, potassium, and calcium ions across the cell membrane, and by the relative conductances of the membrane to these ions.

- The resting membrane potential is very close to the potassium equilibrium potential (calculated from Nernst equation) because the relative conductance of potassium is much higher than the relative conductances of sodium and calcium in the resting cell.

- Ions move across the cell membrane through ion-selective channels, which have open (activated) and closed (inactivated) states that are regulated by either membrane voltage or by receptor-coupled mechanisms.

- Concentrations of sodium, potassium, and calcium across the cell membrane are maintained by the $Na^+/K^+$-ATPase pump, the $Na^+/Ca^{++}$ exchanger, and the $Ca^{++}$-ATPase pump.

- Nonpacemaker cardiac action potentials are characterized as having very negative resting potentials (approximately −90 mV), a rapid phase 0 depolarization produced primarily by a transient increase in sodium conductance, and a prolonged plateau phase (phase 2) generated primarily by inward calcium currents through L-type calcium channels; increased potassium conductance repolarizes the cells during phase 3.

- Pacemaker action potentials (e.g., those found in SA nodal cells) spontaneously depolarize during phase 4, owing in part to special pacemaker currents ($I_f$). Upon reaching the threshold for action potential generation, calcium conductance increases as L-type calcium channels become activated, which causes depolarization (phase 0). As the calcium channels close, potassium conductance increases and the cell repolarizes (phase 3).

- At rest, SA nodal pacemaker activity is strongly influenced by vagal activity (vagal tone), which significantly reduces the intrinsic SA nodal firing rate. Pacemaker activity is increased by sympathetic activation and vagal inhibition.

- Conduction of action potentials within the heart is primarily cell-to-cell, although specialized conduction pathways exist within the heart that ensure rapid distribution of the conducted action potentials. Conduction velocity is increased by activation of sympathetic nerves and decreased by parasympathetic activation.

- The low conduction velocity within the AV node ensures sufficient time for atrial contraction to contribute to ventricular filling.

- Cells located within the AV node and ventricular conducting system can also serve as pacemakers if the SA node fails or conduction is blocked between the atria and ventricles (AV block).

- The ECG evaluates rhythm and conduction by examining the appearance (amplitude, duration, and shape) of specific waveforms that represent atrial depolarization (P wave), ventricular depolarization (QRS complex), and ventricular repolarization (T wave).

- Different ECG leads view the electrical activity of the heart from different angles. Each limb lead can be represented by an electrical axis on a frontal plane from which the direction of depolarization and repolarization vectors within the heart can be determined using standard rules of interpretation (e.g., a wave of depolarization traveling toward a positive electrode produces a positive voltage in the ECG). Chest leads ($V_1$ to $V_6$) measure the electrical activity in a horizontal plane that is perpendicular to the frontal plane.

For each question, choose the one best answer:

1. Which one of the following depolarizes the resting membrane potential in a cardiac myocyte?
   a. Decreased calcium conductance
   b. Decreased sodium conductance
   c. Increased potassium conductance
   d. Inhibition of the sarcolemmal $Na^+/K^+$-ATPase

2. In nonnodal cardiac tissue, fast sodium channels are inactivated
   a. During phase 0.
   b. When the h-gates open.
   c. By slow depolarization of the cell.
   d. More slowly than L-type calcium channels are inactivated.

3. The relative potassium conductance is highest during which of the following phases of a ventricular action potential?
   a. Phase 0
   b. Phase 2
   c. Early phase 3
   d. Late phase 4

4. The rate of sinoatrial (SA) nodal action potential firing increases during exercise. Which of the following mechanisms can cause this increase in rate?
   a. β-adrenoceptor activation increasing "funny" currents ($I_f$)
   b. Decreasing the slope of phase 4 by vagal (parasympathetic) activation
   c. Inactivation of fast sodium channels
   d. Increased potassium conductance during phase 4

5. The normal sequence of conduction within the heart is
   a. SA node → atrioventricular (AV) node → bundle of His → bundle branches → Purkinje fibers
   b. SA node → bundle of His → AV node →bundle branches → Purkinje fibers
   c. AV node → SA node → bundle of His → bundle branches → Purkinje fibers
   d. SA node → AV node → bundle of His → Purkinje fibers → bundle branches

6. A patient is found to have a PR interval that is >0.2 seconds. Which of the following interventions would most likely reduce the PR interval?
   a. Blocking β-adrenoceptors
   b. Blocking muscarinic ($M_2$) receptors
   c. Blocking L-type calcium channels
   d. Enhancing vagal nerve activity

7. In a normal ECG,
   a. The PR interval is >0.2 seconds.
   b The ST segment represents the duration of the ventricular action potential.
   c. The T wave represents ventricular repolarization.
   d. The duration of the QRS is >0.2 seconds.

8. A patient is found to have normal QRS but inverted T waves in leads II, III, and $aV_F$. Which of the following is the most likely explanation for these findings?
   a. The direction of ventricular repolarization is reversed from normal.
   b. The polarity of the recording electrodes is reversed.
   c. Ventricular depolarization and repolarization are occurring in opposite directions.
   d. Ventricular depolarization is abnormal.

9. The following ECG results are obtained from a patient: The QRS is equally biphasic in lead II (no net deflection), and the QRS has a net positive voltage in lead $aV_L$. What is the approximate mean electrical axis?

    a. −30°
    b. 0°
    c. +60°
    d. +120°

10. An ECG rhythm strip shows a complete dissociation between P waves and QRS complexes. The atrial rate is 95 beats/min and regular, and the ventricular rate is about 60 beats/min and regular. The QRS complexes are of normal shape and duration. This ECG represents

    a. First-degree AV nodal block.
    b. Second-degree AV nodal block.
    c. Third-degree AV nodal block.
    d. Premature ventricular complexes.

## ANSWERS TO REVIEW QUESTIONS

1. The correct answer is "d" because the sarcolemmal $Na^+/K^+$-ATPase is an electrogenic pump that generates hyperpolarizing currents; inhibition of this pump results in depolarization. Furthermore, inhibition of the pump leads to an increase in intracellular sodium and a decrease in intracellular potassium, both of which cause depolarization. Choices "a" and "b" are incorrect because decreased calcium and sodium conductance reduces the inward movement of positive charges that normally depolarize the membrane. Choice "c" is incorrect because increased potassium conductance hyperpolarizes the membrane (see Equation 2-4).

2. The correct answer is "c" because slow depolarization leads to closure of the h-gates, which inactivates the fast sodium channels. Choice "a" is incorrect because the m-gates open at the onset of phase 0, which activates the fast sodium channels. Choice "b" is incorrect because it is the closure of the h-gates that inactivates the channel. Choice "d" is incorrect because L-type (long-lasting) calcium channels have a prolonged phase of activation before they become inactivated.

3. The correct answer is "d" because the membrane potential during phase 4 is primarily determined by the high potassium conductance. Choices "a," "b,"

and "c" are incorrect because the overall potassium conductance is reduced during phases 0 through 2, and it begins to recover only during early phase 3.

4. The correct answer is "a" because one effect of β-adrenoceptor activation is to increase $I_f$, which enhances the rate of spontaneous depolarization. Choice "b" is incorrect because vagal stimulation reduces pacemaker firing rate, in part, by decreasing the slope of phase 4. Choice "c" is incorrect because fast sodium channels do not play a role in SA nodal action potentials; inward calcium currents are responsible for phase 0. Choice "d" is incorrect because increasing potassium conductance during phase 4 hyperpolarizes the cell so it takes longer to reach threshold.

5. The correct sequence of activation and conduction within the heart is choice "a".

6. The correct answer is "b" because acetylcholine released by the vagus nerve binds to $M_2$ receptors, which decreases AV nodal conduction velocity and increases the PR interval. Removal of vagal tone through the use of a muscarinic receptor antagonist (e.g., atropine) leads to an increase in conduction velocity. Choice "a" is incorrect because blocking β-adrenoceptors would decrease the influence of sympathetic nerves on the AV node and lead to a decrease in conduction velocity.

Choice "c" is incorrect because L-type calcium channel blockers reduce conduction velocity by decreasing the rate of calcium entry into the cells during depolarization, which decreases the slope of phase 0 in AV nodal cells, thereby decreasing conduction velocity. Choice "d" is incorrect because enhancing vagal activity decreases AV nodal conduction velocity and increases the PR interval.

7. The correct answer is "c" because the T wave represents repolarization of the ventricular muscle. Choice "a" is incorrect because the normal PR interval is between 0.12 and 0.20 seconds. Choice "b" is incorrect because the duration of the ventricular action potential is most closely associated with the QT interval. Choice "d" is incorrect because the duration of the QRS complex is normally <0.1 seconds.

8. The correct answer is "a" because the T wave is normally positive when the last cells that depolarize are the first to repolarize. When the direction of repolarization is reversed, the T wave becomes inverted. Choice "b" is incorrect because accidental reversal of the electrode polarity would lead to an inverted QRS and inverted T wave. Choice "c" is incorrect because when depolarization and repolarization occur in opposite directions (which is normal), both the QRS and T wave are upright. Choice "d" is incorrect because the QRS, which represents ventricular depolarization, is normal.

9. The correct answer is "a" because when lead II is biphasic, the mean electrical axis must be perpendicular to that lead, and therefore it is either −30° or +150°. Because $aV_L$ is positive, the mean electrical axis must be −30° because that is the axis for $aV_L$. All the other choices are therefore incorrect.

10. The correct answer is "c" because a complete dissociation between P waves and QRS complexes indicates a complete (third-degree) AV nodal block. Furthermore, the rate of ventricular depolarizations and the normal shape and duration of the QRS complexes suggest that the pacemaker driving ventricular depolarization lies within the AV node or bundle of His so that conduction follows normal ventricular pathways. Choice "a" is incorrect because a first-degree AV nodal block increases only the PR interval. Choice "b" is incorrect because all of the QRS complexes would still be preceded by a P wave in a second-degree block. Choice "d" is incorrect because premature ventricular complexes normally have an irregular discharge rhythm and the QRS is abnormally shaped and has a longer-than-normal duration.

## ANSWERS TO PROBLEMS AND CASES

### PROBLEM 2-1
Using Equation 2-1, the membrane potential (actually, the equilibrium potential for potassium) with 4 mM external potassium would be −96 mV. Solving the equation for 40 mM external potassium results in a membrane potential of −35 mV. This is the membrane potential predicted by the Nernst equation assuming that no other ions contribute to the membrane potential (see Equation 2-3). This calculation also neglects any contribution of electrogenic pumps to the membrane potential. Nevertheless, a high concentration of external potassium causes a large depolarization, as predicted by the Nernst equation.

### PROBLEM 2-2
Because phase 0 of myocyte action potentials is generated by activation of fast sodium channels, partial inactivation of these channels would decrease the upstroke velocity of phase 0 (decrease the slope of phase 0). Partial

inactivation also would decrease the maximal degree of depolarization. These changes in phase 0 would reduce the conduction velocity within the ventricle. Blockade of fast sodium channels is the primary mechanism of action of Class I antiarrhythmic drugs such as quinidine and lidocaine.

### CASE 2-1

Reentry requires that cells can be prematurely reexcited by action potentials emerging from adjacent conducting pathways. By increasing the ERP of these cells, the action potential emerging from adjacent pathways may encounter tissue that is still refractory and therefore unexcitable, thereby preventing or abolishing reentry.

### CASE 2-2

Sympathetic nerve activity increases conduction velocity within the AV node (positive dromotropic effect). This effect on the AV node is mediated by norepinephrine binding to β-adrenoceptors within the nodal tissue. A β-blocker would remove this sympathetic influence and slow conduction within the AV node, which might prolong the PR interval.

Therefore, taking the patient off the β-blocker might improve AV nodal conduction and thereby decrease the PR interval to within the normal range (0.12 to 0.20 seconds).

### CASE 2-3

The QRS complex has no net voltage in lead I (i.e., equally positive and negative voltages), which indicates that the mean electrical axis is perpendicular (90°) to lead I (see Rule 3); therefore, it is either at −90° or +90° because the axis for lead I is 0° by definition. Because the QRS is positive in leads II and III, the mean electrical axis must be oriented toward the positive electrode on the left leg, which is used for leads II and III. Therefore, the mean electrical axis cannot be −90°, but is instead +90°. Both $aV_L$ and $aV_R$ leads would have net negative QRS voltages because the direction of the mean electrical axis is away from these two leads, which are oriented at −30° and −150°, respectively (see Fig. 2.19). Furthermore, the net negative deflections in these two augmented leads would be of equal magnitude because each lead axis differs from the mean electrical axis by the same number of degrees.

---

### SUGGESTED RESOURCES

Dubin D. Rapid Interpretation of EKGs. 6th Ed. Tampa: Cover Publishing, 2000.

Katz AM. Physiology of the Heart. 4th Ed. Philadelphia: Lippincott Williams & Wilkins, 2006.

Lilly LS. Pathophysiology of Heart Disease. 5th Ed. Philadelphia: Lippincott Williams & Wilkins, 2011.

Opie LH. The Heart: Physiology from Cell to Circula tion. 4th Ed. Philadelphia: Lippincott Williams & Wilkins, 2004.

# CELLULAR STRUCTURE AND FUNCTION

CHAPTER

Understanding the concepts presented in this chapter will enable the student to:

1. Describe the structure and function of the following cellular components of cardiac myocytes: sarcolemma, intercalated disks, transverse (T)-tubules, myofilaments, sarcomeres, sarcoplasmic reticulum, and terminal cisternae.

2. List the steps of excitation–contraction coupling, and describe the cellular mechanisms involved in its regulation.

3. List in order of preference the metabolic substrates used by the heart, and summarize the importance of oxidative metabolism relative to anaerobic metabolism.

4. Describe the major histological structures of a muscular artery and the function of these structures.

5. Contrast the organization of actin and myosin in vascular smooth muscle with the organization of these myofilaments in cardiac myocytes.

6. Describe the mechanisms and regulation of vascular smooth muscle contraction and relaxation.

7. Compare the major G-protein signal transduction pathways of cardiac muscle and vascular smooth muscle and how these pathways regulate contraction.

8. Describe the effects of endothelial-derived nitric oxide (NO), prostacyclin ($PGI_2$), and endothelin-1 (ET-1) on vascular function.

## INTRODUCTION

Many different cell types are associated with the cardiovascular system. This chapter examines the structure and function of three major types of structural cells that serve important roles in cardiovascular function: cardiac myocytes, vascular smooth muscle, and vascular endothelium.

## CARDIAC CELL STRUCTURE AND FUNCTION

### Myocytes and Sarcomeres

Cardiac myocytes represent a type of striated muscle, so called because crossbands or cross striations are observed microscopically.

Although cardiac muscle shares some structural and functional similarities with skeletal muscle, it has several important differences. Cardiac myocytes are generally single nucleated and have a diameter of approximately 25 μm and a length of about 100 μm in the ventricle (atrial myocytes are smaller). In contrast, although some types of skeletal muscle myocytes may have a similar diameter, their cell lengths run the entire length of the muscle and therefore can be many centimeters long. Cardiac myocytes form a branching network of cells that is sometimes referred to as a **functional syncytium**, which results from a fusion of cells. Individual myocytes connect to each other by way of specialized cell membranes called **intercalated disks**. **Gap junctions** within these intercellular regions

**41**

serve as low-resistance pathways between cells, permitting cell-to-cell conduction of electrical (ionic) currents. Therefore, if one cardiac myocyte is electrically stimulated, cell-to-cell conduction ensures that the electrical impulse will travel to all of the interconnected myocytes. This arrangement allows the heart to contract as a unit (i.e., as a syncytium). In contrast, individual skeletal muscle cells are innervated by motor neurons, which utilize neuromuscular transmission to activate individual muscle fibers to contract. No cell-to-cell electrical conduction occurs in skeletal muscle.

The cardiac myocyte is composed of bundles of myofibrils that contain myofilaments (Fig. 3.1). When myocytes are viewed microscopically, distinct repeating lines and bands can be seen, each of which represents different myofilament components. The segment between two **Z-lines** represents the basic contractile unit of the myocyte, the **sarcomere.** The length of each sarcomere under physiologic conditions ranges from about 1.6 to 2.2 μm in human hearts. As described later and in Chapter 4, the length of the sarcomere is an important determinant of the force of myocyte contraction.

The sarcomere contains **thick** and **thin filaments**, which represent about 50% of the cell volume (see Fig. 3.1). Thick filaments are comprised of myosin, whereas thin filaments contain actin and other associated proteins. Chemical interactions between the actin and myosin filaments during the process of excitation–contraction coupling (see the next section) cause the sarcomere to shorten as the myosin and actin filaments slide past each other, thereby shortening the distance between the Z-lines. Within the sarcomere, a large, filamentous protein called **titin** exists. It connects the myosin filament to the Z-lines, which helps to keep the thick filament centered within the sarcomere. Because of its elastic properties, titin plays an important role in the passive mechanical properties of the heart (see Chapter 4). In addition to titin, myosin, and actin, a number of other proteins form the cytoskeleton of myocytes, connecting the internal and external cell components.

**Myosin** is a large molecular weight protein. Within each sarcomere, myosin molecules are bundled together so that there are about 300 molecules of myosin per thick filament. Each myosin molecule contains two heads,

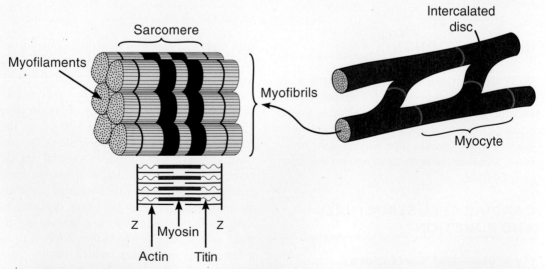

■ **FIGURE 3.1** Structure of cardiac myocytes. Myocytes are joined together by intercalated disks to form a functional syncytium (right side of the figure). Myocytes are composed of myofibrils, each of which contains myofilaments that are composed largely of actin (thin filaments) and myosin (thick filaments) (left side of the figure). Myosin is anchored to the Z-line by the protein titin. The sarcomere, or basic contractile unit, lies between two Z-lines.

which serve as the site of myosin adenosine triphosphatase (**myosin ATPase**), an enzyme that hydrolyzes adenosine triphosphate (ATP). ATP is required for the cross-bridge formation between the thick and thin filaments. The molecule's heads interact with a binding site on actin (Fig. 3.2). Regulatory subunits (myosin light chains) that can alter the ATPase activity when phosphorylated are associated with each myosin head.

Each thick filament is surrounded by a hexagonal arrangement of six thin filaments. The thin filaments are composed of actin, tropomyosin, and troponin (Fig. 3.2). **Actin** is a globular protein arranged as a chain of repeating globular units, forming two helical strands. Interdigitated between the actin strands are rod-shaped proteins called **tropomyosin**. Each tropomyosin molecule is associated with seven actin molecules. Attached to the tropomyosin at regular intervals is the troponin regulatory complex, made up of three subunits: **troponin-T** (TN-T), which attaches to the tropomyosin; **troponin-C** (TN-C), which serves as a binding site for $Ca^{++}$ during excitation–contraction coupling; and **troponin-I** (TN-I), which inhibits myosin binding to actin. The troponin complex holds tropomyosin in position to prevent binding of myosin heads to actin. When $Ca^{++}$ binds to TN-C, a conformational change occurs in the troponin complex such that the troponin–tropomyosin complex moves away from the myosin-binding site on the actin, thereby making the actin accessible to the myosin head for binding. When $Ca^{++}$ is removed from the TN-C, the troponin–tropomyosin complex resumes its inactivated position, thereby inhibiting myosin–actin binding. As a clinical aside, both TN-I and TN-T are used as diagnostic markers for myocardial infarction because of their release into the circulation when myocytes die.

## Excitation–Contraction Coupling

### TRANSVERSE TUBULES AND THE SARCOPLASMIC RETICULUM

The coupling between myocyte action potentials and contraction is called excitation–contraction coupling. To understand this process, the internal structure of the myocyte needs to be examined in more detail. The sarcolemmal membrane of the myocyte surrounds the bundle of myofibrils and has deep invaginations called **transverse (T) tubules** (Fig. 3.3), particularly in ventricular myocytes. The T tubules, being a part of the external sarcolemma, are open to the external environment of the cell. This permits ions to exchange between extracellular and intracellular compartments to occur deep within the myocyte during electrical depolarization and repolarization of the myocyte. Within the cell, and in close association with the T tubules, is an extensive, branching tubular network called the **sarcoplasmic reticulum** that surrounds the myofilaments. The primary function of this structure is to regulate intracellular calcium concentrations, which is involved with contraction and relaxation. **Terminal cisternae** are end pouches of the

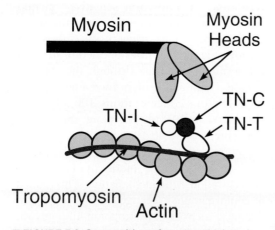

■ **FIGURE 3.2** Composition of cardiac thick and thin myofilaments. The thick filaments are composed of myosin molecules, with each molecule having two myosin heads, which serve as the site of the myosin ATPase. Thin filaments are composed of actin, tropomyosin, and regulatory proteins (troponin complex, TN) having three subunits: TN-T (binds to tropomyosin), TN-C (binds to calcium ions), and TN-I (inhibitory troponin, which inhibits myosin binding to actin). Calcium binding to TN-C produces a conformation change in the troponin–tropomyosin complex that exposes a myosin-binding site on the actin, leading to ATP hydrolysis. For simplicity, this figure shows only one actin strand and its associated tropomyosin filament.

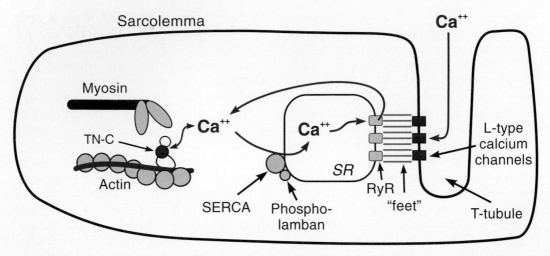

■ **FIGURE 3.3** Role of calcium (*Ca++*) in cardiac excitation–contraction coupling. During action potentials, Ca++ enters cell through L-type Ca++ channels. This so-called trigger Ca++ is sensed by the "feet" of the calcium-release channel (ryanodine receptor, *RyR*) of the sarcoplasmic reticulum (*SR*), which releases Ca++ into the cytoplasm. This Ca++ binds to troponin-C (*TN-C*), inducing a conformational change in the troponin–tropomyosin complex so that movement of the troponin–tropomyosin complex exposes a myosin-binding site on actin, leading to ATP hydrolysis and movement of actin relative to myosin. Ca++ is resequestered into the SR by an ATP-dependent Ca++ pump, sarcoendoplasmic reticulum calcium ATPase (*SERCA*) that is inhibited by phospholamban. Not shown are Ca++ pumps that remove Ca++ from the cell.

sarcoplasmic reticulum that are adjacent to the T tubules. Between the terminal cisternae and the T tubules are electron-dense regions called **feet** that are believed to sense calcium between the T tubules and the terminal cisternae. Closely associated with the sarcoplasmic reticulum are large numbers of mitochondria, which provide the energy necessary for myocyte contraction.

## CALCIUM CYCLING AND THE FUNCTION OF REGULATORY PROTEINS

When an action potential causes depolarization of a myocyte (see Chapter 2), it initiates **excitation–contraction coupling**. When the myocyte is depolarized, calcium ions enter the cell during the action potential through long-lasting (L-type) calcium channels located on the external sarcolemma and T tubules (see Fig. 3.3). It is important to note that a relatively small amount of calcium enters the cell during depolarization. By itself, this calcium influx does not significantly increase intracellular calcium concentrations except in local regions just inside the sarcolemma. This calcium is sensed by the "feet" of the calcium-release channels (**ryanodine**

**receptors**, or **ryanodine-sensitive calcium-release channels**) associated with the terminal cisternae. This triggers the subsequent release of large quantities of calcium stored in the terminal cisternae through the calcium-release channels, which increases intracellular calcium concentrations 100-fold, from about $10^{-7}$ to $10^{-5}$ M. Therefore, the calcium that enters the cell during depolarization is sometimes referred to as "**trigger calcium.**"

The free calcium binds to TN-C in a concentration-dependent manner. This induces a conformational change in the regulatory complex such that the troponin–tropomyosin complex moves away from and exposes a myosin-binding site on the actin molecule. The binding of the myosin head to the actin results in ATP hydrolysis, which supplies energy so that a conformational change can occur in the actin–myosin complex. This results in a movement ("ratcheting") between the myosin heads and the actin. The actin and myosin filaments slide past each other, thereby shortening the sarcomere length (this is referred to as the **sliding filament theory** of muscle contraction) (Fig. 3.4). Ratcheting cycles will occur as long as the cytosolic calcium remains elevated. Toward the end of the myocyte action potential, calcium entry into the cell diminishes and the sarcoplasmic reticulum sequesters calcium by an ATP-dependent calcium pump, sarcoendoplasmic reticulum calcium ATPase (**SERCA**; see Fig. 3-3). As intracellular calcium concentration declines, calcium dissociates from TN-C, which causes a conformational change in the troponin–tropomyosin complex; this again leads to troponin–tropomyosin inhibition of the actin-binding site. At the end of the cycle, a new ATP binds to the myosin head, displacing the adenosine diphosphate, and the initial sarcomere length is restored. Thus, ATP is required both for providing the energy of contraction and for relaxation. In the absence of sufficient ATP as occurs during cellular hypoxia, cardiac muscle contraction and relaxation will be impaired. The events associated with excitation–contraction coupling are summarized in Table 3-1.

## Regulation of Contraction (Inotropy)

Several cellular mechanisms regulate contraction (Fig. 3.5). Most of these mechanisms

| TABLE 3-1 | SUMMARY OF EXCITATION–CONTRACTION COUPLING |
|---|---|

1. Ca$^{++}$ enters cell during depolarization and triggers release of Ca$^{++}$ by terminal cisternae.

2. Ca$^{++}$ binds to TN-C, inducing a conformational change in the troponin complex.

3. Myosin heads bind to actin, leading to cross-bridge movement (requires ATP hydrolysis) and reduction in sarcomere length.

4. Ca$^{++}$ is resequestered by sarcoplasmic reticulum by the SERCA pump.

5. Ca$^{++}$ is removed from TN-C, and myosin unbinds from actin (requires ATP); this allows the sarcomere to resume its original, relaxed length.

ATP, adenosine triphosphate; SERCA, sarcoendoplasmic reticulum calcium ATPase; TN-C, troponin-C.

ultimately affect calcium handling by the cell. Changes in contraction resulting from altered calcium handling and myosin ATPase activity are referred to as inotropic changes (**inotropy**). Inotropy is modulated by (1) calcium entry

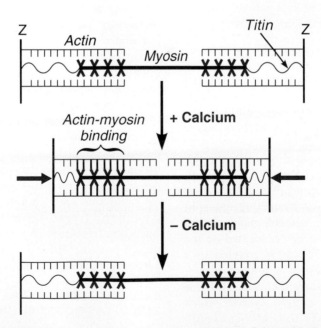

■ **FIGURE 3.4** Sarcomere shortening and the sliding filament theory. Calcium binding to TN-C permits actin–myosin binding (cross-bridge formation) and ATP hydrolysis. This results in the thin filaments sliding over the myosin during cross-bridge cycling, thereby shortening the sarcomere (distance between Z-lines). Removal of calcium from the TN-C inhibits actin–myosin binding so that cross-bridge cycling ceases and the sarcomere resumes its relaxed length.

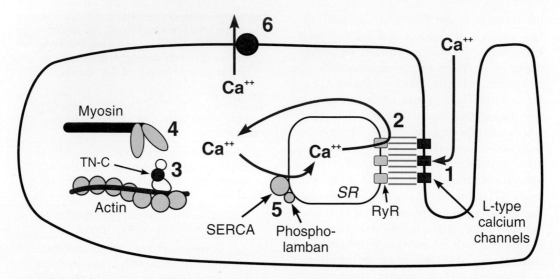

■ **FIGURE 3.5** Intracellular mechanisms regulating inotropy. Inotropy can be increased by increasing Ca$^{++}$ influx through L-type Ca$^{++}$ channels (site 1); increasing release of Ca$^{++}$ by the sarcoplasmic reticulum (*SR*) (site 2); increasing troponin-C (*TN-C*) affinity for Ca$^{++}$ (site 3); increasing myosin–ATPase activity through phosphorylation of myosin heads (site 4); increasing sarcoendoplasmic reticulum calcium ATPase (*SERCA*) activity by phosphorylation of phospholamban (site 5); or inhibiting Ca$^{++}$ efflux across the sarcolemma (site 6).

into the cell through L-type calcium channels; (2) calcium release by the sarcoplasmic reticulum; (3) calcium binding to TN-C; (4) myosin phosphorylation; (5) SERCA activity; and (6) calcium efflux across the sarcolemma.

### CALCIUM ENTRY INTO MYOCYTES

The amount of calcium that enters the cell during depolarization (Fig. 3.5, site 1) is regulated largely by phosphorylation of the L-type calcium channel. The primary mechanism for this regulation involves cyclic adenosine monophosphate (**cAMP**), the formation of which is coupled to β-adrenoceptors (Fig. 3.6). Norepinephrine released by sympathetic nerves, or circulating epinephrine released by the adrenal glands, binds primarily to β$_1$-adrenoceptors located on the sarcolemma. This receptor is coupled to a specific guanine nucleotide-binding regulatory protein (**stimulatory G-protein**; Gs-protein), that activates adenylyl cyclase, which in turn hydrolyzes ATP to cAMP. The cAMP acts as a second messenger to activate **protein kinase A** (cAMP-dependent protein kinase, PK-A), which is capable of phosphorylating

different sites within the cell. One important site of phosphorylation is the L-type calcium channel. Phosphorylation increases the permeability of the channel to calcium, thereby increasing calcium influx during action potentials. This increase in trigger calcium enhances calcium release by the sarcoplasmic reticulum, thereby increasing inotropy. Therefore, norepinephrine and epinephrine are positive inotropic agents.

Another G-protein, the **inhibitory G-protein** (Gi-protein), inhibits adenylyl cyclase and decreases intracellular cAMP. Therefore, activation of this pathway decreases inotropy. This pathway is coupled to muscarinic receptors (M$_2$) that bind acetylcholine released by parasympathetic (vagal) nerves within the heart. Adenosine receptors (A$_1$) also are coupled to the Gi-protein. Therefore, acetylcholine and adenosine are negative inotropic agents.

### CALCIUM RELEASE BY THE SARCOPLASMIC RETICULUM

Enhanced calcium release by the sarcoplasmic reticulum also can increase inotropy (Fig. 3.5, site 2). During β-adrenoceptor and cAMP

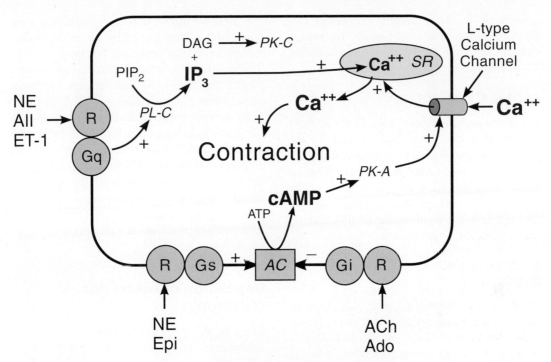

■ **FIGURE 3.6** Signal transduction pathways regulating cardiac myocyte contraction. The two major pathways involve formation of either cyclic adenosine monophosphate (*cAMP*) or inositol 1,4,5-triphosphate (*IP$_3$*), both of which affect Ca$^{++}$ release by sarcoplasmic reticulum and therefore affect contraction. *R*, receptor; *Gs*, stimulatory G-protein; *Gi*, inhibitory G-protein; *Gq*, phospholipase C-coupled G-protein; *AC*, adenylyl cyclase; *PL-C*, phospholipase C; *PIP$_2$*, phosphatidylinositol 4,5-bisphosphate; *DAG*, diacylglycerol; *PK-C*, protein kinase C; *PK-A*, protein kinase A; *SR*, sarcoplasmic reticulum; *ATP*, adenosine triphosphate; *NE*, norepinephrine; *AII*, angiotensin II; *ET-1*, endothelin-1; *Epi*, epinephrine; *ACh*, acetylcholine; *Ado*, adenosine.

activation, PK-A phosphorylates sites on the sarcoplasmic reticulum, leading to an increase in calcium release.

Besides the cAMP pathway, a second pathway within myocytes can affect calcium release by the sarcoplasmic reticulum, although this pathway appears to be less important physiologically than the cAMP/PK-A pathway. This second pathway involves a class of G-proteins (**Gq-proteins**; Fig. 3.6) that are associated with α$_1$-adrenoceptors (bind norepinephrine), angiotensin II receptors (AT$_1$), and endothelin-1 receptors (ET$_A$). Activation of these receptors stimulates **phospholipase C** to form inositol triphosphate (**IP$_3$**) from phosphatidylinositol 4,5-bisphosphate (PIP$_2$), which stimulates calcium release by the sarcoplasmic reticulum.

### CALCIUM BINDING TO TN-C

Another mechanism by which inotropy can be modulated is by altered binding of calcium to TN-C (Fig. 3.5, site 3). The binding of calcium to TN-C is determined by the free intracellular concentration of calcium and the binding affinity of TN-C to calcium. The greater the intracellular calcium concentration, the more the calcium that is bound to TN-C, and the more the force that is generated between actin and myosin. Increasing the affinity of TN-C for calcium increases binding at any given calcium concentration, thereby increasing force generation. Acidosis, which occurs during myocardial hypoxia, has been shown to decrease TN-C affinity for calcium. This may be one mechanism by which acidosis decreases the force of contraction.

Changes in calcium sensitivity may explain in part how increases in sarcomere length (also known as preload; see Chapter 4) leads to an increase in force generation. It appears that increased preload increases calcium sensitivity of TN-C, thereby increasing calcium binding. The mechanism by which changes in length increase calcium affinity by TN-C is unknown.

## MYOSIN ATPASE ACTIVITY

The myosin heads have sites (myosin light chains) that can be phosphorylated by the enzyme myosin light chain kinase (Fig. 3.5, site 4). Increased cAMP is known to be associated with increased phosphorylation of the myosin heads, which may increase inotropy. The physiologic significance of this mechanism, however, is uncertain.

## CALCIUM UPTAKE BY SARCOPLASMIC RETICULUM

In addition to influencing relaxation, increasing calcium transport into the sarcoplasmic reticulum by the SERCA pump can indirectly increase the amount of calcium released by the sarcoplasmic reticulum (Fig. 3.5, site 5). PK-A phosphorylation of phospholamban, which removes the inhibitory effect of phospholamban on SERCA, increases the rate of calcium transport into the sarcoplasmic reticulum. SERCA activity can also be stimulated by increased intracellular calcium caused by increased calcium entry into the cell or decreased cellular efflux. Enhanced sequestering of calcium by the sarcoplasmic reticulum increases subsequent release of calcium by the sarcoplasmic reticulum, thereby increasing inotropy. Because the SERCA pump requires ATP, hypoxic conditions that reduce ATP production by the cell can diminish the pump activity, thereby reducing subsequent release of calcium by the sarcoplasmic reticulum and decreasing inotropy.

## REGULATION OF CALCIUM EFFLUX FROM THE MYOCYTE

The final mechanisms that can modulate inotropy are the sarcolemmal $Na^+/Ca^{++}$ exchange pump and the ATP-dependent calcium pump (Fig. 3.5, site 6). As described in Chapter 2, these pumps transport calcium out of the cell, thereby preventing the cell from becoming overloaded with calcium. If calcium extrusion is inhibited, the rise in intracellular calcium can increase inotropy because more calcium is available to be taken up by the sarcoplasmic reticulum and subsequently released.

Digoxin and related cardiac glycosides inhibit the $Na^+/K^+$-ATPase, which increases intracellular $Na^+$ (see Chapter 2). This leads to an increase in intracellular $Ca^{++}$ through the $Na^+/Ca^{++}$ exchange pump, leading to enhanced inotropy. Cellular hypoxia also decreases the activity of the $Na^+/K^+$-ATPase pump, as well as the $Ca^{++}$-ATPase pump, by reducing ATP availability. This leads to calcium accumulation in the cell; however, inotropy is not increased, in part, because the lack of ATP decreases myosin ATPase activity.

# Regulation of Relaxation (Lusitropy)

The rate of myocyte relaxation (**lusitropy**) is determined by the ability of the cell to rapidly reduce the intracellular concentration of calcium following its release by the sarcoplasmic reticulum. This reduction in intracellular calcium causes calcium that is bound to TN-C to be released, thereby permitting the troponin–tropomyosin complex to resume its resting, inactivated conformation.

Several intracellular mechanisms help to regulate lusitropy, most of which influence intracellular calcium concentrations.

1. The rate at which calcium enters the cell at rest and during action potentials influences intracellular concentrations. Under some pathologic conditions (e.g., myocardial ischemia), the cell becomes more permeable to calcium, leading to "calcium overload," which impairs relaxation.
2. The rate with which calcium leaves the cell through the sarcolemmal calcium ATPase pump and the $Na^+/Ca^{++}$ exchange pump (see Chapter 2) affects intracellular concentrations. Inhibiting these transport systems can cause intracellular calcium concentrations to increase sufficiently to impair relaxation.
3. The activity of the SERCA pump, which pumps calcium back into the sarcoplasmic reticulum, has a major role in determining

intracellular calcium concentrations. Lusitropy can be increased by increasing SERCA activity through phosphorylation of phospholamban, a regulatory protein associated with SERCA. Phosphorylation of phospholamban removes its inhibitory effect on SERCA. This is a normal physiologic mechanism in response to β-adrenoceptor stimulation, which increases cAMP and PK-A, the latter of which phosphorylates phospholamban. Impairment of the activity of the SERCA pump, as occurs in some forms of heart failure, causes intracellular calcium concentrations to rise, leading to impaired relaxation.

4. The binding affinity of TN-C for calcium also influences lusitropy. Calcium binding to TN-C can be modulated by PK-A phosphorylation of TN-I. This increases calcium dissociation from TN-C, thereby increasing relaxation. The increased lusitropy caused by β-adrenoceptor stimulation may be partly related to TN-I phosphorylation. Some drugs used to increase the force of contraction (inotropic drugs) do so by increasing TN-C affinity for calcium. Although this may increase inotropy, it also may lead to reduced lusitropy because the calcium is more tightly bound to the TN-C.

---

**PROBLEM 3-1**

Describe the mechanisms by which norepinephrine, after being released by sympathetic nerve activation, increases myocardial inotropy and lusitropy. Note that norepinephrine primarily binds to $\beta_1$-adrenoceptors, although it also can bind to $\alpha_1$-adrenoceptors.

---

## Cardiac Myocyte Metabolism

The maintenance of ionic pumps and other transport systems in living cells requires significant amounts of energy, primarily in the form of ATP. Cardiac myocytes have an exceptionally high metabolic rate because their primary function is to contract repetitively. Unlike skeletal muscle, in which contraction is often intermittent and relatively

short, cardiac muscle contracts one to three times per second throughout life. Repetitive cycles of contraction and relaxation require an enormous amount of ATP, which the heart must produce aerobically. This is why cardiac myocytes contain such large numbers of mitochondria. In the absence of oxygen, myocytes can contract for no more than a minute. Unlike some types of skeletal muscle fibers (e.g., fast twitch, glycolytic), cardiac myocytes have only a limited anaerobic capacity for meeting ATP requirements. This limited anaerobic capacity coupled with a high use of ATP explains why cellular ATP concentrations fall and contractions weaken so rapidly under hypoxic conditions.

Unlike many other cells in the body, cardiac myocytes can use a variety of substrates to regenerate ATP oxidatively. For example, in an overnight fasted state, the heart uses primarily fatty acids (~60%) and carbohydrates (~40%). Following a high-carbohydrate meal, the heart can adapt to using carbohydrates (primarily glucose) almost exclusively. Lactate can be used in place of glucose, and it becomes an important substrate during exercise when circulating concentrations of lactate increase. The heart also can use amino acids and ketones (e.g., acetoacetate) instead of fatty acids.

Myocyte ATP use and oxygen consumption increase dramatically when the frequency of contraction (i.e., heart rate) and the force of contraction are increased. Under these conditions, more oxygen must be delivered to the heart by the coronary circulation to support myocyte metabolic demands. As Chapter 8 discusses, biochemical signals from the myocytes dilate the coronary blood vessels to supply additional blood flow and oxygen to meet greater oxygen demands. This ensures that the heart is able to generate ATP by aerobic mechanisms.

## VASCULAR STRUCTURE AND FUNCTION

Large blood vessels, both arterial and venous, are composed of three layers—intima, media, and adventitia (Fig. 3.7). The **intima**, or innermost layer, is composed of a single layer

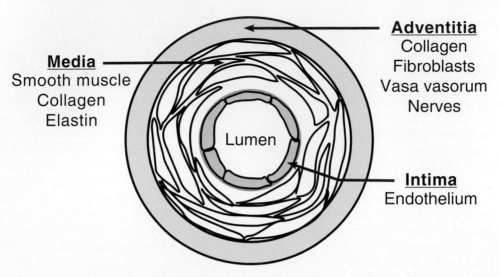

■ **FIGURE 3.7** Blood vessel components. Blood vessels, except capillaries and small postcapillary venules, are composed of three layers: intima, media, and adventitia. Capillaries and small postcapillary venules do not have media and adventitia. The primary components are given for each layer.

of thin endothelial cells, which are separated from the media by a basal lamina. In larger vessels, a region of connective tissue also exists between the endothelial cells and the basal lamina. The **media** contains smooth muscle cells, imbedded in a matrix of collagen, elastin, and various glycoproteins. Depending on the size of the vessel, there may be several layers of smooth muscle cells, some arranged circumferentially and others arranged helically along the longitudinal axis of the vessel. The smooth muscles cells are organized so that their contraction reduces the vessel diameter. The ratio of smooth muscle, collagen, and elastin, each of which has different elastic properties, determines the overall mechanical properties of the vessel. For example, the aorta has a large amount of elastin, which enables it to passively expand and contract as blood is pumped into it from the heart. This mechanism enables the aorta to dampen the arterial pulse pressure (see Chapter 5). In contrast, smaller arteries and arterioles have a relatively large amount of smooth muscle, which is required for these vessels to contract and thereby regulate arterial blood pressure and organ blood flow. The outermost layer, or **adventitia**, is separated from the media by the external elastic lamina.

The adventitia contains collagen, fibroblasts, blood vessels (vasa vasorum found in large vessels), lymphatics, and autonomic nerves (primarily sympathetic adrenergic). The smallest vessels, capillaries, are composed of endothelial cells and a basal lamina; they are devoid of smooth muscle.

## Vascular Smooth Muscle Cells

### CELLULAR STRUCTURE OF VASCULAR SMOOTH MUSCLE

Vascular smooth muscle cells are typically 5 to 10 μm in diameter and vary from 50 to 300 μm in length. Numerous small invaginations (**caveolae**) found in the cell membrane significantly increase the surface area of the cell (Fig. 3.8). The sarcoplasmic reticulum is poorly developed compared with the sarcoplasmic reticulum found in cardiac myocytes. Contractile proteins (actin and myosin) are present; however, the actin and myosin in smooth muscle are not organized into distinct bands of repeating units as they are in cardiac and skeletal muscle. Instead, bands of actin filaments are joined together and anchored by **dense bodies** within the cell or **dense bands** on the inner surface of the sarcolemma, which function like Z-lines in cardiac myocytes. Each myosin filament is

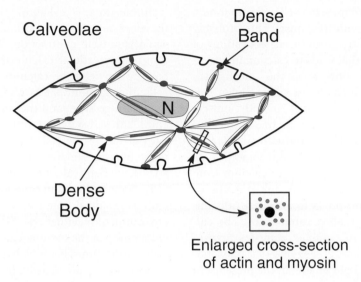

Calveolae

Dense
Band

N

Dense
Body

Enlarged cross-section
of actin and myosin

■ **FIGURE 3.8** Vascular smooth muscle cell structure. Actin and myosin filaments are connected by dense bodies and dense bands. Each myosin filament is surrounded by several actin filaments. *N,* nucleus.

surrounded by several actin filaments. Similar to cardiac myocytes, vascular smooth muscle cells are electrically connected by **gap junctions.** These low-resistance intercellular connections allow propagated responses along the length of the blood vessels. For example, electrical depolarization and contraction of a local site on an arteriole can result in depolarization at a distant site along the same vessel, indicating cell-to-cell propagation of the depolarizing currents.

## VASCULAR SMOOTH MUSCLE CONTRACTION

Contractile characteristics and the mechanisms responsible for contraction differ considerably between vascular smooth muscle and cardiac myocytes. Vascular smooth muscle tonic contractions are slow and sustained, whereas cardiac muscle contractions are rapid and relatively short (a few hundred milliseconds). In blood vessels, the smooth muscle is normally in a partially contracted state, which determines the resting tone or diameter of the vessel. This tonic contraction is determined by stimulatory and inhibitory influences acting on the vessel. As described in later chapters, the most important of these are sympathetic adrenergic nerves, circulating

hormones (e.g., epinephrine, angiotensin II), substances released by the endothelium lining the vessel, and vasoactive substances released by the tissue surrounding the blood vessel.

Vascular smooth muscle contraction can be initiated by electrical, chemical, and mechanical stimuli. Electrical depolarization of the vascular smooth muscle cell membrane using electrical stimulation elicits contraction primarily by opening voltage-dependent calcium channels (L-type calcium channels), which causes an increase in the intracellular concentration of calcium. Membrane depolarization can also occur through changes in ion concentrations (e.g., depolarization induced by high concentrations of extracellular potassium) or by the receptor-coupled opening of ion channels, particularly calcium channels.

Many different chemical stimuli, such as norepinephrine, epinephrine, angiotensin II, vasopressin, endothelin-1, and thromboxane $A_2$ can elicit contraction. Each of these substances binds to specific receptors on the vascular smooth muscle cell. Different signal transduction pathways converge to increase intracellular calcium, thereby eliciting contraction.

Mechanical stimuli in the form of passive stretching of smooth muscle in some arteries can cause a contraction that originates from the smooth muscle itself and is therefore termed a **myogenic response**. This probably results from stretch-induced activation of ionic channels that leads to calcium influx.

Figure 3.9 illustrates the mechanism by which an increase in intracellular calcium stimulates vascular smooth muscle contraction. An increase in free intracellular calcium can result from either increased entry of calcium into the cell through L-type calcium channels or release of calcium from internal stores (e.g., sarcoplasmic reticulum). The free calcium binds to a special calcium-binding protein called **calmodulin**. The calcium–calmodulin complex activates **myosin light chain kinase**, an enzyme that phosphorylates **myosin light chains** in the presence of ATP. Myosin light chains are regulatory subunits found on the myosin heads. Myosin light chain phosphorylation leads to cross-bridge formation between the myosin heads and the actin filaments, thus leading to smooth muscle contraction.

Intracellular calcium concentrations, therefore, are very important in regulating smooth muscle contraction. The concentration of intracellular calcium depends on the balance between the calcium that enters the cells, the calcium that is released by intracellular storage sites, and the movement of calcium either back into intracellular storage sites or out of the cell. Calcium is resequestered by the sarcoplasmic reticulum by an ATP-dependent calcium pump similar to the SERCA pump found in cardiac myocytes. Calcium is removed from the cell to the external environment by either an ATP-dependent calcium pump or the sodium–calcium exchanger, as in cardiac muscle (see Chapter 2).

Several signal transduction mechanisms modulate intracellular calcium concentration and therefore the state of vascular tone. This section describes three different pathways: (1) $IP_3$ via Gq-protein activation of phospholipase C; (2) cAMP via Gs-protein activation of adenylyl cyclase; and (3) cyclic guanosine

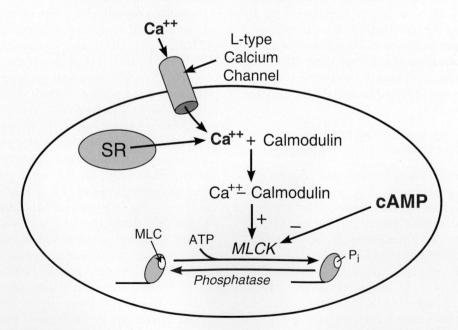

■ **FIGURE 3.9** Regulation of vascular smooth muscle contraction by myosin light chain kinase (*MLCK*). Increased intracellular calcium, by either increased entry into the cell (through L-type Ca++ channels) or release from the sarcoplasmic reticulum (*SR*), forms a complex with calmodulin, activating MLCK, which phosphorylates myosin light chains (*MLC*), causing contraction. Cyclic adenosine monophosphate (*cAMP*) inhibits MLCK, thereby causing relaxation. Dephosphorylation of myosin light chains by MLC phosphatase also produces relaxation. *ATP*, adenosine triphosphate; $P_i$, phosphate group.

monophosphate (cGMP) via nitric oxide (NO) activation of guanylyl cyclase (Fig. 3.10).

The $IP_3$ pathway in vascular smooth muscle is similar to that found in the heart. Norepinephrine and epinephrine (via $\alpha_1$-adrenoceptors), angiotensin II (via $AT_1$ receptors), endothelin-I (via $ET_A$ receptors), vasopressin (via $V_1$ receptors) and acetylcholine (via $M_3$ receptors) activate phospholipase C through the Gq-protein, causing the formation of $IP_3$ from $PIP_2$. $IP_3$ then directly stimulates the sarcoplasmic reticulum to release calcium. The formation of diacylglycerol from $PIP_2$ activates protein kinase C, which can modulate vascular smooth muscle contraction as well via protein phosphorylation.

Receptors coupled to the Gs-protein stimulate adenylyl cyclase, which catalyzes the formation of cAMP. In vascular smooth muscle, unlike cardiac myocytes, an increase in cAMP by a $\beta_2$-adrenoceptor agonist such

as isoproterenol causes relaxation. The mechanism for this process is cAMP inhibition of myosin light chain kinase (see Fig. 3.9), which decreases myosin light chain phosphorylation, thereby inhibiting the interactions between actin and myosin. Adenosine and prostacyclin ($PGI_2$) also activate Gs-protein through their receptors, leading to an increase in cAMP and smooth muscle relaxation. Epinephrine binding to $\beta_2$-adrenoceptors relaxes vascular smooth muscle through the Gs-protein.

A third important mechanism for regulating vascular smooth muscle contraction is the NO–cGMP system. Many endothelial-dependent vasodilator substances (e.g., acetylcholine, bradykinin, substance P), when bound to their respective endothelial receptors, stimulate the conversion of L-arginine to NO by activating NO synthase. The NO diffuses from the endothelial cell to the vascular

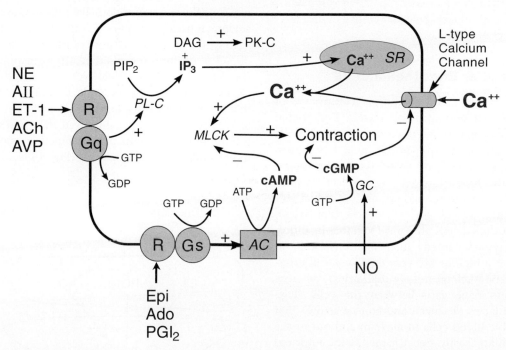

■ **FIGURE 3.10** Receptors and signal transduction pathways that regulate vascular smooth muscle contraction. *R*, receptor; *Gs*, stimulatory G-protein; *Gq*, phospholipase C-coupled G-protein; *AC*, adenylyl cyclase; *PL-C*, phospholipase C; *PIP₂*, phosphatidylinositol 4,5-bisphosphate; *IP₃*, inositol triphosphate; *DAG*, diacylglycerol; *PK-C*, protein kinase C; *SR*, sarcoplasmic reticulum; *MLCK*, myosin light chain kinase; *Ado*, adenosine; *PGI₂*, prostacyclin; *Epi*, epinephrine; *NO*, nitric oxide; *GC*, guanylyl cyclase; *AII*, angiotensin II; *ET-1*, endothelin-1; *NE*, norepinephrine; *ACh*, acetylcholine; *AVP*, arginine vasopressin; *GDP*, guanosine diphosphate; *GTP*, guanosine triphosphate; *ATP*, adenosine triphosphate; *cAMP*, cyclic adenosine monophosphate; *cGMP*, cyclic guanosine monophosphate.

smooth muscle cells, where it activates guanylyl cyclase, increases cGMP formation, and causes smooth muscle relaxation. The precise mechanisms by which cGMP relaxes vascular smooth muscle are unclear; however, cGMP can activate a cGMP-dependent protein kinase, inhibit calcium entry into the vascular smooth muscle, activate K$^+$ channels causing cellular hyperpolarization, stimulate myosin light chain phosphatase, and decrease IP$_3$.

### PROBLEM 3-2

Intracellular cAMP is degraded by a phosphodiesterase enzyme. Milrinone, a drug sometimes used in the treatment of acute heart failure, is a phosphodiesterase inhibitor that increases cardiac inotropy and relaxes blood vessels by inhibiting the degradation of cAMP. Explain why an increase in cAMP in cardiac muscle increases the force of contraction, whereas an increase in cAMP in vascular smooth muscle cells diminishes the force of contraction.

## Vascular Endothelial Cells

The vascular endothelium is a thin layer of cells that line all blood vessels. Endothelial cells are flat, single-nucleated, elongated cells that are 0.2 to 2.0 μm thick and 1 to 20 μm across (varying by vessel type). Depending on the type of vessel (e.g., arteriole versus capillary) and tissue location (e.g., renal glomerular versus skeletal muscle capillaries), endothelial cells are joined together by different types of intercellular junctions. Some of these junctions are very tight (e.g., all arteries and skeletal muscle capillaries), whereas others have gaps between the cells (e.g., capillaries in spleen and bone marrow) that enable blood cells to move in and out of the capillary easily. See Chapter 8 for information about different types of capillaries and endothelium.

Endothelial cells have several important functions, including

1. Serving as a barrier for the exchange of fluid, electrolytes, macromolecules, and cells between the intravascular and extravascular space (see Chapter 8)
2. Regulating smooth muscle function through the synthesis of several different vasoactive substances, the most important of which are NO, PGI$_2$, and endothelin-1
3. Modulating platelet aggregation primarily through biosynthesis of NO and PGI$_2$
4. Modulating leukocyte adhesion and transendothelial migration through the biosynthesis of NO and the expression of surface adhesion molecules

Vascular endothelial cells continuously produce NO. This basal NO production can be enhanced by (1) specific agonists (e.g., acetylcholine, bradykinin) binding to endothelial receptors; (2) increased shearing forces acting on the endothelial surface (e.g., as occurs with increased blood flow); and (3) cytokines such as tumor necrosis factor and interleukins, which are released by leukocytes during inflammation and infection. NO, although very labile, rapidly diffuses out of endothelial cells to cause smooth muscle relaxation or inhibit platelet aggregation in the blood. Both of these actions of NO result from increased cGMP formation (see Fig. 3.10). Endothelial NO also inhibits the expression of adhesion molecules involved in attaching leukocytes to the endothelial surface. Therefore, endothelial-derived NO relaxes smooth muscle, inhibits platelet function, and inhibits inflammatory responses (Fig. 3.11).

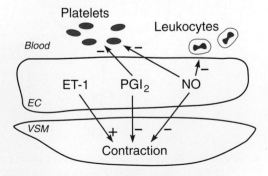

■ **FIGURE 3.11** Endothelial cell (*EC*) production of nitric oxide (*NO*), prostacyclin (*PGI₂*), and endothelin-1 (*ET-1*) stimulates (+) or inhibits (−) vascular smooth muscle (*VSM*) contraction, platelet aggregation and adhesion, and leukocyte–endothelial cell adhesion.

In addition, endothelial cells synthesize endothelin-1 (ET-1), a powerful vasoconstrictor (see Fig. 3.11). Synthesis is stimulated by angiotensin II, vasopressin, thrombin, cytokines, and shearing forces, and it is inhibited by NO and $PGI_2$. ET-1 leaves the endothelial cell and can bind to receptors ($ET_A$) on vascular smooth muscle, which causes calcium mobilization and smooth muscle contraction. The smooth muscle actions of ET-1 occur through activation of the $IP_3$ signaling pathway (see Fig. 3.10).

$PGI_2$ is a product of arachidonic acid metabolism within endothelial cells. The two primary roles of $PGI_2$ formed by endothelial cells are smooth muscle relaxation and inhibition of platelet aggregation (see Fig. 3.11), both of which are induced by the formation of cAMP (see Fig. 3.10).

The importance of normal endothelial function is made clear from examining how endothelial dysfunction contributes to disease states. For example, endothelial damage and dysfunction occur in atherosclerosis,

hypertension, diabetes, and hypercholesterolemia. Endothelial dysfunction results in less NO and $PGI_2$ production, which causes vasoconstriction, loss of vasodilatory capacity, thrombosis, and vascular inflammation. Evidence exists that enhanced ET-1 production contributes to hypertension and other vascular disorders. Physical damage to the endothelium at the capillary level increases capillary permeability (see Chapter 8), which leads to increased capillary fluid filtration and tissue edema.

### PROBLEM 3-3

When acetylcholine is infused into normal coronary arteries, the vessels dilate; however, if the vessel is diseased and the endothelium damaged, acetylcholine can cause vasoconstriction. Explain why acetylcholine can have opposite effects on vascular function depending on the integrity of the vascular endothelium.

### SUMMARY OF IMPORTANT CONCEPTS

- The basic contractile unit of a cardiac myocyte is the sarcomere, which contains thick filaments (myosin) and thin filaments (actin, troponin, and tropomyosin) that are involved in muscle contraction.

- Excitation–contraction coupling is initiated by depolarization of the cardiac myocyte, and is controlled by changes in intracellular calcium, which binds to regulatory proteins on the thin filaments; ATP is required for contraction and relaxation.

- Relaxation of cardiac myocytes (lusitropy) is primarily regulated by the reuptake of calcium into the sarcoplasmic reticulum by the SERCA pump.

- The contractile function of cardiac myocytes requires large amounts of

ATP, which is generated primarily by oxidative metabolism of fatty acids and carbohydrates, although the heart is flexible in its use of substrates and can also metabolize amino acids, ketones, and lactate.

- Arteries and veins are arranged as three layers: adventitia, media, and intima. Autonomic nerves and small blood vessels (vasa vasorum in large vessels) are found in the adventitia; vascular smooth muscle is found in the media; and the intima is lined by the endothelium.

- Vascular smooth muscle contains actin and myosin; however, these components are not arranged in the same repetitive pattern as that found in cardiac myocytes. Unlike cardiac muscle

*(Continued)*

contraction, vascular smooth muscle contraction is slow and sustained.

- Cardiac muscle contraction is regulated by various substances that bind to receptors coupled to G-proteins. Vascular smooth muscle contraction/ relaxation is additionally regulated by NO/cGMP-dependent pathways. All these pathways largely affect

contraction/relaxation primarily by regulating intracellular calcium.

- The vascular endothelium synthesizes nitric oxide and prostacyclin, both of which relax vascular smooth muscle. Endothelin-1, which is also synthesized by the endothelium, contracts vascular smooth muscle.

## REVIEW QUESTIONS

For each question, choose the one best answer:

1. Which of the following is common to both cardiac myocytes and vascular smooth muscle cells?

   a. Dense bodies
   b. Myosin light chain kinase
   c. Terminal cisternae
   d. T tubules

2. Thick filaments within cardiac myocytes contain

   a. Actin.
   b. Myosin.
   c. Tropomyosin.
   d. Troponin.

3. During excitation–contraction coupling in cardiac myocytes,

   a. Calcium binds to myosin causing ATP hydrolysis.
   b. Calcium binds to troponin-I.
   c. Myosin heads bind to actin.
   d. SERCA pumps calcium out of the sarcoplasmic reticulum.

4. Cardiac inotropy is enhanced by

   a. Agonists coupled to Gi-protein.
   b. Decreased calcium binding to troponin-C.
   c. Decreased release of calcium by terminal cisternae.
   d. Protein kinase A phosphorylation of L-type calcium channels.

5. Vascular smooth muscle contraction is enhanced by

   a. Activation of myosin light chain kinase.
   b. Activation of myosin light chain phosphatase.
   c. Calcium binding to troponin-C.
   d. Dephosphorylation of myosin light chains.

6. Angiotensin II causes contraction of vascular smooth muscle by

   a. Activating Gs-protein.
   b. Increasing cAMP.
   c. Increasing IP3.
   d. Inhibiting release of calcium by sarcoplasmic reticulum.

7. A patient in circulatory shock is treated with norepinephrine to raise arterial pressure by stimulating the heart through β-adrenoceptor activation and constricting blood vessels through $\alpha_1$-adrenoceptor activation. The cardiac and vascular effects can be explained by

   a. Increased cardiac cAMP and increased vascular cGMP.
   b. Increased cardiac cAMP and increased vascular $IP_3$.
   c. Increased cardiac and vascular cAMP.
   d. Increased cardiac $IP_3$ and increased vascular cAMP.

8. A patient with a complaint of leg pain is found to have a blood clot in a large artery in his leg; he is subsequently diagnosed with peripheral artery disease. Because peripheral artery disease is associated with endothelial dysfunction, which of the following could have contributed to the formation of the blood clot?

   a. Increased endothelial production of nitric oxide and prostacyclin.
   b. Diminished endothelial production of cGMP.
   c. Increased endothelial production of prostacyclin and decreased production of endothelin-1.
   d. Decreased endothelial production of nitric oxide.

## ANSWERS TO REVIEW QUESTIONS

1. The correct answer is "b" because myosin light chain kinase is involved in myosin phosphorylation in both types of muscle. Choice "a" is incorrect because dense bodies are specialized regions found only within vascular smooth muscle cells where bands of actin filaments are joined together. Choices "c" and "d" are incorrect because these structures are found in cardiac muscle cells, not smooth muscle cells.

2. The correct answer is "b" because myosin is the major component of the thick filament. Choices "a," "c," and "d" are incorrect because they are all components of the thin filament.

3. The correct answer is "c" because a myosin-binding site is exposed on the actin after calcium binds to TN-C. Choices "a" and "b" are incorrect because calcium binds to TN-C, not myosin or TN-I. Choice "d" is incorrect because SERCA pumps calcium back into the sarcoplasmic reticulum.

4. The correct answer is "d" because phosphorylation of the L-type calcium channels by protein kinase A increases the permeability of the channel to calcium, thereby permitting more calcium to enter the cell during depolarization, which triggers the release of calcium by the sarcoplasmic reticulum. Choice "a" is incorrect because Gi-protein activation decreases cAMP formation, thereby decreasing inotropy. Choice "b" is incorrect because calcium binding to TN-C enhances inotropy. Choice "c" is

incorrect because it is the calcium that is released by the terminal cisternae of the sarcoplasmic reticulum that binds to TN-C leading to contraction.

5. The correct answer is "a" because myosin light chain kinase activation by calcium–calmodulin phosphorylates myosin light chains, which induces contraction. Choices "b" and "d" are incorrect because myosin light chain phosphatase activation dephosphorylates the myosin light chains, which causes relaxation. Choice "c" is incorrect because there is no troponin C in vascular smooth muscle.

6. The correct answer is "c" because angiotensin II receptors $(AT_1)$ are coupled to the Gq-protein and activates phospholipase C, which increases $IP_3$. Choice "a" is incorrect because angiotensin II activates the Gq-protein, not the Gs-protein. Choice "b" is incorrect because the Gq-protein stimulates $IP_3$ formation, not cAMP. Choice "d" is incorrect because the increase in $IP_3$ stimulates calcium release from the sarcoplasmic reticulum.

7. The correct answer is "b" because cardiac β-adrenoceptors are coupled to the Gs-protein and cAMP formation, and the vascular $α_1$-adrenoceptors are coupled to the Gq-protein and $IP_3$ formation. Choice "a" is incorrect because cGMP is increased by nitric oxide in blood vessels, not by Gq-protein activation. Choice "c" is incorrect because vascular $α_1$-adrenoceptors are not coupled to the Gs-protein. Choice "d" is incorrect because vascular cAMP is

not increased by Gq-proteins linked to $\alpha_1$-adrenoceptors, and $\beta$-adrenoceptors in the heart are not coupled to $IP_3$; however, $IP_3$ may increase in the heart because norepinephrine also binds to cardiac $\alpha_1$-adrenoceptors.

8. The correct answer is "d" because endothelial-derived nitric oxide normally inhibits platelet aggregation and clot formation; therefore, decreased nitric oxide

production can lead to clot formation. Choice "a" is incorrect because the production of nitric oxide and prostacyclin are decreased when the endothelium is damaged or dysfunctional. Choice "b" is incorrect because decreased endothelial cGMP does not affect platelet function. Choice "c" is incorrect because dysfunctional endothelium results in decreased prostacyclin production.

## ANSWERS TO PROBLEMS AND CASES

### PROBLEM 3-1

Sympathetic nerve stimulation releases norepinephrine, which binds to $\beta_1$-adrenoceptors and $\alpha_1$-adrenoceptors found on cardiac myocytes. $\beta_1$-adrenoceptor activation stimulates cAMP production through the Gs-protein. cAMP production activates protein kinase A (PK-A), which phosphorylates L-type calcium channels, leading to an increase in calcium influx during the action potential. Increased calcium influx triggers increased calcium release by the sarcoplasmic reticulum, leading to increased calcium binding by TN-C. Calcium binding increases myosin ATPase activity and force generation. PK-A also phosphorylates phospholamban and removes its inhibition of SERCA, which leads to increased calcium reuptake by the sarcoplasmic reticulum and increases the rate of relaxation, or lusitropy. Increased calcium within the sarcoplasmic reticulum subsequently enhances the release of calcium from the sarcoplasmic reticulum. In addition, PK-A may phosphorylate sites on the sarcoplasmic reticulum to enhance calcium release. PK-A phosphorylation of TN-I also may contribute to enhanced lusitropy by altering TN-C affinity for calcium. Although physiologically less important than the $\beta_1$-adrenoceptor-Gs protein pathway, norepinephrine binding to $\alpha_1$-adrenoceptors increases the formation of $IP_3$ via Gq-protein and phospholipase C activation, which stimulates the release of calci-

um from the sarcoplasmic reticulum, leading to an increase in inotropy.

### PROBLEM 3-2

Increasing cAMP in the heart activates protein kinase A, which phosphorylates different sites within the cells (see the answer to Problem 3-1). Phosphorylation enhances calcium influx into the cell and calcium release by the sarcoplasmic reticulum, leading to an increase in inotropy. In vascular smooth muscle, myosin light chain kinase, when activated by calcium–calmodulin, phosphorylates myosin light chains to stimulate smooth muscle contraction. cAMP inhibits myosin light chain kinase; therefore, an increase in cAMP by a phosphodiesterase inhibitor such as milrinone inhibits the myosin light chain kinase, thereby reducing smooth muscle contraction.

### PROBLEM 3-3

Acetylcholine has two effects on blood vessels. When acetylcholine binds to $M_2$ receptors on the vascular endothelium, it stimulates the formation of nitric oxide (NO) by NO synthase. The NO can then diffuse from the endothelial cell into the adjacent smooth muscle cells, where it activates guanylyl cyclase to form cGMP. Increased cGMP relaxes vascular smooth muscle cells by inhibiting calcium entry into the cell and by other mechanisms. Acetylcholine, however, also can bind to $M_3$ receptors located on the smooth muscle. This activates the $IP_3$ pathway and stimulates calcium release by the sarcoplasmic reticulum, which leads to increased smooth muscle contraction.

If the endothelium is intact, stimulation of the NO–cGMP pathway dominates over the actions of the $IP_3$ pathway; therefore, acetylcholine normally causes vasodilation.

## SUGGESTED RESOURCES

Goldstein MA, Schroeter JP. Ultrastructure of the heart. In: Page E, Fozzard HA, Solaro RJ, eds. Handbook of Physiology, vol 1. Bethesda: American Physiological Society, 2002; 3–74.

Katz AM. Physiology of the Heart. 4th Ed. Philadelphia: Lippincott Williams & Wilkins, 2006.

Moss RL, Buck SH. Regulation of cardiac contraction by calcium. In: Page E, Fozzard HA, Solaro RJ, eds. Handbook of Physiology, vol 1. Bethesda: American Physiological Society, 2002; 420–454.

Opie LH. The Heart: Physiology from Cell to Circulation. 4th Ed. Philadelphia: Lippincott Williams & Wilkins, 2004.

Rhodin JAG. Architecture of the vessel wall. In: Bohr DF, Somlyo AP, Sparks HV, eds. Handbook of Physiology, vol 2. Bethesda: American Physiological Society, 1980; 1–31.

Sanders KM. Invited review: mechanisms of calcium handling in smooth muscles. J Appl Physiol 2001;91:1438–1449.

Somlyo AV: Ultrastructure of vascular smooth muscle. In: Bohr DF, Somlyo AP, Sparks HV, eds. Handbook of Physiology, vol 2. Bethesda: American Physiological Society, 1980; 33–67.

# CARDIAC FUNCTION

Understanding the concepts presented in this chapter will enable the student to:

1. Describe the basic anatomy of the heart, including the names of vessels entering and leaving the heart, cardiac chambers, and heart valves; trace the flow of blood through the heart.

2. Describe the changes in cardiac pressures and volumes, and associated electrical events and heart sounds, that occur during one cardiac cycle.

3. Draw and label ventricular pressure–volume loops derived from ventricular pressure and volume changes during the cardiac cycle.

4. Calculate stroke volume, cardiac output, and ejection fraction from ventricular end-diastolic and end-systolic volumes and heart rate.

5. Describe the factors that determine or modify ventricular preload, afterload, and inotropy.

6. Show how changes in preload, afterload, and inotropy affect ventricular end-diastolic volume, end-systolic volume, and stroke volume by using Frank-Starling curves and ventricular pressure–volume loops.

7. Describe how changes in preload, afterload, and inotropy alter the length-tension and force–velocity relationships for cardiac muscle.

8. Calculate myocardial oxygen consumption given coronary blood flow, and coronary arterial and venous oxygen contents.

9. Explain how changes in stroke volume, stroke work, afterload, heart rate, and inotropy affect myocardial oxygen consumption.

## INTRODUCTION

The heart is a specialized muscular organ that rhythmically contracts and pumps blood from the low-pressure venous side to the high-pressure arterial side of the circulation. Efficient pumping occurs because of the orderly contraction sequence of the different heart chambers and the presence of valves within the heart that ensure a unidirectional flow of blood. This chapter describes the basic anatomy of the heart—its chambers, valves, and vessels entering and leaving the heart—and the sequence of electrical and mechanical events that occur during a cycle of contraction and relaxation. It then describes the mechanisms that regulate cardiac output, particularly those mechanisms that influence the amount of blood ejected into the aorta with each contraction of the left ventricle. The last section of this chapter discusses the relationship between myocardial oxygen consumption and the mechanical activity of the heart.

## CARDIAC ANATOMY

### Functional Anatomy of the Heart

The heart consists of four chambers: **right atrium**, right ventricle, left atrium, and left ventricle (Fig. 4.1). The **right atrium** receives blood

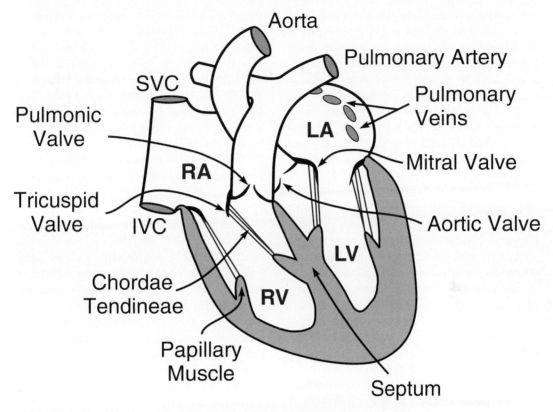

■ **FIGURE 4.1** Anatomy of the heart. *SVC*, superior vena cava; *IVC*, inferior vena cava; *RA*, right atrium; *RV*, right ventricle; *LA*, left atrium; *LV*, left ventricle.

from the **superior and inferior vena cavae**, which carry blood returning from the systemic circulation. The right atrium is a highly distensible chamber that can easily expand to accommodate the venous return at a low pressure (0 to 4 mm Hg). Blood flows from the right atrium, across the **tricuspid valve** (right atrioventricular [AV] valve), and into the right ventricle. The free wall of the **right ventricle** wraps around part of the larger and thicker left ventricle. The outflow tract of the right ventricle is the **pulmonary artery**, which is separated from the ventricle by the semilunar **pulmonic valve**. Blood returns to the heart from the lungs via four **pulmonary veins** that enter the **left atrium**. Blood flows from the left atrium, across the **mitral valve** (left AV valve), and into the left ventricle. The **left ventricle** has a thick muscular wall that allows it to generate high pressures during contraction. The left ventricle ejects blood across the **aortic valve** and into the **aorta**.

The tricuspid and mitral valves have fibrous strands (**chordae tendineae**) on their leaflets that attach to **papillary muscles** located on the respective ventricular walls. The papillary muscles contract when the ventricles contract. This generates tension on the valve leaflets via the chordae tendineae, preventing the valves from bulging back and leaking blood into the atria (i.e., preventing regurgitation) as the ventricles develop pressure. The semilunar valves (pulmonic and aortic) do not have analogous attachments.

## Autonomic Innervation

Autonomic innervation of the heart plays an important role in regulating cardiac function. The heart is innervated by parasympathetic (vagal) and sympathetic efferent fibers (see Chapter 6 for details on the origin of these autonomic nerves). The right vagus nerve preferentially innervates the sinoatrial (SA) node, whereas the left vagus nerve innervates the AV node; however, significant overlap can occur in the anatomical distribution. Atrial muscle is also innervated by vagal efferents; the ventricular myocardium is only sparsely innervated by vagal efferents. Sympathetic efferent nerves are present throughout the atria (especially in the SA node) and ventricles, and in the conduction system of the heart.

Vagal activation of the heart decreases heart rate (negative **chronotropy**), decreases conduction velocity (negative **dromotropy**), and decreases contractility (negative **inotropy**) of the heart. Vagal-mediated inotropic influences are moderate in the atria and relatively weak in the ventricles. Activation of the sympathetic nerves to the heart increases heart rate, conduction velocity, and inotropy. Sympathetic influences are pronounced in both the atria and ventricles.

As Chapter 6 describes in more detail, the heart also contains vagal and sympathetic afferent nerve fibers that relay information from stretch and pain receptors. The stretch receptors are involved in feedback regulation of blood volume and arterial pressure, whereas the pain receptors produce chest pain when activated during myocardial ischemia.

## THE CARDIAC CYCLE

### Cardiac Cycle Diagram

To understand how cardiac function is regulated, one must know the sequence of mechanical events during a complete cardiac cycle and how these mechanical events relate to the electrical activity of the heart. The cardiac cycle diagram in Figure 4.2 (sometimes called the Wiggers diagram) depicts changes in the left side of the heart (left ventricular pressure and volume, left atrial pressure, and aortic pressure) as a function of time. Although not shown in this figure, pressure and volume changes in the right side of the heart (right atrium and ventricle and pulmonary artery) are qualitatively similar to those in the left

side. Furthermore, the timing of mechanical events in the right side of the heart is very similar to that of the left side. The main difference is that the pressures in the right side of the heart are much lower than those found in the left side. For example, the right ventricular pressure typically changes from about 0 to 4 mm Hg during filling to a maximum of 25 to 30 mm Hg during contraction.

A catheter can be placed in the ascending aorta and left ventricle to obtain the pressure and volume information shown in the cardiac cycle diagram and to measure simultaneous changes in aortic and intraventricular pressure as the heart beats. This catheter can also be used to inject a radiopaque contrast agent into the left ventricular chamber. This permits fluoroscopic imaging (contrast ventriculography) of the ventricular chamber, from which estimates of ventricular volume can be obtained; however, real-time echocardiography and nuclear imaging of the heart are more commonly used to obtain clinical assessment of volume and function.

In the following discussion, a complete cardiac cycle is defined as the cardiac events initiated by the P wave in the electrocardiogram (ECG) and continuing until the next P wave. The cardiac cycle is divided into two general categories: systole and diastole. **Systole** refers to events associated with ventricular contraction and ejection. **Diastole** refers to the rest of the cardiac cycle, including ventricular relaxation and filling. The cardiac cycle is further divided into seven phases, beginning when the P wave appears. These phases are atrial systole, isovolumetric contraction, rapid ejection, reduced ejection, isovolumetric relaxation, rapid filling, and reduced filling. The events associated with each of these phases are described below.

### Phase 1. Atrial Systole: AV Valves Open; Aortic and Pulmonic Valves Closed

The P wave of the ECG represents electrical depolarization of the atria, which initiates contraction of the atrial musculature. As the atria contract, the pressures within the atrial

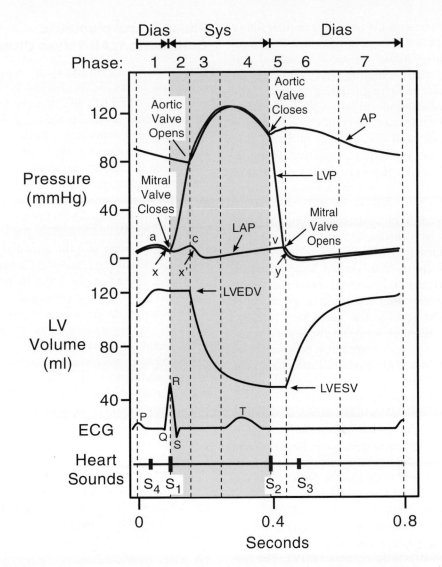

**■ FIGURE 4.2** Cardiac cycle. The seven phases of the cardiac cycle are (1) atrial systole; (2) isovolumetric contraction; (3) rapid ejection; (4) reduced ejection; (5), isovolumetric relaxation; (6) rapid filling; and (7) reduced filling. *Sys,* systole; *Dias,* diastole; *AP,* aortic pressure; *LVP,* left ventricular pressure; *LAP,* left atrial pressure; *a, a* wave; *c, c* wave; *v, v* wave; *x, x* descent; *x', x'* descent; *y, y* descent; *LV,* left ventricle; *ECG,* electrocardiogram; *LVEDV,* left ventricular end-diastolic volume; *LVESV,* left ventricular end-systolic volume, $S_1$-$S_4$, four heart sounds.

chambers increase; this drives blood from the atria, across the open AV valves, and into the ventricles. Retrograde atrial flow back into the vena cava and pulmonary veins is impeded by the inertial effect of venous return and by the wave of contraction throughout the atria, which has a "milking effect." Atrial contraction produces a small transient increase in left and right atrial pressure that is called the "*a* wave." The *a* wave is also reflected proximally

into the venous vessels (i.e., pulmonary veins and vena cava). On the right side of the heart, this produces the "*a* wave" of the jugular pulse. This can be observed when a person is recumbent and the jugular vein in the neck expands with blood, which permits pulsations to be visualized.

Atrial contraction normally accounts for only about 10% of left ventricular filling when a person is at rest and the heart rate is low, because most of the ventricular filling occurs before the atria contract. Therefore, ventricular filling is mostly passive and depends on the venous return. However, at high heart rates (e.g., during exercise), the period of diastolic filling is shortened considerably (because overall cycle length is decreased), and the amount of blood that enters the ventricle by passive filling is reduced. Under these conditions, the relative contribution of atrial contraction to ventricular filling increases greatly and may account for up to 40% of ventricular filling. In addition, atrial contribution to ventricular filling is enhanced by an increase in the force of atrial contraction caused by sympathetic nerve activation. Enhanced ventricular filling owing to increased atrial contraction is sometimes referred to as the "atrial kick." During atrial fibrillation (see Chapter 2), the contribution of atrial contraction to ventricular filling is lost. This leads to inadequate ventricular filling, particularly when ventricular rates increase during physical activity.

After atrial contraction is complete, the atrial pressure begins to fall, which causes a slight pressure gradient reversal across the AV valves. This fall in atrial pressure following the peak of the a-wave is termed the "*x* descent." As the pressures within the atria fall, the AV valves float upward (preposition) before closure.

At the end of this phase, which represents the end of diastole, the ventricles are filled to their **end-diastolic volume (EDV)**. The left ventricular EDV (typically about 120 mL) is associated with end-diastolic pressures of about 8 mm Hg. The right ventricular end-diastolic pressure is typically about 4 mm Hg.

A heart sound is sometimes heard during atrial contraction (**Fourth Heart Sound**, $S_4$). The sound is caused by vibration of the ventricular wall as blood rapidly enters the ventricle during atrial contraction. This sound generally is noted when the ventricle compliance is reduced (i.e., "stiff" ventricle), as occurs in ventricular hypertrophy (described later in this chapter). The sound is commonly present in older individuals because of changes in ventricular compliance.

## Phase 2. Isovolumetric Contraction: All Valves Closed

This phase of the cardiac cycle, which is the beginning of systole, is initiated by the QRS complex of the ECG, which represents ventricular depolarization. As the ventricles depolarize, myocyte contraction leads to a rapid increase in intraventricular pressure. The abrupt rise in pressure causes the AV valves to close as the intraventricular pressure exceeds atrial pressure. Contraction of the papillary muscles with their attached chordae tendineae prevents the AV valve leaflets from bulging back or prolapsing into the atria and becoming incompetent (i.e., "leaky"). Closure of the AV valves results in the **First Heart Sound** ($S_1$). This heart sound is generated when sudden closure of the AV valves results in oscillation of the blood, which causes vibrations (i.e., sound waves) that can be heard with a stethoscope overlying the heart. The first heart sound is normally split (~0.04 second) because mitral valve closure precedes tricuspid closure; however, because this very short time interval normally cannot be perceived through a stethoscope, only a single sound is heard.

During the time between the closure of the AV valves and the opening of the aortic and pulmonic semilunar valves, ventricular pressures rise rapidly without a change in ventricular volumes (i.e., no ejection of blood into the aorta or pulmonary artery occurs). Ventricular contraction, therefore, is said to be "isovolumic" or "isovolumetric" during this phase. During this phase, some individual fibers shorten when they contract, whereas others generate force without shortening or can be mechanically stretched as they are contracting because of nearby contracting cells. Ventricular chamber geometry changes considerably as the heart becomes more spheroid in shape, although the volume does not change. Early in this phase, the rate of pressure development becomes maximal. The maximal rate of pressure development, abbreviated "dP/dt max," is the maximal slope of the ventricular pressure tracing plotted against time during isovolumetric contraction.

Atrial pressures transiently increase during this phase owing to continued venous return and possibly to bulging of AV valves back into the atrial chambers, which results in a "*c wave*" noted in the atria and their proximal veins (e.g., in the jugular vein).

## Phase 3. Rapid Ejection: Aortic and Pulmonic Valves Open; AV Valves Remain Closed

When the intraventricular pressures exceed the pressures within the aorta and pulmonary artery, the aortic and pulmonic valves open and blood is ejected out of the ventricles. Ejection occurs because the total energy of the blood within the ventricle exceeds the total energy of blood within the aorta. The total energy of the blood is the sum of the pressure energy and the kinetic energy; the latter is related to the square of the velocity of the blood flow. In other words, ejection occurs because an energy gradient is present (mostly owing to pressure energy) that propels blood into the aorta and pulmonary artery. During this phase, ventricular pressure normally exceeds outflow tract pressure by only a few millimeters of mercury (mm Hg). Although blood flow across the valves is high, the relatively large valve opening (i.e., providing low resistance) requires only a few mm Hg of a pressure gradient to propel flow across the valve. Maximal outflow velocity is reached early in the ejection phase, and maximal (systolic) aortic and pulmonary artery pressures are achieved, which are typically about 120 and 25 mm Hg in the aorta and pulmonary artery, respectively.

While blood is being ejected and ventricular volumes decrease, the atria continue to fill with blood from their respective venous inflow tracts. Although atrial volumes are increasing, atrial pressures initially decrease (*x' descent*) as the base of the atria is pulled downward, expanding the atrial chambers.

No heart sounds are ordinarily heard during ejection. *The opening of healthy valves is silent.* The presence of a sound during ejection (i.e., ejection murmurs) indicates valve disease or intracardiac shunts (see Chapter 9).

## Phase 4. Reduced Ejection: Aortic and Pulmonic Valves Open; AV Valves Remain Closed

Approximately 150 to 200 milliseconds after the QRS, ventricular repolarization (T wave) occurs. This causes ventricular active tension to decrease (i.e., muscle relaxation occurs) and the rate of ejection (ventricular emptying) to fall. Ventricular pressure falls slightly below outflow tract pressure; however, outward flow still occurs owing to kinetic (or inertial) energy of the blood that helps to propel the blood into the aorta and pulmonary artery. Atrial pressures gradually rise during this phase owing to continued venous return into the atrial chambers. The end of this phase concludes systole.

## Phase 5. Isovolumetric Relaxation: All Valves Closed

As the ventricles continue to relax and intraventricular pressures fall, a point is reached at which the total energy of blood within the ventricles is less than the energy of blood in the outflow tracts. When this total energy gradient reversal occurs, the aortic and pulmonic valves to abruptly close. At this point, systole ends and diastole begins. Valve closure causes the **Second Heart Sound** ($S_2$), which is physiologically and audibly split because the aortic valve closes before the pulmonic valve. Normally, little or no blood flows backward into the ventricles as these valves close. Valve closure is associated with a characteristic notch (**incisura**) in the aortic and pulmonary artery pressure tracings. Unlike in the ventricles, where pressure rapidly falls, the decline in aortic and pulmonary artery pressures is not abrupt because of potential energy stored in their elastic walls and because systemic and pulmonic vascular resistances impede the flow of blood into distributing arteries of the systemic and pulmonary circulations.

Ventricular volumes remain constant (isovolumetric) during this phase because all valves are closed. The residual volume of blood that remains in a ventricle after ejection is called the **end-systolic volume (ESV)**. For the left ventricle, this is approximately 50 mL of blood. The difference between the EDV (120 mL) and the ESV (50 mL) represents the stroke volume (SV) of the ventricle, which is about 70 mL. In a normal ventricle, about 60% or more of the EDV is ejected. The SV (EDV − ESV) divided by the EDV is called the **ejection fraction** (EF) of the ventricle, which normally is >0.55 (or 55%). Although ventricular volume does not change during isovolumetric relaxation, atrial volumes and pressures continue to increase owing to venous return.

## Phase 6. Rapid Filling: AV Valves Open; Aortic and Pulmonic Valves Closed

When the ventricular pressures fall below atrial pressures, the AV valves open and ventricular filling begins. Initially, the ventricles are still relaxing, which causes intraventricular pressures to continue to fall by several mm Hg despite ongoing ventricular filling. The rate of initial filling is enhanced by the fact that atrial volumes are maximal just prior to AV valve opening. Once the valves open, the elevated atrial pressures coupled with declining ventricular pressures (ventricular diastolic suction) and the low resistance of the opened AV valves results in rapid, passive filling of the ventricles. Once the ventricles are fully relaxed, their pressure begins to rise as they fill.

The opening of the AV valves causes a rapid fall in atrial pressures. The peak of the atrial pressure just before the valve opens is the "**v wave**." This peak is followed by the "**y descent**" as blood leaves the atria. The v wave and y descent are transmitted into the proximal venous vessels such as the jugular vein on the right side of the heart and pulmonary veins on the left side. Clinically, changes in atrial pressures and jugular pulses are useful in the diagnosis of altered cardiac function (see Chapter 9).

If the AV valves are functioning normally, no prominent sounds will be heard during filling. When a **Third Heart Sound** ($S_3$) is audible during ventricular filling, it may represent tensing of chordae tendineae and the AV ring, which is the connective tissue support for the valve leaflets. This $S_3$ heart sound is normal in children, but it is considered pathologic in adults because it is often associated with ventricular dilation.

## Phase 7. Reduced Filling: AV Valves Open; Aortic and Pulmonic Valves Closed

No clear demarcation exists between the phases of rapid and reduced ventricular filling. The reduced filling phase is the period during diastole when passive ventricular filling is nearing completion. This is sometimes referred to as the period of **ventricular diastasis**. As the ventricles continue to fill with blood and expand, they become less compliant (i.e., "stiffer"). This causes the intraventricular pressures to rise, as described later in this chapter. Increased intraventricular pressure reduces the pressure gradient across the AV valve (the pressure gradient is the difference between the atrial and ventricular pressure) so that the rate of filling declines, even though atrial pressures continue to increase slightly as venous blood continues to flow into the atria. Aortic pressure and pulmonary arterial pressure continue to fall during this period as blood flows into the systemic and pulmonary circulations.

It is important to note that Figure 4.2 depicts the cardiac cycle at a relatively low heart rate (75 beats/min). At low heart rates, the length of time allotted to diastole is relatively long, which lengthens the time of the reduced filling phase. High heart rates reduce the overall cycle length and are associated with reductions in the duration of both systole and diastole, although diastole shortens much more than systole. Without compensatory mechanisms, this cycle length reduction would lead to less ventricular filling (i.e., reduced EDV). Compensatory mechanisms are important for maintaining adequate ventricular filling during exercise (see Chapter 9).

## Summary of Intracardiac Pressures

It is important to know normal values of intracardiac pressures, as well as the pressures within the veins and arteries entering and leaving the heart, because abnormal pressures can be used to diagnose certain types of cardiac disease and dysfunction. Figure 4.3 summarizes normal, typical pressures in an adult

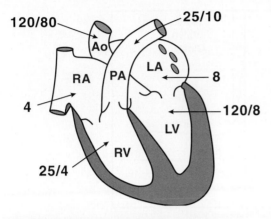

**■ FIGURE 4.3** Summary of normal pressures within the cardiac chambers and great vessels. The higher of the two pressure values (expressed in mm Hg) in the right ventricle (*RV*), left ventricle (*LV*), pulmonary artery (*PA*), and aorta (*Ao*) represent the normal peak pressures during ejection (systolic pressure), whereas the lower pressure values represent normal end of diastole pressure (ventricles) or the lowest pressure (diastolic pressure) found in the PA and Ao. Pressures in the right atrium (*RA*) and left atrium (*LA*) represent average values during the cardiac cycle.

heart. Note that the pressures on the right side of the heart are considerably lower than those on the left side of the heart, and that the pulmonary circulation has low pressures compared to the systemic arterial system. The pressures shown for the right and left atria indicate an average atrial pressure during the cardiac cycle—atrial pressures change by several mm Hg as they fill and contract.

## Ventricular Pressure–Volume Relationship

Although measurements of pressures and volumes over time can provide important insights into ventricular function, pressure–volume loops provide another powerful tool for analyzing the cardiac cycle, particularly ventricular function.

Pressure–volume loops (Fig. 4.4, bottom panel) are generated by plotting left ventricular pressure against left ventricular volume at many time points during a complete cardiac cycle (Fig. 4.4, top panel). In Figure 4.4, the letters represent the periods of ventricular filling (a), isovolumetric contraction (b),

ventricular ejection (c), and isovolumetric relaxation (d). The EDV is the maximal volume achieved at the end of filling, and ESV is the minimal volume (i.e., residual volume) of the ventricle found at the end of ejection. The width of the loop, therefore, represents the difference between EDV and ESV, which is the SV. The area within the pressure–volume loop is the **ventricular stroke work**.

The filling phase moves along the **end-diastolic pressure–volume relationship** (EDPVR), or passive filling curve for the ventricle. The slope of the EDPVR at any point along the curve is the reciprocal of ventricular compliance, as described later in this chapter.

The maximal pressure that can be developed by the ventricle at any given left ventricular volume is described by the **end-systolic pressure–volume relationship** (ESPVR). The pressure–volume loop, therefore, cannot cross over the ESPVR, because the ESPVR defines the maximal pressure that can be generated at any given volume under a given inotropic state, as described later in this chapter.

The changes in pressures and volumes described in the cardiac cycle diagram and by the pressure–volume loop are for normal adult hearts at resting heart rates. Pressure–volume loops appear very differently in the presence of valve disease and heart failure as described in Chapter 9.

## CARDIAC OUTPUT

The primary function of the heart is to impart energy to blood to generate and sustain an arterial blood pressure sufficient to adequately perfuse organs. The heart achieves this by contracting its muscular walls around a closed chamber to generate sufficient pressure to propel blood from the left ventricle, through the aortic valve, and into the aorta. Each time the left ventricle contracts, a volume of blood is ejected into the aorta. This SV, multiplied by the number of beats per minute (heart rate, HR), equals the cardiac output (CO) (Equation 4-1).

**Eq. 4-1** $\qquad CO = SV \cdot HR$

Therefore, changes in either SV or heart rate alter cardiac output.

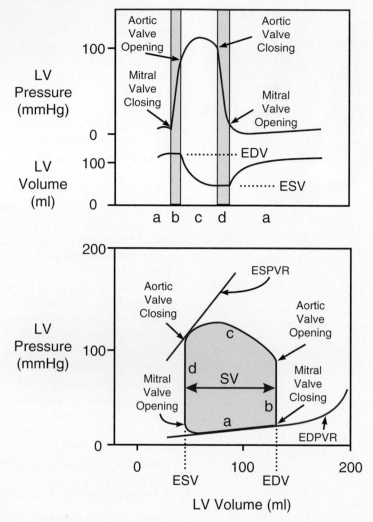

■ **FIGURE 4.4** Ventricular pressure–volume loops. The left ventricular pressure–volume loop (**bottom panel**) is generated by plotting ventricular pressure against ventricular volume at many different corresponding points during a single cardiac cycle (**upper panel**). *a*, ventricular filling; *b*, isovolumetric contraction; *c*, ventricular ejection; *d*, isovolumetric relaxation; *EDV* and *ESV*, left ventricular end-diastolic and end-systolic volumes, respectively; *EDPVR*, end-diastolic pressure–volume relationship; *ESPVR*, end-systolic pressure–volume relationship; *SV*, stroke volume (EDV – ESV).

The units for cardiac output are expressed as either milliliters/minute (mL/min) or liters/min. The units for SV are mL/beat, and the units for heart rate are beats/min. In a resting adult, cardiac output typically ranges from 5 to 6 L/min. Sometimes cardiac output is expressed as a **cardiac index**, which is the cardiac output divided by the estimated body surface area (BSA) in square meters. Several different formulas can be used to estimate BSA. One formula is BSA (m²) equals the square root of the (height [cm] times weight [kg] divided by 3600); BSA = $(cm \cdot kg/3600)^{1/2}$ (Mosteller formula). Calculating the cardiac index normalizes cardiac output to individuals of different size. A normal range for cardiac index is 2.6 to 4.2 L/min/m².

### PROBLEM 4-1

Calculate left ventricular SV in milliliters/beat when the cardiac output is 8.8 L/min and the heart rate is 110 beats/min.

## Measurement of Cardiac Output

In experimental settings, cardiac output can be measured by electromagnetic or Doppler flowmeters placed around the pulmonary artery. Obviously, this approach cannot be used in humans; therefore, indirect techniques are used. The most commonly used is the thermodilution technique, which uses a special multilumen, thermistor-tipped catheter (Swan-Ganz) that is inserted into the pulmonary artery from a peripheral vein. A cold saline solution of known temperature and volume is injected into the right atrium from a proximal port on the catheter. The cold injectate mixes into the blood and cools the blood, which then passes through the right ventricle and into the pulmonary artery. The thermistor at the catheter tip measures the blood temperature, and a cardiac output computer is used to calculate flow (cardiac output). Doppler echocardiography can be used to estimate real-time changes in flow within the heart, pulmonary artery, or ascending aorta. Echocardiography and various radionuclide techniques can also be used to measure changes in ventricular dimensions during the cardiac cycle in order to calculate SV, which, when multiplied by heart rate, gives cardiac output. Although used less frequently, the Fick method permits time-averaged cardiac output (CO; mL/min) calculations from measurements of arterial and venous blood oxygen content ($CaO_2$ and $CvO_2$, respectively; mL $O_2$/mL blood), and whole body oxygen consumption ($\dot{V}O_2$; mL $O_2$/min). This method is based on the following relationship (Fick Principle):

$$CO = \frac{\dot{V}O_2}{(CaO_2 - CvO_2)}$$

## Influence of Heart Rate and Stroke Volume on Cardiac Output

Although cardiac output is determined by both heart rate and SV, changes in heart rate are generally more important quantitatively in producing changes in cardiac output. For example, heart rate may increase by 100% to 200% during exercise, whereas SV may increase by <50%. These changes in heart rate are brought about primarily by changes in sympathetic and parasympathetic nerve activity at the SA node (see Chapter 2).

A change in heart rate does not necessarily result in a proportionate change in cardiac output. The reason is that changes in heart rate can inversely affect SV. For example, doubling heart rate from 70 to 140 beats/min by pacemaker stimulation alone does not double cardiac output because SV falls when heart rate is elevated. This occurs because the ventricular filling time decreases as the length of diastole shortens, thereby resulting in less ventricular filling. However, when normal physiological mechanisms during exercise cause the heart rate to double, cardiac output more than doubles because SV actually increases. This increase in SV, despite the elevation in heart rate, is brought about by several mechanisms acting on the heart and systemic circulation (see Chapter 9). When these mechanisms fail, SV cannot be maintained at elevated heart rates. Therefore, it is important to understand the mechanisms that regulate SV because impaired SV regulation can lead to a state of heart failure and limited exercise capacity (see Chapter 9).

## EFFECTS OF PRELOAD ON STROKE VOLUME

**Preload** *is the initial stretching of the cardiac myocytes prior to contraction; therefore, it is related to the sarcomere length at the end of diastole.* Sarcomere length cannot be determined in the intact heart, so indirect indices of preload, such as ventricular EDV or pressure, must be used. These measures of preload are not ideal because they may not always reflect sarcomere length because of changes in the structure and mechanical properties of the heart. Despite these limitations, *acute changes* in end-diastolic pressure and volume are useful indices for examining the effects of acute preload changes on SV.

## Effects of Ventricular Compliance on Preload

As the ventricle fills with blood, the pressure generated at a given volume is determined by the **compliance** of the ventricle, in which compliance is defined as *the ratio of a change in volume divided by a change in pressure*. Normally, compliance curves are plotted with volume on the Y-axis and pressure on the X-axis, so that the compliance is the slope of the line at any given pressure (i.e., the slope of the tangent at a particular point on the line). For the ventricle, however, it is common to plot pressure versus volume (Fig. 4.5) and to refer to this pressure–volume relationship as the filling curve for the ventricle. Plotted in this manner, the slope of the tangent at a given point on the curve is the reciprocal of the compliance. Therefore, the steeper the slope of the pressure–volume relationship, the lower the compliance. This means that the ventricle becomes "stiffer" when the slope of the passive filling curve is greater; therefore, compliance and stiffness are reciprocally related.

The relationship between pressure and volume is nonlinear in the ventricle (as in most biological tissues); therefore, compliance decreases with increasing pressure or volume. When pressure and volume are plotted as in Figure 4.5, we find that the slope of the filling curve (the EDPVR described in Fig. 4.4) increases at higher volumes; that

is, the ventricle becomes less compliant or "stiffer" at higher volumes.

Ventricular compliance is determined by the physical properties of the tissues making up the ventricular wall and the state of ventricular relaxation. For example, in ventricular hypertrophy, the increased muscle thickness decreases the ventricular compliance; therefore, ventricular end-diastolic pressure is higher for any given EDV. This is shown in Figure 4-5, in which the filling curve of the hypertrophied ventricle shifts upward and to the left. From a different perspective, for a given end-diastolic pressure, a less compliant ventricle will have a smaller EDV (i.e., filling will be decreased). If ventricular relaxation (lusitropy) is impaired, as occurs in some forms of diastolic ventricular failure (see Chapter 9), the functional ventricular compliance will be reduced. This will impair ventricular filling and increase end-diastolic pressure. If the ventricle becomes chronically dilated, as occurs in other forms of heart failure, the filling curve shifts downward and to the right. This enables a dilated heart to have a greater EDV without causing a large increase in end-diastolic pressure.

The length of a sarcomere prior to contraction, which represents its preload, depends on

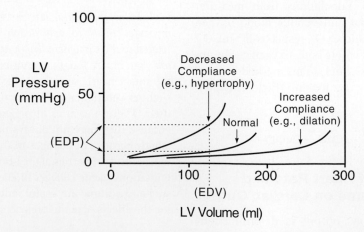

■ **FIGURE 4.5** Left ventricular compliance (or filling) curves. The slope of the tangent of the passive pressure–volume curve at a given volume represents the reciprocal of the ventricular compliance. The slope of the normal compliance curve is increased by a decrease in ventricular compliance (e.g., ventricular hypertrophy), whereas the slope of the compliance curve is reduced by an increase in ventricular compliance (e.g., ventricular dilation). Decreased compliance increases the end-diastolic pressure (*EDP*) at a given end-diastolic volume (*EDV*), whereas increased compliance decreases EDP at a given EDV. *LV*, left ventricle.

the ventricular EDV. This, in turn, depends on the ventricular end-diastolic pressure and compliance. Although end-diastolic pressure and EDV are sometimes used as indices of preload, care must be taken when interpreting the significance of these values in terms of how they relate to the preload of individual sarcomeres. An elevated end-diastolic pressure may be associated with sarcomere lengths that are increased, decreased, or unchanged, depending on the ventricular volume and compliance at that volume. For example, a stiff, hypertrophied ventricle may have an elevated end-diastolic pressure with a reduced EDV owing to the reduced compliance. Because the EDV is reduced, the sarcomere length will be reduced despite the increase in end-diastolic pressure. As another example, a larger than normal EDV may not be associated with an increase in sarcomere length if the ventricle is chronically dilated and structurally remodeled such that new sarcomeres have been added in series, thus maintaining normal individual sarcomere lengths.

## Effects of Preload on Tension Development (Length–Tension Relationship)

We have seen how ventricular EDV, which is determined by ventricular end-diastolic

pressure and ventricular compliance, can alter the preload on sarcomeres in cardiac muscle cells. This change in preload will alter the ability of the myocyte to generate force when it contracts. The **length–tension relationship** examines how changes in the initial length of a muscle (i.e., preload) affect the ability of the muscle to develop force (tension). To illustrate this relationship, a piece of cardiac muscle (e.g., papillary muscle) is isolated and placed within an in vitro bath containing an oxygenated, physiologic salt solution. One end of the muscle is attached to a force transducer to measure tension, and the other end is attached to an immovable support rod (Fig. 4.6, left side). The end that is attached to the force transducer is movable so that the initial length (preload) of the muscle can be fixed at a desired length. The muscle is then electrically stimulated to contract; however, the length is not permitted to change and therefore the contraction is isometric.

If the muscle is stimulated to contract at a relatively short initial length (low preload), a characteristic increase in tension (termed "active" tension) will occur, lasting about 200 milliseconds (Fig. 4.6, right side, curve *a*). By stretching the muscle to a longer initial length, the passive tension will be increased prior to stimulation. The amount of passive tension depends on the

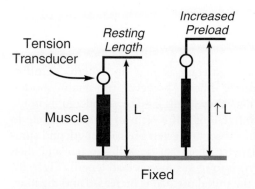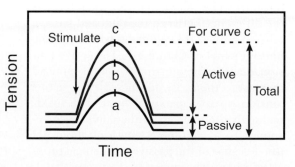

■ **FIGURE 4.6** Effects of increased preload on tension development by an isolated strip of cardiac muscle. The left side shows how muscle length and tension are measured in vitro. The bottom of the muscle strip is fixed to an immovable rod, whereas the top of the muscle is connected to a tension transducer and a movable bar that can be used to adjust initial muscle length (*L*). The right side shows how increased preload (initial length) increases both passive and active (developed) tension. The greater the preload, the greater the active tension generated by the muscle.

elastic modulus ("stiffness") of the tissue. The elastic modulus of a tissue is related to the ability of a tissue to resist deformation; therefore, the higher the elastic modulus, the "stiffer" the tissue. When the muscle is stimulated at the increased preload, there will be a larger increase in active tension (curve *b*) than had occurred at the lower preload. If the preload is again increased, there will be a further increase in active tension (curve *c*). Therefore, *increases in preload lead to an increase in active tension.* Not only is the magnitude of active tension increased, but also the rate of active tension development (i.e., the maximal slope with respect to time of the tension curve during contraction). The duration of contraction and the time-to-peak tension, however, are not changed.

If the results shown in Figure 4.6 are plotted as tension versus initial length (preload), a length–tension diagram is generated (Fig. 4.7). In the top panel, the passive tension curve is the tension that is generated as the muscle is stretched prior to contraction. Points *a*, *b*, and *c* on the passive curve correspond to the passive tensions and initial preload lengths for curves *a*, *b*, and *c* in Figure 4.6 prior to contraction. The total tension curve represents the maximal tension that occurs during contraction at different initial preloads. The total tension curve is the sum of the passive tension and the additional tension generated during contraction (active tension). The active tension, therefore, is the difference between the total and passive tension curves; it is plotted separately in the bottom panel of Figure 4-7. The active tension diagram demonstrates that as preload increases, there is an increase in active tension up to a maximal limit. The maximal active tension in cardiac muscle corresponds to a sarcomere length of about 2.2 μm. Because of the passive mechanical properties of cardiac myocytes, their length seldom exceeds 2.2 μm at maximal ventricular EDVs.

This discussion described how changes in preload affect the force generated by cardiac muscle fibers during isometric contractions

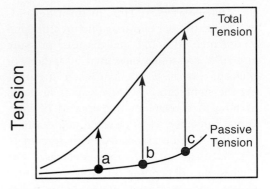

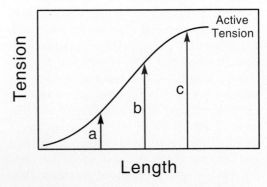

■ **FIGURE 4.7** Length–tension relationship for cardiac muscle undergoing isometric contraction. The **top panel** shows that increasing the preload length from points *a* to *c* increases the passive tension. Furthermore, increasing the preload increases the total tension during contraction as shown by *arrows a, b,* and *c,* which correspond to active tension changes depicted by curves a, b, and c in Figure 4.6. The length of the arrow is the active tension, which is the difference between the total and passive tensions. The **bottom panel** shows that the active tension increases to a maximum value as preload increases.

(i.e., with no change in length). Cardiac muscle fibers, however, normally shorten when they contract (i.e., undergo isotonic contractions). If a strip of cardiac muscle in vitro is set at a given preload length and stimulated to contract, it will shorten and then return to its resting preload length (Fig. 4.8). If the initial preload is increased and the muscle stimulated again, it will ordinarily shorten to the same minimal length, albeit at a higher velocity of shortening.

The length–tension relationship, although usually used to describe the contraction of

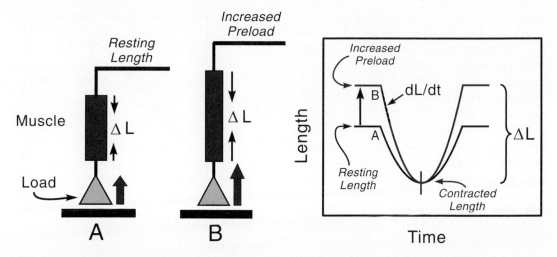

■ **FIGURE 4.8** Effects of increased initial muscle length (increased preload) on muscle shortening (isotonic contractions). The **left panel** shows a muscle lifting a load (afterload) at two different preload lengths (*A* and *B*). The **right panel** shows how increasing the preload leads to increased shortening (Δ*L*) and increased velocity of shortening (dL/dt; change in length with respect to time). The muscle shortens to the same minimal length when preload is increased.

isolated muscles, can be applied to the whole heart. By substituting ventricular volume for length and ventricular pressure for tension, the length–tension relationship becomes a pressure–volume relationship for the ventricle. This can be done because a quantitative relationship exists between tension and pressure and between length and volume that is determined by the geometry of the ventricle. Figure 4.9 shows that as ventricular EDV increases, an increase in isovolumet-

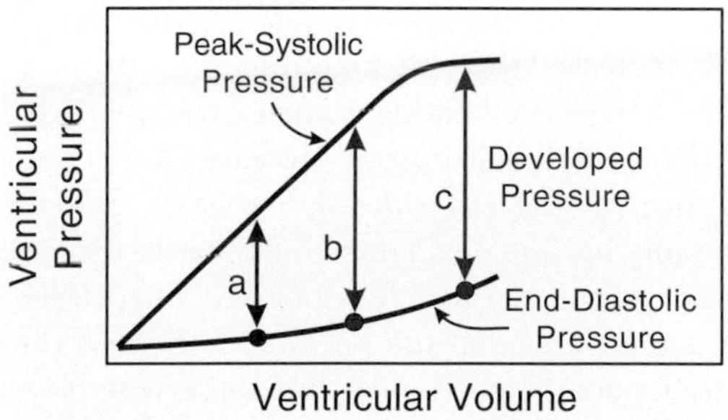

■ **FIGURE 4.9** Effects of increasing ventricular volume (preload) on ventricular pressure development. Increasing ventricular volume from *a* to *c* and then stimulating the ventricle to contract isovolumetrically increases the developed pressure and the peak-systolic pressure.

ric ventricular pressure development occurs during ventricular contraction, analogous to what is observed with a single papillary muscle (see Fig. 4.7). This can be observed experimentally in the ventricle by occluding the aorta during ventricular contraction at different ventricular volumes and measuring the peak systolic pressure generated by the ventricle under this isovolumetric condition. The peak systolic pressure curve is analogous to the ESPVR shown in Figure 4.4 because this is the maximal pressure that can be generated by the ventricle at a given ventricular volume.

What mechanisms are responsible for the increase in force generation with increased preload in the heart? In the past, it was thought that changes in active tension caused by altered preload could be explained by the overlap of actin and myosin and therefore by a change in the number of actin and myosin cross bridges formed (see Chapter 3). However, unlike skeletal muscle that can operate under a very wide range of sarcomere lengths (1.3 to 3.5 μm), the intact heart under physiologic conditions operates within a narrow range of sarcomere lengths (1.6 to 2.2 μm). These and other observations have led to the concept of **length-dependent activation**. Experimental evidence supports three possible explanations. First, studies have shown that increased sarcomere length sensitizes the regulatory protein troponin C to calcium without necessarily increasing intracellular release of calcium. This increases calcium binding by troponin C, leading to an increase in force generation as described in Chapter 3. A second explanation is that fiber stretching alters calcium homeostasis within the cell so that increased calcium is available to bind to troponin C. A third explanation is that as a myocyte (and sarcomere) lengthens, the diameter must decrease because the volume has to remain constant. It has been proposed that this would bring the actin and myosin molecules closer to each other (decreased lateral spacing), which would facilitate their interactions.

## Effects of Venous Return on Stroke Volume (Frank-Starling Mechanism)

Altered preload is an important mechanism by which the ventricle changes its force of contraction and therefore its SV. When venous return to the heart is increased, ventricular filling increases, and therefore its preload. This stretching of the myocytes causes an increase in force generation, which enables the heart to eject the additional venous return and thereby increase SV. This is called the **Frank-Starling mechanism** in honor of the scientific contributions of Otto Frank (late 19th century) and Ernest Starling (early 20th century). Another term for this mechanism is "Starling's law of the heart." In summary, *the Frank-Starling mechanism states that increasing venous return and ventricular preload leads to an increase in SV.* Figure 4.10 shows the Frank-Starling relationship for the left ventricle. Assume that the left ventricle is normally operating at an end-diastolic pressure of 8 mm Hg and is ejecting an SV of 70 mL (Point A). If the

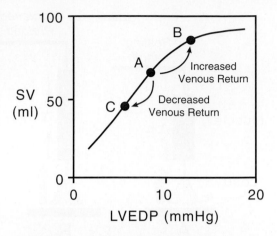

■ **FIGURE 4.10** Frank-Starling mechanism. Increasing venous return to the left ventricle increases left ventricular end-diastolic pressure (*LVEDP*) by increasing ventricular volume; this increased preload increases stroke volume (*SV*) from point *A* (normal operating point) to *B*. Decreasing venous return decreases preload and stroke volume (point *C*).

venous return to the heart is increased and the end-diastolic pressure is increased, this will lead to an increase in SV (Point B). A decrease in venous return (Point C) would result in less ventricular filling, leading to a lower end-diastolic pressure and a reduced SV along this Frank-Starling curve.

The Frank-Starling mechanism plays an important role in balancing the output of the two ventricles. For example, when venous return increases to the right side of the heart during physical activity, the Frank-Starling mechanism enables the right ventricular SV to increase, thereby matching its output to the increased venous return. The increased right ventricular output increases the venous return to the left side of the heart, and the Frank-Starling mechanism operates to increase the output of the left ventricle. This mechanism ensures that the outputs of the two ventricles are matched over time; otherwise blood volume would shift between the pulmonary and systemic circulations.

This analysis using Frank-Starling curves shows how changes in venous return and ventricular preload lead to changes in SV. These

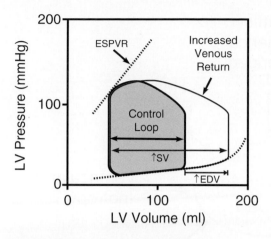

■ **FIGURE 4.11** Effects of increasing venous return on left ventricular (*LV*) pressure-volume loops. This diagram shows the acute response to an increase in venous return. It assumes no cardiac or systemic compensation and that aortic pressure remains unchanged. Increased venous return increases end-diastolic volume (*EDV*), but it normally does not change ESV; therefore, stroke volume (*SV*) is increased. *ESPVR*, end-systolic pressure-volume relationship.

curves, however, do not show how changes in venous return affect end-diastolic and end-systolic volumes. These changes in ventricular volumes are best illustrated by using pressure–volume diagrams.

When venous return is increased, increased filling of the ventricle occurs along its passive filling curve (Fig. 4.11). This leads to an increase in EDV. If the ventricle now contracts at this increased preload, and the aortic pressure is held constant, the ventricle will empty to the same ESV, and therefore, SV will be increased. This is shown as an increase in the width of the pressure–volume loop. The ventricle ejects to the same ESV because, as shown in Figure 4.8, increasing preload leads to a more rapid fiber shortening, and the fiber shortens to the same minimal length at the end of contraction. The normal ventricle, therefore, is capable of increasing its SV to match an increase in venous return. The increase in the area within the pressure–volume loop, which represents the ventricular stroke work, will also be increased.

## Factors Determining Ventricular Preload

Ventricular filling, and therefore preload of the right ventricle, is altered by several factors (Fig. 4.12).

1. **Venous Pressure.** An increase in venous blood pressure outside of the right atrium increases right ventricular preload. This venous pressure is determined by venous blood volume and compliance (see Chapter 5). For example, reduced venous compliance brought about by contraction of the venous smooth muscle increases venous pressure. Venous blood volume, particularly in the thoracic (central) compartment, is influenced by the total blood volume (regulated by the kidneys) and the rate of venous return into the thoracic compartment.

2. **Ventricular Compliance.** The compliance of the ventricle determines the EDV for any given intraventricular filling pressure. Therefore, the greater the compliance, the greater the ventricular filling at a given filling pressure.

3. **Heart Rate.** Through its influence on filling time, heart rate and ventricular filling are inversely related.

4. **Atrial Contraction.** At resting heart rates, atrial contraction normally has only a small influence on ventricular preload because most of ventricular filling occurs passively. An increase in the force of atrial contraction caused by sympathetic activation, for example, can significantly enhance ventricular filling. This becomes especially important for maintaining preload at high heart rates when there is less time for diastolic filling of the right ventricle.

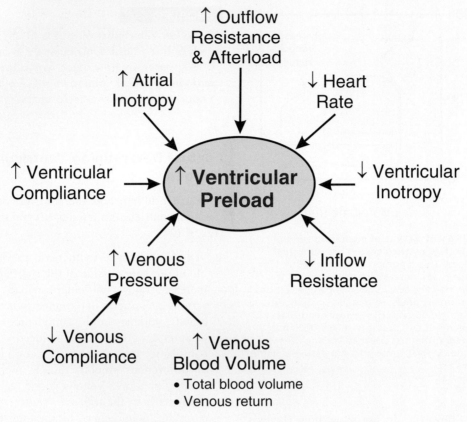

**■ FIGURE 4.12** Factors that increase ventricular preload.

5. **Inflow Resistance.** Elevated inflow resistance (e.g., tricuspid valve stenosis; see Chapter 9) reduces the rate of ventricular filling and therefore decreases ventricular preload.

6. **Outflow Resistance.** An increase in outflow resistance, as caused by pulmonic valve stenosis (see Chapter 9) or elevated pulmonary artery pressure (pulmonary hypertension), impairs the ability of the right ventricle to empty, leading to an increase in preload.

7. **Ventricular Inotropy.** In ventricular systolic failure (see Chapter 9), when ventricular inotropy is diminished, the ventricular preload increases because of the inability of the ventricle to eject normal volumes of blood. This causes blood to back up in the ventricle and proximal venous circulation.

Left ventricular preload is determined by the same factors as for right ventricular preload, except that the venous pressure is pulmonary venous pressure instead of central (or thoracic) venous pressure, the inflow resistance is the mitral valve, and the outflow resistance is the aortic valve and aortic pressure.

---

**CASE 4-1**

Echocardiography reveals that the left ventricle of a chronically hypertensive patient is significantly hypertrophied. Using left ventricular pressure–volume loops, describe how end-diastolic pressure and volume and SV will be altered by the hypertrophy. Assume no change in heart rate, inotropy, or aortic pressure.

# EFFECTS OF AFTERLOAD ON STROKE VOLUME

**Afterload** *is the "load" against which the heart must contract to eject blood.* A major component of the afterload for the left ventricle is the aortic pressure, or the pressure the ventricle must overcome to eject blood. The greater the aortic pressure, the greater the afterload on the left ventricle. For the right ventricle, the pulmonary artery pressure represents the major afterload component.

Ventricular afterload, however, involves factors other than the pressure that the ventricle must develop to eject blood. One way to estimate the afterload on the individual cardiac fibers within the ventricle is to examine **ventricular wall stress** ($\sigma$), which is proportional to the product of the intraventricular pressure (P) and ventricular radius (r), divided by the wall thickness (h) (Equation 4-2). This relationship for wall stress assumes that the ventricle is a sphere. The determination of actual wall stress is complex and must consider not only ventricular geometry, but also muscle fiber orientation. Nonetheless, Equation 4-2 helps to illustrate the factors that contribute to wall stress and therefore afterload on the muscle fibers.

**Eq. 4-2**
$$\sigma \propto \frac{P \cdot r}{h}$$

Wall stress can be thought of as the average tension that individual muscle fibers within the ventricular wall must generate to shorten against the developed intraventricular pressure. At a given intraventricular pressure, wall stress is increased by an increase in radius (ventricular dilation). Therefore, afterload is increased whenever intraventricular pressures are elevated during systole and by ventricular dilation. On the other hand, a thickened, hypertrophied ventricle will have reduced wall stress and afterload on individual fibers. Ventricular wall hypertrophy can be thought of as an adaptive mechanism by which the ventricle is able to offset the increase in wall stress that accompanies increased ventricular systolic pressures or ventricular dilation.

# Effects of Afterload on the Velocity of Fiber Shortening (Force–Velocity Relationship)

Afterload influences the contraction of cardiac muscle fibers. Increased afterload decreases the velocity of fiber shortening, whereas decreased afterload increases the velocity of shortening. This inverse relationship between afterload and velocity of fiber shortening is basis for the **force–velocity relationship**. To illustrate this, a papillary muscle is placed in an in vitro bath, set at a fixed initial length and passive tension (preload), and a load is attached to one end (Fig. 4.13, left panel). When the muscle is stimulated to contract, the fiber first generates active tension isometrically, that is, active tension is developed with no change in length (right panel, *a* to *b*). Once the developed tension exceeds the load imposed on the muscle, the muscle fiber begins to shorten, and the tension remains constant and equal to the load that is being lifted (*b* to *c*). The maximal velocity of shortening (rate of shortening) occurs shortly after the muscle begins to shorten. The muscle continues to shorten until the muscle begins to relax. When active tension falls below the load (point *c*), the muscle resumes its resting length and tension (i.e., preload) (point *c*). Active tension continues to fall isometrically (*c* to *d*) until only the passive tension remains (point *d*).

If this experiment with the papillary muscle were repeated with increasing loads, a decrease would occur in both the maximal velocity of fiber shortening (maximal slope of line) and the degree of shortening, as shown in Figure 4.14. Plotting the maximal velocity of shortening against the load that the muscle fiber must shorten against (i.e., the afterload) generates an inverse relationship between velocity of shortening and afterload (force–velocity relationship; Fig. 4.15). In other words, *the greater the afterload, the slower the velocity of shortening.*

To further illustrate the force–velocity relationship, consider the following example. If a person holds a 2-lb dumbbell at their side while standing, and then contracts their biceps muscle at maximal effort, the weight will be lifted at a relatively high velocity as the biceps muscle shortens. If the weight is increased to 20 lb, and the weight once again is lifted at maximal effort,

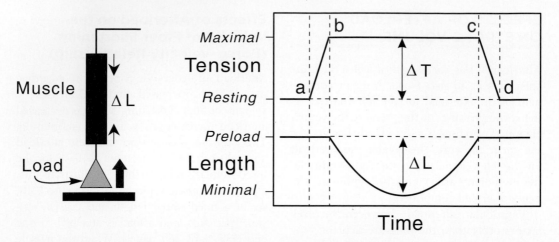

■ **FIGURE 4.13** Cardiac muscle isotonic contractions. The **left panel** shows how muscle length and tension are measured in vitro. The lower end of the muscle is attached to a weight (load) that is lifted up from an immovable platform as the muscle develops tension and shortens ($\Delta L$). A bar attached to the top of the muscle can be moved to adjust initial muscle length (preload). The **right panel** shows changes in tension and length during contraction. The periods from *a* to *b* and from *c* to *d* represent periods of isometric contraction and relaxation, respectively. Muscle shortening ($\Delta L$) occurs between *b* and *c*, which occurs when the developed tension ($\Delta T$) exceeds the load.

the velocity will be slower. Higher weights further reduce the velocity until the weight can no longer be lifted and the contraction of the biceps muscle becomes isometric. The x-intercept in the force–velocity diagram (see Fig. 4.15) is the point at which the afterload is so great that the muscle fiber cannot shorten. The x-intercept therefore represents the maximal isometric force. The y-intercept represents an extrapolated value for the maximal velocity ($V_{max}$) that would be achieved if there was no afterload. The value is extrapolated because it cannot be measured experimentally (a muscle will not contract in the absence of any load).

$V_{max}$ represents the intrinsic capability of the muscle fiber to generate force independent of load, and therefore changes when inotropy is altered, as discussed later in this chapter.

It is important to note that a cardiac muscle fiber does not operate on a single force–velocity curve (Fig. 4.16). As previously

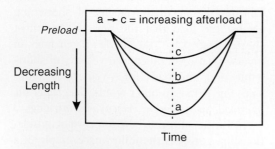

■ **FIGURE 4.14** Effects of afterload on myocyte shortening. Increased afterload (curves *a* to *c*) decreases the degree of muscle shortening and maximal velocity of shortening at a given preload, which is measured as the change in length over time shortly after muscle begins to shorten.

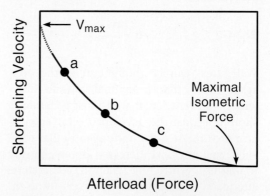

■ **FIGURE 4.15** Force–velocity relationship. Increased afterload (which requires increased force generation) decreases velocity of shortening by the muscle fiber. The x-intercept represents the maximal isometric force that occurs when the load exceeds the muscle's force-generating capacity, thus preventing muscle shortening; the y-intercept represents the maximal velocity of shortening ($V_{max}$) extrapolated to zero load. Points *a, b,* and *c* represent the maximal shortening velocity generated in Figure 4.14 for three increasing afterloads.

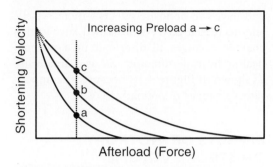

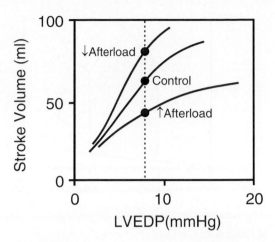

■ **FIGURE 4.16** Effects of increasing preload (shift from curve *a* to *c*) on the force–velocity relationship. At a given afterload (vertical dashed line), increasing the preload increases the velocity of shortening. Furthermore, increasing the preload shifts the x-intercept to the right, which represents an increase in isometric force generation. Note that y-intercept, which is the maximal velocity of shortening ($V_{max}$) extrapolated to zero load, does not change with increasing preload.

■ **FIGURE 4.17** Effects of afterload on Frank-Starling curves. An increase in afterload shifts the Frank-Starling curve downward, whereas a decrease in afterload shifts the Frank-Starling curve upward. Therefore, at a given preload (*vertical dashed line*) increased afterload decreases stroke volume, and decreased afterload increases stroke volume.

discussed, changes in preload also affect the velocity of fiber shortening (see Fig. 4.8). If preload is increased, a cardiac muscle fiber will have a greater velocity of shortening at a given afterload. This occurs because the length–tension relationship requires that as the preload is increased, there is an increase in active tension development. Once the fiber begins to shorten, an increased preload with an increase in tension-generating capability causes a greater shortening velocity. In other words, increasing the preload enables the muscle to contract faster against a given afterload; this shifts the force–velocity relationship to the right (see Fig. 4.16). Note that increasing the preload increases the maximal isometric force (x-intercept) as well as the shortening velocity at a given afterload (*a* to *b* to *c*). Changes in preload, however, do not alter $V_{max}$. Therefore, *an increase in preload on a cardiac myocyte can help to offset the reduction in velocity that occurs when afterload is increased.*

## Effects of Afterload on Frank-Starling Curves

We have just seen how an increase in afterload at a given preload decreases the velocity and extent of fiber shortening. This being the case, we should expect ventricular SV to be

reduced, and indeed, this is what occurs, as shown in Figure 4.17. An increase in afterload rotates the Frank-Starling curve down and to the right. Therefore, at a given preload (left ventricular end-diastolic pressure [LVEDP] in Fig. 4.17), an increase in afterload decreases SV. Conversely, decreasing afterload shifts the curves up and to the left, thereby increasing the SV at a given preload. As discussed in Chapter 9, reducing ventricular afterload in heart failure patients is an important therapeutic approach to enhance SV.

## Effects of Afterload on Pressure–Volume Loops

The effects of afterload on ventricular function can be depicted using ventricular pressure–volume loops as shown in Figure 4.18. Increasing afterload by increasing aortic pressure at a constant preload (EDV) causes a decrease in SV (width of the loop) and an increase in ESV. The ventricle will generate increased pressure to overcome the elevated aortic pressure, but at the cost of a reduced SV. A reduction in afterload

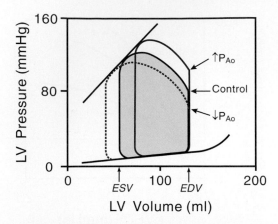

■ **FIGURE 4.18** Effects of changes in afterload (aortic pressure) on steady-state left ventricular (*LV*) pressure–volume loops. Increased aortic pressure ($\uparrow P_{Ao}$; solid red loop) decreases stroke volume (width of loop) and increases end-systolic volume (*ESV*), whereas decreased aortic pressure ($\downarrow P_{Ao}$; dashed red loop) increases stroke volume and decreases end-systolic volume. Preload and inotropy are held constant in this illustration.

will have the opposite effects—increased SV and decreased ESV. As described later in this chapter, changes in afterload in a normal, healthy heart do not affect SV as dramatically as shown in Figure 4.18 because of compensatory changes in preload (EDV).

## EFFECTS OF INOTROPY ON STROKE VOLUME

### Effects of Inotropy on Length–Tension Relationship

Ventricular SV is altered not only by changes in preload and afterload, but also by changes in ventricular **inotropy** (sometimes referred to as contractility). *Changes in inotropy are caused by cellular mechanisms that regulate*

---

**CASE 4-2**

A 67-year-old male patient is diagnosed with left ventricular failure 4 months following an acute myocardial infarction. One of the drugs he is given for treatment acts as a systemic arterial vasodilator. Using Frank-Starling curves and left ventricular pressure-volume loops, explain how decreasing afterload will improve left ventricular EF.

---

*the interaction between actin and myosin independent of changes in sarcomere length* (see Chapter 3). Therefore, an increase in inotropy augments the force of myocyte contraction independent of changes in either preload or afterload, although changes in inotropy may result in secondary changes in preload and afterload. For example, if isolated cardiac muscle is exposed to norepinephrine, it increases active tension development at any initial preload length as shown by the length–tension relationship (Fig. 4.19). This occurs because the norepinephrine binds to $\beta_1$-adrenoceptors, increasing calcium entry into the cell and calcium release by the sarcoplasmic reticulum during contraction (see Chapter 3). Because the increase in active tension occurs at a given preload length, the inotropic response exhibits **length-independent activation**.

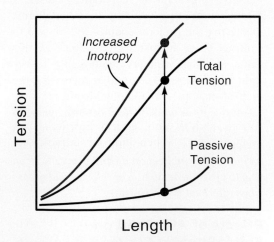

■ **FIGURE 4.19** Effects of increased inotropy on the length–tension relationship for cardiac muscle. Increasing inotropy (e.g., by stimulating the cardiac muscle with norepinephrine) shifts the total tension curve upward, which increases active tension development (*vertical arrows*) at any given preload length.

## Effects of Inotropy on Force–Velocity Relationship

Changes in inotropy also alter the force–velocity relationship. If the inotropic state of the myocyte is increased, the force–velocity curve exhibits an upward parallel shift, resulting in an increase in both $V_{max}$ (y-intercept) and maximal isometric force (x-intercept) (Fig. 4.20). The increase in velocity at any given afterload (*a* to *b* to *c*) results from the increased inotropy enhancing force generation by the actin and myosin filaments and increasing the rate of cross-bridge turnover. The increase in $V_{max}$ represents an increased intrinsic capability of the muscle fiber to generate force independent of load. In contrast, changes in preload do not alter $V_{max}$ (see Fig. 4-16).

## Effects of Inotropy on Frank-Starling Curves

The change in velocity of muscle shortening associated with a change in inotropy results in an increase in SV at any given preload and afterload and therefore causes the Frank-Starling curve to shift up or down (Fig. 4.21). If, at a given preload, inotropy is enhanced, SV will increase. Conversely, a decrease in inotropy at a given preload will decrease SV.

## Effects of Inotropy on Pressure-Volume Loops

The increased velocity of fiber shortening that occurs with increased inotropy causes an increased rate of ventricular pressure development (dP/dt), which increases ejection velocity and SV, and reduces ESV, as shown in Figure 4.22. When inotropy is increased, the ESPVR is shifted to the left and becomes steeper because the ventricle can generate increased pressure at any given volume. The ESPVR sometimes is used experimentally to define the inotropic state of the ventricle. It is analogous to the upward shift that occurs in the total tension curve in the length–tension relationship (Fig. 4.19) when inotropy increases. Conversely, a decrease in inotropy (decreased ESPVR slope) decreases the rate of ejection and SV, which leads to an

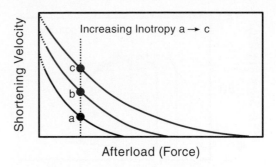

**■ FIGURE 4.20** Effects of increasing inotropy (parallel shift from curve *a* to *c*) on the force–velocity relationship. Increased inotropy increases the velocity of shortening at any given afterload (*vertical dashed line*), and increases $V_{max}$ (y-intercept). Furthermore, increased inotropy increases maximal isometric force (x-intercept).

increase in ESV. As described later in this chapter, changes in inotropy in a normal, healthy heart will also lead to secondary changes in preload and afterload that are not shown in Figure 4.22.

Changes in inotropy change the **ejection fraction**, which is defined as the SV divided by the EDV. In Figure 4.22, this would be represented by the ratio of the width of the pressure–volume loop divided by the EDV. A normal EF is >0.55 (or 55%). Increasing

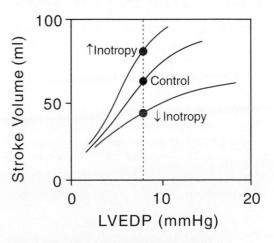

**■ FIGURE 4.21** Effects of inotropy on Frank-Starling curves. An increase in inotropy shifts the Frank-Starling curve upward, whereas a decrease in inotropy shifts the Frank-Starling curve downward. Therefore, at a given preload (*vertical dashed line*), increased inotropy increases stroke volume, and decreased inotropy decreases stroke volume.

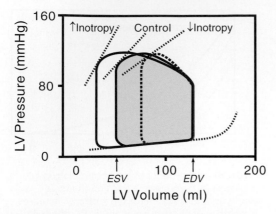

■ **FIGURE 4.22** Effects of increasing inotropy on steady-state left ventricular pressure–volume loops. Increased inotropy shifts the ESPVR (see Fig. 4.4) up and to the left, thereby increasing stroke volume and decreasing end-systolic volume (*ESV*). Decreased inotropy shifts the end-diastolic pressure–volume relationship down and to the right, thereby decreasing stroke volume and increasing end-systolic volume. *LV*, left ventricle. Preload and aortic pressure are held constant in this illustration.

inotropy increases EF, whereas decreasing inotropy decreases EF. Therefore, *EF often is used as a clinical index for evaluating the inotropic state of the heart.*

## Factors Influencing Inotropic State

Several factors influence ventricular inotropy (Fig. 4.23); the most important of these is the activity of sympathetic nerves. Sympathetic nerves, by releasing norepinephrine that binds to $\beta_1$-adrenoceptors on myocytes, serve a prominent role in ventricular and atrial inotropic regulation (see Chapter 3). Elevated levels of circulating catecholamines (epinephrine and norepinephrine) have positive inotropic effects similar to sympathetic activation. In humans and some other mammalian hearts, an abrupt increase in afterload can cause a modest increase in ino-tropy (**Anrep effect**) by a mechanism that is not fully understood. In addition, an increase in heart rate can cause a positive inotropic effect (also termed the **Bowditch effect**, treppe, or frequency-dependent activation). This latter phenomenon probably is due to an inability of the $Na^+/K^+$-ATPase to keep up with the sodium influx at the higher frequency of action potentials at elevated heart rates, leading to an accumulation of intracellular calcium via the sodium–calcium exchanger (see Chapter 2).

Increased inotropy brought about by sympathetic activation and increased heart rate is particularly important during exercise (see Chapter 9) because it helps to maintain SV at high heart rates. Recall that increased heart rate alone decreases SV because reduced diastolic filling time decreases EDV. When inotropic state increases at the same time, this decreases ESV to help maintain SV despite reduced EDV.

Systolic failure that results from cardiomyopathy, ischemia, valve disease, arrhythmias, and other conditions is characterized by a loss of intrinsic inotropy (see Chapter 9). Furthermore, there are many inotropic drugs that are used clinically to increase inotropy in acute and chronic heart failure. These drugs include digoxin (inhibits sarcolemmal $Na^+/K^+$-ATPase), $\beta$-adrenoceptor agonists (e.g., dopamine, dobutamine, epinephrine, isoproterenol), and cAMP-dependent phosphodiesterase inhibitors (e.g., milrinone).

Although the above discussion focuses on the regulation of ventricular inotropy, it is important to note that many of these same factors influence atrial inotropy. Unlike the ventricles, the atria are richly innervated with parasympathetic nerves (vagal efferents), and activation of this autonomic pathway decreases atrial inotropy.

## Cellular Mechanisms of Inotropy

As previously stated, inotropy can be thought of as a **length-independent activation** of the

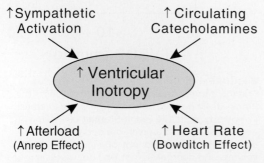

■ **FIGURE 4.23** Factors that increase inotropy.

contractile proteins. Any cellular mechanism that ultimately alters myosin ATPase activity at a given sarcomere length alters force generation and therefore can be considered an inotropic mechanism. Most of the signal transduction pathways that regulate inotropy involve $Ca^{++}$ (see Chapter 3 for details). Briefly, the following calcium-related intracellular mechanisms play an important role in regulating inotropy:

1. Increasing $Ca^{++}$ influx across the sarcolemma during the action potential
2. Increasing the release of $Ca^{++}$ by the sarcoplasmic reticulum
3. Sensitizing troponin C to $Ca^{++}$

## INTERDEPENDENCE OF PRELOAD, AFTERLOAD, AND INOTROPY

Previous discussion focused on the independent effects of preload, afterload, and inotropy on ventricular function; however, it is important to understand that these determinants of ventricular function are also interdependent. For example, a change in preload leads to secondary changes in afterload that can alter the initial response to the change in preload. Furthermore, a change in afterload leads to changes in preload, and a change in inotropy can alter both preload and afterload.

Let us first consider how ventricular responses to a change in preload can be modified by secondary changes in afterload. Similar to Figure 4.11, panel A of Figure 4.24 (solid red loop) shows that the independent effect of an increase in preload (EDV) is an increase in SV (width of pressure–volume loop) without a change in ESV. However, because SV is increased, cardiac output is increased, and this will likely lead to an increase in arterial pressure, which increases afterload. Furthermore, the increase in EDV increases ventricular wall stress (see Equation 4-2), which represents an increase in afterload. Therefore, a change in preload is normally accompanied by a secondary change in afterload. If afterload increases when there is an increase in preload (dashed red loop), then this will lead

to a small increase in ESV that will partially attenuate the increase in SV brought about by the increased preload as shown in Figure 4.24 (panel A). The increased preload still results in an increase in SV, but the increase is less than what would have occurred had the afterload not increased.

An increase in afterload, as previously discussed, leads to a decrease in SV and an increase in ESV as shown in Figure 4.24 (panel B, solid red loop). However, because the ESV is increased, changes in afterload produce secondary changes in preload (dashed red loop). The increased ESV inside the ventricle is added to the venous return, thereby increasing EDV. After several beats, a steady state is achieved in which the increase in ESV is greater than the secondary increase in EDV so that the difference between the two—the SV—is decreased (i.e., the width of the pressure–volume loop is decreased). This increase in preload secondary to an increase in afterload activates the Frank-Starling mechanism, which partially compensates for the reduction in SV caused by the initial increase in afterload.

The direct, independent effects of an increase inotropy are an increase in SV and a decrease in ESV (Fig. 4.24, panel C, solid red line). However, the increased SV increases cardiac output and arterial pressure, which increases afterload on the ventricle (dashed red line). Increased afterload tends to increase ESV, which partially offsets the effects of increased inotropy on ESV. With a decrease in ESV from control, less blood remains in the ventricle that can be added to the venous return, so the EDV will be smaller, although this will be partially offset by the tendency of the increased afterload to increase EDV. After a new steady state is reached following the increase in inotropy, the net effect of these changes is an increase in SV, which is accompanied by a reduction in ESV and a smaller reduction in EDV.

The interactions between preload, afterload, and inotropy can also be visualized using Frank-Starling curves (Fig. 4.25). In this figure, the left ventricle under control conditions has a SV of 60 mL at an end-diastolic pressure (index of preload) of about 8 mm Hg. Decreasing the afterload or

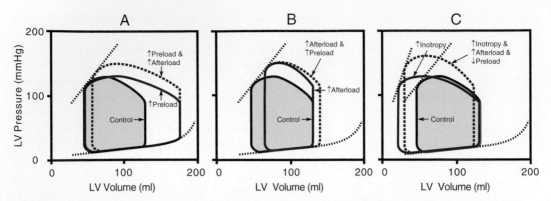

■ **FIGURE 4.24** Interdependent effects of changes in preload, afterload, and inotropy on left ventricular pressure–volume loops. **Panel A** shows effects of increasing preload (end-diastolic volume) with and without a secondary increase in afterload (aortic pressure). **Panel B** shows the effects of increasing afterload with and without a secondary increase in preload. **Panel C** shows the effects of increasing inotropy with and without secondary changes in preload and afterload.

---

**CASE 4-3**

A patient suddenly goes into sinus tachycardia, which reduces ventricular filling time. This also causes a fall in arterial pressure. Using left ventricular pressure–volume loops, describe how the tachycardia and hypotension likely alters ventricular function. Assume no changes in inotropy.

---

increasing the inotropy causes an upward shift in the Frank-Starling curve. The heart responds by increasing the SV while, at the

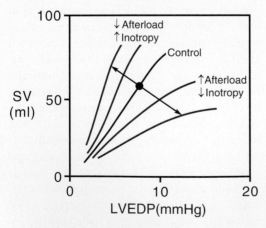

■ **FIGURE 4.25** Frank-Starling curves showing interactions between preload, afterload, and inotropy. Increased afterload or decreased inotropy shifts the Frank-Starling curve down and to the right, whereas the decreased afterload or increased inotropy shift the curve upward and to the left. The diagonal arrows show how changes in afterload and inotropy change both stroke volume (SV) and preload (*LVEDP*, left ventricular end-diastolic pressure).

same time, decreasing the end-diastolic pressure (i.e., there is a diagonal shift in the operating point between the curves). With an increase in afterload or a decrease in inotropy, the Frank-Starling curves shifts downward, leading to a fall in SV and a secondary increase in EDV.

These interactions between changes in preload, afterload, and inotropy will be discussed further in Chapter 9 in the context of cardiac disorders such as heart failure and valve disease.

## MYOCARDIAL OXYGEN CONSUMPTION

Changes in SV, whether caused by changes in preload, afterload, or inotropy, alter the oxygen consumption of the heart. Changes in heart rate likewise affect myocardial oxygen consumption. The contracting heart consumes a considerable amount of oxygen because of its need to regenerate the large amount of ATP hydrolyzed during contraction and relaxation. Therefore, any change in myocardial function that affects either the generation of force by myocytes or their frequency of contraction will alter oxygen consumption. In addition, even in noncontracting cells, ATP utilized by ion pumps and other transport functions requires oxygen for the resynthesis of ATP.

## How Myocardial Oxygen Consumption is Determined

Oxygen consumption is defined as the volume of oxygen consumed per min (e.g., mL $O_2$/min) and is sometimes expressed per 100 g of tissue weight (mL $O_2$/min per 100 g). The myocardial oxygen consumption ($M\dot{V}O_2$) can be calculated by knowing the coronary blood flow (CBF) and the arterial and venous oxygen contents ($CaO_2$ and $CvO_2$) according to the following equation that uses the **Fick principle**:

**Eq. 4-3**     $M\dot{V}O_2 = CBF \cdot (CaO_2 - CvO_2)$

Myocardial oxygen consumption, therefore, is equal to the CBF multiplied by the amount of oxygen extracted from the blood (the arterial–venous oxygen difference). The content of oxygen in blood is usually expressed as mL $O_2$/100 mL blood (or, vol % $O_2$). The oxygen content of arterial blood is normally about 20 mL $O_2$/100 mL blood. To calculate the myocardial oxygen consumption in the correct units, mL $O_2$/100 mL blood is converted to mL $O_2$/mL blood; with this conversion, the arterial oxygen content is 0.2 mL $O_2$/mL blood. For example, if CBF is 80 mL/min per 100 g, the $CaO_2$ is 0.2 mL $O_2$/mL blood and $CvO_2$ is 0.1 mL $O_2$/mL blood, then $M\dot{V}O_2$ = 8 mL $O_2$/min per 100 g. This value of myocardial oxygen consumption is typical for what is found in a heart contracting at resting heart rates against normal aortic pressures. During heavy exercise, myocardial oxygen consumption can increase to 70 mL $O_2$/min per 100 g, or more. If contractions are arrested (e.g., by depolarization of the heart with a high concentration of potassium chloride), the myocardial oxygen consumption decreases to about 2 mL $O_2$/min per 100 g. This value represents the energy costs of cellular functions not associated with contraction. Therefore, myocardial oxygen consumption varies considerably depending on the state of mechanical activity.

Although myocardial oxygen consumption can be calculated as described above, generally it is not feasible to measure CBF and coronary venous oxygen content except in experimental studies. CBF can be measured by placing flow probes on coronary arteries or a thermodilution catheter within the coronary sinus. Arterial oxygen content can be taken from a peripheral artery, but the venous oxygen content has to be obtained from the coronary sinus by inserting a catheter into the right atrium and then into the coronary sinus.

Indirect indices of myocardial oxygen consumption have been developed to estimate myocardial oxygen consumption when it is not feasible to measure it. Although no index has proven to be satisfactory over a wide range of physiologic conditions, one simple index sometimes used in clinical studies is the **pressure–rate product** (also called the double product). This index can be measured noninvasively by multiplying heart rate and systolic arterial pressure (mean arterial pressure sometimes is used instead of systolic arterial pressure). The pressure–rate product assumes that the pressure generated by the ventricle is not significantly different than the aortic pressure (i.e., there is no aortic valve stenosis). Experiments have shown that a reasonable correlation exists between changes in the pressure–rate product and myocardial oxygen consumption. For example, if arterial pressure, heart rate, or both become elevated, oxygen consumption will increase.

---

**PROBLEM 4-3**

In an experimental study, administration of an inotropic drug is found to increase CBF from 50 to 150 mL/min and increase the arterial–venous oxygen difference ($CaO_2 - CvO_2$) from 10 to 14 mL $O_2$/100 mL blood. Calculate the percent increase in myocardial oxygen consumption ($M\dot{V}O_2$) caused by infusion of this drug.

## Factors Influencing Myocardial Oxygen Consumption

Part of the difficulty in finding a suitable index of oxygen consumption is that several factors determine myocyte oxygen consumption, including frequency of contraction, inotropic state, afterload, and preload (Table 4-1). For example, doubling heart rate approximately doubles oxygen consumption, because myocytes are generating twice the number of tension cycles per minute. Increasing inotropy increases oxygen consumption because both the rate of tension development and the magnitude of tension are increased, and they both are associated with increased ATP hydrolysis and oxygen consumption. An increase in afterload likewise increases oxygen consumption because it increases the tension that must be developed by myocytes. Increasing SV by increasing preload (EDV) also increases oxygen consumption.

Quantitatively, increased preload has less impact on oxygen consumption than does an increase in afterload (e.g., aortic pressure). To understand why, we need to examine the relationship between wall stress, pressure, and radius of the ventricle. As discussed earlier (see Equation 4-2), ventricular wall stress ($\sigma$) is proportional to the intraventricular pressure (P) multiplied by the ventricular internal radius (r) and divided by the wall thickness (h).

$$\sigma \propto \frac{P \cdot r}{h}$$

Wall stress is related to the tension an individual myocyte must develop during contraction to generate a given ventricular pressure. At a given radius and wall thickness, a myocyte

| TABLE 4-1 FACTORS INCREASING MYOCARDIAL OXYGEN CONSUMPTION |
| --- |
| ↑ Heart rate |
| ↑ Inotropy |
| ↑ Afterload |
| ↑ Preload[1] |

[1]Changes in preload affect oxygen consumption much less than do changes in the other factors.

must generate increased contractile force (i.e., wall stress) to develop a higher pressure. The contractile force must be increased even further to generate the same elevated pressure if the ventricular radius is increased. For example, if the ventricle is required to generate 50% more pressure than normal to eject blood because of elevated aortic pressure, the wall stress that individual myocytes must generate will be increased by approximately 50%. This will increase the oxygen consumption of these myocytes by about 50% because changes in oxygen consumption are closely related to changes in wall stress. As a second example, if the radius of the ventricle is increased by 50%, the wall stress needed by the myocytes to eject blood at a normal pressure will be increased by about 50%. On the other hand, if the ventricular EDV is increased by 50% and the pressure and wall thickness remain unchanged, the wall stress will be increased by only about 14%. The reason for this is that a large change in ventricular volume (V) requires only a small change in radius (r). If we assume that the shape of the ventricle is a sphere, then

$$V = \frac{4}{3} \pi \cdot r^3$$

By rearranging this relationship, we find that

$$r \propto \sqrt[3]{V}$$

Substituting this into the wall stress equation results in

**Eq. 4-4**   $\sigma \propto \dfrac{P \cdot \sqrt[3]{V}}{h}$

Although no single acceptable model for the shape of the ventricle exists because its shape changes during contraction, a sphere serves as a convenient model for illustrating why changes in volume have a relatively small affect on wall stress and oxygen consumption. Using this model, Equation 4-4 shows that increasing the EDV by 50% (by a factor of 1.5) represents only a 14% (cube root of 1.5) increase in wall stress at a given ventricular pressure, whereas a 50% increase in pressure increases wall stress by 50%. Therefore, increasing pressure by a given percentage increases wall stress about four times more than the same change in volume.

Relating the wall stress equation to oxygen consumption helps to explain why increases in pressure generation have a much greater influence on oxygen consumption than a similar percentage increase in ventricular preload. It is important, however, not to use the wall stress equation to estimate oxygen demands by the whole heart. The reason for this is that wall stress estimates the tension required by individual myocytes to generate pressure as they contract. This wall stress, in large part, determines the oxygen consumption of individual myocytes, but oxygen consumption of the whole heart is the sum of the oxygen consumed by all of the myocytes. A hypertrophied ventricle with a thicker wall, which has reduced wall stress, will not have a reduction in overall oxygen consumption as suggested by Equation 4-4. In fact, because of its greater muscle mass, oxygen consumption may be significantly increased in a hypertrophied heart, particularly if its efficiency is impaired by disease. A less efficient heart performs less work per unit oxygen consumed (i.e., it generates less pressure and SV).

The concepts described above have implications for treating patients with coronary artery disease (CAD). For example, drugs that decrease afterload, heart rate, and inotropy are particularly effective in reducing myocardial oxygen consumption and relieving symptoms of chest pain (i.e., angina), which results from inadequate oxygen delivery relative to the oxygen demands of the myocardium. CAD patients are counseled to avoid activities such as lifting heavy weights that lead to large increases in arterial blood pressure. In contrast, CAD patients are often encouraged to participate in exercise programs such as walking that utilize preload and SV changes to augment cardiac output by the Frank-Starling mechanism. It is important to minimize stressful situations in these patients because stress causes sympathetic activation of the heart and vasculature that increases heart rate, inotropy, and afterload, all of which lead to significant increases in oxygen demand by the heart.

## SUMMARY OF IMPORTANT CONCEPTS

- The cardiac cycle is divided into two general phases: diastole and systole. Diastole refers to the period of time that the ventricles are undergoing relaxation and filling with blood from the atria. Ventricular filling is primarily passive, although atrial contraction has a variable effect on the final extent of ventricular filling (EDV). Systole represents the time when the ventricles are contracting and ejecting blood (SV). The volume of blood remaining in the ventricle at the end of ejection is the ESV.

- Normal heart sounds ($S_1$ and $S_2$) originate from abrupt closure of heart valves.

- Ventricular SV is the difference between the end-diastolic and end-systolic volumes. Ventricular ejection fraction (EF) is calculated as the SV divided by the EDV.

- Cardiac output is normally influenced more by changes in heart rate than by changes in SV; however, impaired regulation of SV can have a significant adverse affect on cardiac output, as occurs during heart failure.

- Ventricular preload is related to the extent of ventricular filling (EDV) and the sarcomere length. Increased preload increases the force of contraction and SV.

*(Continued)*

- Ventricular afterload can be estimated by ventricular wall stress, which is the product of ventricular pressure and ventricular radius divided by the ventricular wall thickness. Increased afterload decreases the velocity of fiber shortening during contraction, which decreases the SV.

- Inotropy is the property of a cardiac myocyte that enables it to alter its tension development independent of changes in preload length. Increased inotropy enhances active tension development by individual muscle fibers and increases ventricular pressure development, ejection velocity, and SV at a given preload and afterload.

- Preload, afterload, and inotropy are interdependent, meaning that a change in one usually leads to secondary changes in the others.

- Myocardial oxygen consumption can be calculated using the Fick Principle, in which oxygen consumption equals the product of the CBF and the arteriovenous oxygen difference. Myocardial oxygen consumption is strongly influenced by changes in arterial pressure, heart rate, and inotropy; it is less influenced by changes in SV.

## REVIEW QUESTIONS

For each question, choose the one best answer:

1. During the phase of rapid ventricular filling,

   a. $S_4$ may sometimes be heard.
   b. The aortic valve is open.
   c. The mitral valve is open.
   d. Ventricular pressure is higher than aortic pressure.

2. A patient with valve disease undergoes cardiac catheterization to compare vascular and intracardiac pressures against normal values. Which of the following is found in a heart with normal valve function?

   a. Aortic diastolic pressure is less than pulmonary artery systolic pressure.
   b. Left ventricular end-diastolic pressure is less than mean right atrial pressure.
   c. Mean left atrial pressure is normally greater than mean right atrial pressure by <10 mm Hg.
   d. Pulmonary artery diastolic pressure is less than mean right atrial pressure.

3. Right ventricular preload is increased by which of the following?

   a. Decreased atrial contractility
   b. Decreased blood volume
   c. Decreased heart rate
   d. Decreased ventricular compliance

4. A 78-year-old female patient with a history of left ventricular failure complains of difficulty breathing when lying down. Which of the following occurs to the cardiac muscle fibers that can lead to an increase in right ventricular output and pulmonary congestion when this patient lies down?

   a. Active tension development increases.
   b. Degree of muscle shortening is diminished.
   c. Preload decreases.
   d. Velocity of shortening decreases.

5. Left ventricular end-diastolic pressure is increased by

   a. Decreased afterload.
   b. Decreased venous return.
   c. Increased inotropy.
   d. Ventricular hypertrophy.

6. A 67-year-old male patient complains of excessive shortness of breath during exertion. The report from a follow-up echocardiogram says that his left ventricular stroke volume is 50 mL, with an ejection fraction of 25%. Which of the following statements is true concerning this patient's left ventricle?

   a. End-diastolic volume is elevated above normal.
   b. End-systolic volume is less than normal.
   c. Inotropy is increased.
   d. Preload is reduced.

7. A patient is experiencing an acute hypertensive crisis. This large increase in arterial pressure will have which of the following direct effects on the heart?

   a. Decrease left ventricular end-systolic volume
   b. Decrease the velocity of muscle fiber shortening
   c. Decrease ventricular preload
   d. Increase stroke volume

8. Increasing the inotropic state of the myocardium will

   a. Increase end-systolic volume.
   b. Increase the width of the pressure–volume loop.
   c. Increase ventricular end-diastolic volume.
   d. Shift the force–velocity relationship to the left.

9. If each of the following is increased by 25%, which one would cause the *smallest* change in myocardial oxygen consumption?

   a. Heart rate
   b. Ventricular end-diastolic volume
   c. Mean arterial pressure
   d. Ventricular radius

## ANSWERS TO REVIEW QUESTIONS

1. The correct answer is "c" because the mitral valve is open throughout ventricular filling. Choice "a" is incorrect because $S_4$, when heard, is associated with atrial contraction and frequently is heard in hypertrophied hearts. Choice "b" is incorrect because the aortic valve is open only during ventricular ejection. Choice "d" is incorrect because the ventricular pressure is higher than aortic pressure only during the phase of rapid ejection.

2. The correct answer is "c" because average left atrial pressure is about 8 mm Hg and average right atrial pressure is about 4 mm Hg. Choice "a" is incorrect because aortic diastolic pressure is about 80 mm Hg compared to a pulmonary artery systolic pressure of 25 mm Hg. Choice "b" is incorrect because left atrial and left ventricular end-diastolic pressures are normally higher than their corresponding pressures on the right side of the heart. Choice "d" is incorrect because pulmonary artery diastolic pressure is about 10 mm Hg, whereas right atrial pressure is about 4 mm Hg.

3. The correct answer is "c" because more time is available for filling at reduced heart rates (diastole is lengthened);

therefore, preload is increased at reduced heart rates. Choices "a," "b," and "d" are incorrect because decreased atrial contractility, blood volume, and ventricular compliance lead to reduced ventricular filling and therefore reduced preload.

4. The correct answer is "a" because increased preload resulting from increased venous return when lying down causes length-dependent activation of actin and myosin, which increases active tension development. This is the basis for the Frank-Starling mechanism. Being in heart failure, increased output of the right ventricle may not lead to a corresponding increase in left ventricular stroke, thereby causing pulmonary congestion and difficulty breathing. Choices "b," "c," and "d" are incorrect because decreased muscle shortening, preload, and velocity of shortening all lead to a decrease in stroke volume.

5. The correct answer is "d" because ventricular hypertrophy reduces ventricular compliance, which results in elevated end-diastolic pressures when the ventricle fills. Choice "a" is incorrect because decreased afterload leads to a reduction in end-systolic volume, which results in a secondary fall in end-diastolic volume and pressure. Choice "b" is incorrect because decreased venous return decreases ventricular filling, which decreases ventricular end-diastolic volume and pressure. Choice "c" is incorrect because increased inotropy reduces end-systolic volume, which results in a secondary fall in end-diastolic volume and pressure.

6. The correct answer is "a" because with an ejection fraction (EF) of 25% and a stroke volume (SV) of 50 mL, this patient's end-diastolic volume (EDV) is 200 mL, which is much greater than normal (usually <150 mL). The calculation is based on: EF = (SV/EDV) × 100, and therefore EDV = (SV/EF) × 100 when EF is expressed as a percentage.

Choices "b," "c," and "d" are incorrect because this low EF (normally >55%) indicates ventricular failure (loss of inotropy), which leads to a reduced SV and an elevated end-systolic volume. Preload (end-diastolic volume) is increased (as calculated above) because the elevated end-systolic volume leads to a secondary increase in preload, and because of other compensatory mechanisms discussed in Chapter 9.

7. The correct answer is "b" because an increased arterial pressure increases left ventricular afterload, which decreases the velocity of fiber shortening as shown by the force–velocity relationship. Choices "a," "c," and "d" are incorrect because increased afterload decreases the velocity of fiber shortening, which decreases stroke volume. This leads to an increase in left ventricular end-systolic volume and a secondary increase in preload (end-diastolic volume).

8. The correct answer is "b" because an increase in inotropy increases stroke volume, which is represented by the width of the pressure–volume loop. Choice "a," "c," and "d" are incorrect because increased inotropy causes a parallel, upward shift in the force–velocity relationship, which leads to an increase in velocity of fiber shortening and therefore an increase in stroke volume at any given afterload. Increased stroke volume decreases end-systolic volume and leads to a secondary decrease in left ventricular end-diastolic volume (preload).

9. The correct answer is "b" because an increase in end-diastolic volume will increase stroke volume; however, stroke volume changes are about one-fourth as effective in changing myocardial oxygen consumption as are changes in heart rate, mean arterial pressure, or ventricular radius because of the relationships between oxygen consumption, wall stress, ventricular pressure, and ventricular radius. For this reason, choices "a," "c," and "d" are incorrect.

## ANSWERS TO PROBLEMS AND CASES

### PROBLEM 4-1

Stroke volume equals cardiac output divided by heart rate. Because stroke volume uses milliliters (mL) for units, cardiac output (8.8 L/min) must be expressed in mL/min (8800 mL/min). This value, divided by a heart rate of 110 beats/min, gives a stroke volume of 80 mL/beat.

### PROBLEM 4-2

Because the right ventricular stroke volume is 0.1% greater than the left ventricular stroke volume of 60 mL/beat, the right ventricular stroke volume can be calculated by multiplying 60 times 1.001, which gives a stroke volume of 60.06 mL/beat. The difference in stroke volume between the two ventricles therefore is 0.06 mL/beat. To obtain the difference in total stroke volume over 1 hour when the rate is 75 beats/min, multiply the rate (75 beats/min) × 60 min/h × stroke volume difference (0.06 mL/beat). This calculation yields a value of 270 mL, which represents the increase in pulmonary blood volume that occurs after only 1 hour because of a small imbalance between the outputs of the right and left ventricles.

### PROBLEM 4-3

Myocardial oxygen consumption can be calculated from Equation 4-3, such that

$$\dot{M}VO_2 = CBF \cdot (CaO_2 - CvO_2)$$

The control oxygen consumption is 50 mL/min times the arterial–venous oxygen difference of 0.1 mL $O_2$/mL blood, which equals 5 mL $O_2$/min. Note that the arterial–venous oxygen difference must be converted from mL $O_2$/100 mL blood to mL $O_2$/mL blood. The experimental oxygen consumption is 150 mL/min times 0.14 mL $O_2$/mL blood, which equals 21 mL $O_2$/min. This is a 320% increase in oxygen consumption ($[(21-5)/5] \times 100$).

### CASE 4-1

A hypertrophied ventricle is less compliant. This causes the end-diastolic pressure–volume curve to shift up and to the left, as shown in figure below. This shift reduces the end-diastolic volume and increases the end-diastolic pressure at the end of ventricular filling. The end-systolic volume will be normal unless there is a significant change in inotropy or aortic diastolic pressure (afterload). The width of the pressure–volume loop is narrower; therefore, the stroke volume is reduced.

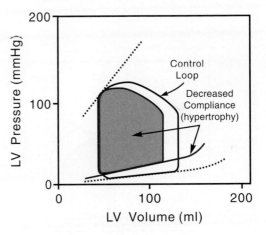

### CASE 4-2

A systemic vasodilator reduces afterload on the left ventricle. This causes the Starling curve to shift up and to the left from its depressed state (because of the loss of inotropy in failure) (Figure A in the next page). This shift increases stroke volume and at the same time reduces preload (end-diastolic pressure) from point A to B. Systemic vasodilation reduces aortic diastolic pressure, which enables the ventricle to eject sooner, more rapidly, and to a smaller end-systolic volume (Figure B in the next page). The reduced end-systolic volume leads to a compensatory decrease in end-diastolic volume; however, the reduction in end-systolic volume is greater than the reduction in end-diastolic volume so that stroke volume is increased. By increasing stroke volume and reducing the end-diastolic volume, the ejection fraction (EF) is increased because it is calculated as stroke volume (SV) divided by end-diastolic volume (EDV) as follows: EF = SV/EDV.

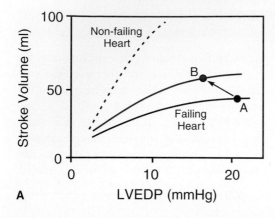

**A**

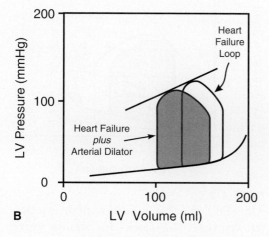

**B**

## CASE 4-3

Reduced ventricular filling time caused by tachycardia leads to a decrease in EDV and SV. This preload change alone, however, will not alter ESV. The addition of a fall in arterial pressure decreases afterload on the ventricle, which independently increases stroke volume and reduces ESV. This can lead to a further decrease in EDV. The net effect of these two conditions will be a large reduction in EDV coupled with a small reduction in ESV, and large fall in stroke volume. Because of the hypotension (both systolic and diastolic), the ejection phase of the pressure–volume loop starts at a lower pressure, and the peak ventricular systolic pressure is also reduced.

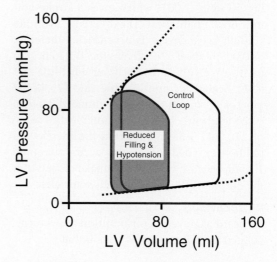

## SUGGESTED RESOURCES

Braunwald E, Ross J, Sonnenblick EH. Mechanisms of Contraction of the Normal and Failing Heart. 2nd Ed. Boston: Little, Brown & Co., 1976.

Covell JW, Ross J. Systolic and diastolic function (mechanics) of the intact heart. In: Page E, Fozzard HA, Solaro RJ, eds. Handbook of Physiology, vol. 1. Bethesda: American Physiological Society, 2002; 741–785.

Fuchs F, Smith SH. Calcium, cross-bridges, and the Frank-Starling relationship. News Physiol Sci 2001;16:5–10.

Katz AM. Physiology of the Heart. 4th Ed. Philadelphia: Lippincott Williams & Wilkins, 2006.

Lilly LS. Pathophysiology of Heart Disease. 5th Ed. Philadelphia: Lippincott Williams & Wilkins, 2011.

Opie LH. The Heart: Physiology from Cell to Circulation. 4th Ed. Philadelphia: Lippincott Williams & Wilkins, 2004.

Sagawa K, Maughan L, Suga H, Sunagawa K. Cardiac Contraction and the Pressure-Volume Relationship. New York: Oxford University Press, 1988.

Solaro, RJ. Integration of Myocyte Response to Ca²⁺ with Cardiac Pump Regulation and Pump Dynamics. Am. J. Physiol. 1999;277(Adv. Physiol. Educ. 22): S155–S163.

# VASCULAR FUNCTION

Understanding the concepts presented in this chapter will enable the student to:

1. Name the different types of vessels constituting the vascular network of the body and describe the general function of each.

2. Describe how changes in cardiac output, systemic vascular resistance, and central venous pressure affect mean arterial pressure.

3. Describe the factors that determine arterial pulse pressure.

4. Describe in quantitative terms how changes in vessel radius, vessel length, blood viscosity, and perfusion pressure affect blood flow.

5. Explain how turbulent flow alters the relationship between pressure and flow.

6. Calculate total resistance from series or parallel resistance networks.

7. Explain why the pressure drop across small arteries and arterioles is much greater than the pressure drop across other vessel types.

8. Define vascular tone and list factors that alter vascular tone.

9. Explain how each of the following affects central venous pressure: blood volume, venous compliance, gravity, respiration, and muscle contraction.

10. Using cardiac and systemic function curves, explain how changes in blood volume, venous compliance, vascular resistance, and cardiac performance influence the equilibrium between right atrial pressure and cardiac output.

## INTRODUCTION

The vascular system serves two basic functions: distribution and exchange. Distribution includes transporting blood to and away from organs. Exchange involves the movement of gases, nutrients, and fluid between the blood and tissues. This chapter focuses on vascular anatomy and the general hemodynamic principles involved in the regulation of blood pressure and the distribution of blood flow in the body. Chapters 6 and 7 describe these physiologic control mechanisms in more detail. The exchange function is described in Chapter 8.

## ANATOMY AND FUNCTION

### Vascular Network

The left ventricle ejects blood into the aorta, which then distributes the blood flow throughout the body using a network of arterial vessels, which branch into successively smaller vessels until they reach the smallest vascular unit, capillaries, within organs and tissues. Capillaries then converge into successively larger vessels (veins), which return the blood to the heart. These vessels are illustrated in Figure 5.1. Table 5–1 summarizes the relative sizes and functions of different blood vessels.

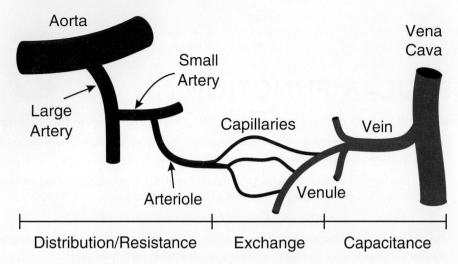

**■ FIGURE 5.1** Major types of blood vessels found within the circulation.

The different types of vessels can be grouped by their primary function: distribution/resistance (aorta, large and small distributing arteries), exchange (capillaries, small venules), and capacitance (large venules, veins, vena cavae).

### DISTRIBUTION/RESISTANCE VESSELS

The **aorta,** besides being the main vessel to distribute blood from the heart to the arterial system, dampens the pulsatile pressure that results from the intermittent ejection of blood from the left ventricle. The dampening is a function of the aortic compliance, which is discussed in more detail later in this chapter. **Large arteries** branching off the aorta

(e.g., carotid, mesenteric, and renal arteries) distribute the blood flow to specific organs or regions of the body. These large arteries, although capable of constricting and dilating, serve no significant role in the regulation of pressure and blood flow under normal physiologic conditions. Once the distributing artery reaches the organ to which it supplies blood, it branches into **small arteries** that distribute blood flow within the organ. These smaller arteries continue branching into smaller and smaller vessels. Once they reach diameters of <200 µm, they are termed **arterioles.** No clear demarcation between small arteries and arterioles exists; therefore, no consensus has been reached regarding the point at

| TABLE 5-1 | SIZE AND FUNCTION OF DIFFERENT TYPES OF BLOOD VESSELS IN THE SYSTEMIC CIRCULATION | |
|---|---|---|
| **VESSEL TYPE** | **DIAMETER (mm)** | **FUNCTION** |
| Aorta | 25 | Pulse dampening and distribution |
| Large arteries | 1.0–10.0 | Distribution |
| Small arteries | 0.2–1.0 | Distribution and resistance |
| Arterioles | 0.01–0.20 | Resistance (pressure/flow regulation) |
| Capillaries | 0.006–0.010 | Exchange |
| Venules | 0.01–0.20 | Exchange, collection, and capacitance |
| Veins | 0.2–10.0 | Capacitance function (blood volume) |
| Vena cava | 35 | Collection |

which a small artery becomes an arteriole. Many investigators speak of different branching orders of arterial vessels within a tissue or organ. Most would agree that arterioles have only a few layers of vascular smooth muscle and are, in general, <200 μm in diameter.

Together, the small arteries and arterioles represent the primary **resistance vessels** that regulate arterial blood pressure and blood flow within organs. Resistance vessels are highly innervated by autonomic nerves (particularly sympathetic adrenergic), and they constrict or dilate in response to changes in nerve activity. The resistance vessels are richly endowed with receptors that bind circulating hormones (e.g., catecholamines, angiotensin II), which can alter vessel diameter (see Chapters 3 and 6). They also respond to various substances (e.g., adenosine, potassium ion, and nitric oxide) produced by the tissue surrounding the vessel or by the vascular endothelium.

### EXCHANGE VESSELS

As arterioles become smaller in diameter (<10 μm), they lose their smooth muscle. Vessels that have no smooth muscle and are composed of only endothelial cells and a basement membrane are termed **capillaries**. Although they are the smallest vessels within the circulation, they have the greatest cross-sectional area because they are so numerous. Because the total blood flow of all capillaries in the body is the same as the flow within the aorta leaving the heart, and because the capillary cross-sectional area is about 1000 times greater than the aorta, the mean velocity of blood flowing within capillaries (~0.05 cm/s) is about 1000-fold less than the velocity in the aorta (~50 cm/s). The reason for this is that flow (F) is the product of mean velocity (V) times cross-sectional area (A) ($F = V \cdot A$). When this expression is rearranged, we find that the mean velocity is inversely proportional to cross-sectional area ($V = F/A$).

Capillaries have the greatest surface area for exchange. Oxygen, carbon dioxide, water, electrolytes, proteins, metabolic substrates and by-products, and circulating hormones are exchanged across the capillary endothelium between the plasma and the surrounding tissue interstitium (see Chapter 8). Capillaries, therefore, are the primary exchange vessels within the body.

When capillaries join together, they form small, postcapillary venules, which are still devoid of smooth muscle. They, like capillaries, serve as exchange vessels for fluid and macromolecules because of their high permeability.

### CAPACITANCE VESSELS

As small postcapillary venules converge and form larger venules, smooth muscle reappears. These vessels, like the resistance vessels, are capable of dilating and constricting. Changes in venular diameter regulate capillary pressure and venous blood volume. Venules converge to form larger veins. Together, venules and veins are the primary capacitance vessels of the body, that is, the site where most of the blood volume is found and regional blood volume is regulated. Constriction of veins decreases venous blood volume and increases venous pressure, which can alter cardiac output by affecting right atrial pressure and ventricular preload. The final venous vessels are the inferior and superior vena cavae, which carry the blood back to the right atrium of the heart.

## Distribution of Pressures and Volumes

Mean blood pressure is highest in the aorta (about 95 mm Hg in a normal adult) and progressively decreases as the blood flows further away from the heart (Fig. 5.2). The reason why pressure falls as blood flows through vessels is because energy is lost as heat owing to friction within the moving blood (related to blood viscosity) and between the blood and the vessel wall. Between any two points along the length of an artery, for example, the drop in pressure (ΔP) is related to the flow (F) and resistance to flow (R) as shown in Equation 5–1.

Eq. 5-1 $$\Delta P = F \cdot R$$

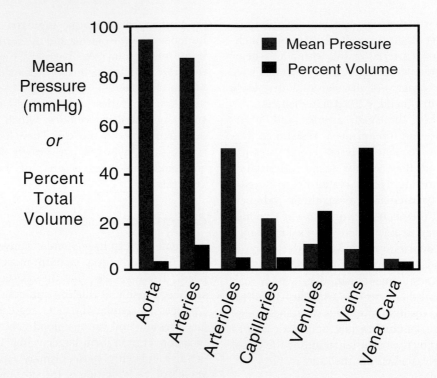

■ **FIGURE 5.2** Distribution of pressures and volumes in the systemic circulation. The greatest pressure drop occurs across small arteries and arterioles; most of the blood volume is found within the veins and venules.

Equation 5–1 is a hydrodynamic form of Ohm law ($\Delta V = I \cdot R$), where the voltage difference ($\Delta V$; analogous to $\Delta P$) is equal to the current (I; analogous to F) times the resistance (R). This equation generally applies in the body when blood is flowing under nonturbulent, laminar flow conditions.

The mean blood pressure does not fall much as the blood flows down the aorta and through large distributing arteries because these vessels have a low resistance relative to their flow, and therefore, little loss of pressure energy ($\Delta P$) occurs along their lengths. In contrast, when the blood flows through the small arteries and arterioles (the primary resistance vessels), there is a large fall in mean arterial blood pressure. The reason is that these vessels, as a group, have a high resistance relative to their flow, and therefore, $\Delta P$ across this group of vessels is large. In fact, approximately 50% to 70% of the pressure drop within the vasculature occurs within the resistance vessels. By the time blood reaches the capillaries, the mean blood pressure may

be 25 to 30 mm Hg, depending on the organ. It is important that the capillary pressure is relatively low; otherwise, large amounts of fluid would leak through the capillaries (and post-capillary venules), causing tissue edema (see Chapter 8). The pressure falls further as blood travels through veins back to the heart; however, the pressure drop is small compared to the pressure drop across the small arteries and arterioles because the resistance of the veins is very low compared to the arterial resistance vessels. Pressure within the thoracic vena cava near the right atrium is very close to zero millimeters of mercury (mm Hg), although it fluctuates by a few mm Hg during the cardiac cycle and because of respiratory activity.

The greatest volume (60% to 80%) of blood within the circulation resides within the venous vasculature. This is why veins are referred to as capacitance vessels. The relative volume of blood between the arterial and venous sides of the circulation can vary considerably depending on total blood volume, intravascular pressures, and vascular compliance as described later in this chapter. Vascular compliance varies depending on the state of venous smooth muscle contraction, which is primarily regulated by sympathetic nerves innervating the veins.

## ARTERIAL BLOOD PRESSURE

Ejection of blood into the aorta by the left ventricle results in a characteristic aortic pressure pulse (Fig. 5.3). The peak pressure of the aortic pulse is termed the **systolic** pressure. Shortly after the peak systolic pressure, there appears a notch (dicrotic notch or incisura) followed by the appearance of a small increase in pressure (dicrotic wave) prior to the pressure falling toward its minimal value, the **diastolic pressure**. The difference between the systolic and diastolic pressures is the aortic **pulse pressure**. If, for example, the systolic pressure is 130 mm Hg and the diastolic pressure is 85 mm Hg, then the pulse pressure is 45 mm Hg. Therefore, any factor that affects either systolic or diastolic pressures affects pulse pressure. The systolic and diastolic pressures are those that are measured with an arm blood pressure cuff (sphygmomanometer). While these values are very important clinically, neither value is the primary pressure that drives blood flow in organs. That pressure is the mean arterial pressure, which is the average pressure over time. This pressure needs to be determined when hemodynamic information is required to assess vascular function.

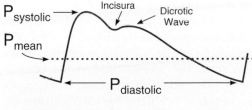

**Pulse Pressure = P$_{systolic}$ − P$_{diastolic}$**

■ **FIGURE 5.3** Pressure pulse within the aorta. The pulse pressure is the difference between the maximal pressure (systolic) and the minimal pressure (diastolic). The mean pressure is approximately equal to the diastolic pressure plus one–third the pulse pressure.

## Mean Arterial Pressure

Because of the shape of the aortic pressure pulse, the value for the **mean pressure** (geometric mean) is less than the arithmetic average of the systolic and diastolic pressures as shown in Figure 5.3. At normal resting heart rates, mean aortic (or arterial) pressure (MAP) can be *estimated* from the diastolic (P$_{dias}$) and systolic (P$_{sys}$) pressures by Equation 5–2:

**Eq. 5-2**  $\text{MAP} \cong P_{dias} + \frac{1}{3}(P_{sys} - P_{dias})$

For example, if systolic pressure is 120 mm Hg and diastolic pressure is 80 mm Hg, the mean arterial pressure will be approximately 93 mm Hg. At high heart rates, however, mean arterial pressure is more closely approximated by the arithmetic average of systolic and diastolic pressure because the shape of the arterial pressure pulse changes (it becomes narrower) as the period of diastole shortens more than does systole. Therefore, to determine mean arterial pressure accurately, analog electronic circuitry or digital techniques are used, usually in conjunction with an indwelling arterial catheter.

No single value exists for normal mean arterial pressure. In infant children, the mean arterial pressure may be only 70 mm Hg, whereas in older adults, mean arterial pressure may be 100 mm Hg. With increasing age, the systolic pressure generally rises more than diastolic pressure; therefore, the pulse pressure increases with age. Small differences exist between men and women, with women having slightly lower pressures at equivalent ages. In adults, arterial pressure is considered normal when the systolic pressure is <120 mm Hg (but > 90 mm Hg) and the diastolic pressure is <80 mm Hg (but > 60 mm Hg), which represents a normal mean pressure of <95 mm Hg. Abnormally low and elevated arterial pressures are discussed in Chapter 9.

What factors determine mean arterial pressure? As blood is pumped into the resistance network of the systemic circulation, pressure is generated within the arterial vasculature. The mean arterial (or aortic) pressure (MAP) is determined by the cardiac output (CO), systemic vascular resistance (SVR), and central venous pressure (CVP) as shown in Equation 5–3.

### Eq. 5-3    MAP = (CO · SVR) + CVP

This equation is based on Equation 5–1, where $\Delta P = F \cdot R$. The $\Delta P$ in Equation 5–3 represents the pressure drop across the entire systemic circulation, which is MAP – CVP; the CO and SVR are the F and R, respectively, of Equation 5–1. Therefore, from Equation 5–3, changes in cardiac output, systemic vascular resistance, or CVP affect mean arterial pressure. If cardiac output and systemic vascular resistance change reciprocally and proportionately, MAP will not change. For example, if cardiac output is reduced by one–half and systemic vascular resistance is doubled, mean arterial pressure will remain unchanged.

Figure 5.4, which is based upon Equation 5–3, shows that as cardiac output is increased, a linear increase occurs in arterial pressure (assuming that resistance and venous pressure remain constant). An increase in systemic vascular resistance (increased slope of the line) results in a greater arterial pressure for any given cardiac output. Conversely, a decrease in resistance results in a lower arterial pressure for any given cardiac output.

Cardiac output, systemic vascular resistance, and venous pressure are constantly changing, and they are interdependent (i.e., changing one variable can change each of the other variables). For example, increasing systemic vascular resistance increases the afterload on the heart, which decreases cardiac output and alters CVP, as described in more detail later in this chapter. Furthermore, extrinsic control mechanisms acting on the heart and circulation can affect these variables. If, for example, cardiac output suddenly falls by 20% (as can occur when standing), mean arterial pressure will not decrease by 20% because the body compensates by increasing systemic vascular resistance through baroreceptor mechanisms to maintain constant pressure (see Chapter 6).

## Aortic Pulse Pressure

As blood flows down the aorta and into distributing arteries, characteristic changes take place in the shape of the pressure wave contour. As the pressure pulse moves away from the heart, the systolic pressure rises, and the diastolic pressure falls. The change in the shape of the pressure pulse is related to a number of factors including (1) decreased compliance of distal arteries and (2) reflective waves, particularly from arterial branch points, which summate with the pulse wave traveling down the aorta and arteries. In addition, mean arterial pressure declines as the pressure pulse travels down distributing arteries owing to the resistance of the arteries; however, the reduction in mean pressure is small (just a few mm Hg) because the distributing arteries have a relatively low resistance. Therefore, the values measured for arterial pressure differ depending on the site of measurement. When the arterial pressure is measured using a sphygmomanometer (i.e., blood pressure cuff) on the upper arm, the pressure measurement represents the pressure within the brachial artery. The measured pressures, however, are not identical with the systolic and diastolic pressures found in the aorta or the pressures measured in other distributing arteries.

The compliance of the aorta and the ventricular stroke volume determine pulse pressure. **Compliance** is defined by the relationship between volume and pressure, in which compliance (C) equals the slope of that

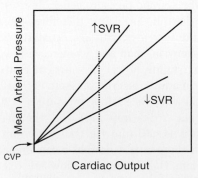

■ **FIGURE 5.4** The relationship between cardiac output (*CO*), systemic vascular resistance (*SVR*), mean arterial pressure (MAP), and central venous pressure (*CVP*). Increasing SVR increases MAP at any given cardiac output (*dotted line*), whereas decreasing SVR decreases MAP at a given cardiac output. This figure is based on Equation 5-3, in which MAP = (CO · SVR) + CVP.

relationship, or the change in volume (ΔV) divided by the change in pressure (ΔP) at a given pressure:

**Eq. 5-4**    $C = \dfrac{\Delta V}{\Delta P}$   or,   $\Delta V = C \cdot \Delta P$

Therefore, a highly compliant vessel will display a relatively small increase in pressure for a given increase in volume. Conversely, a less compliant vessel (i.e., "stiffer" vessel) will display a relatively large increase in pressure for a given increase in volume.

The compliance of a blood vessel is determined in large part by the relative proportion of elastin fibers versus smooth muscle and collagen in the vessel wall (see Fig. 3.7). Elastin fibers offer the least resistance to stretch, whereas collagen offers the greatest resistance. A vessel such as the aorta that has a greater proportion of elastin fibers versus smooth muscle and collagen has a relatively low resistance to stretch and, therefore, has a compliance that is greater than that found in a muscular artery that has more smooth muscle and less elastin.

The relatively high compliance of the aorta dampens the pulsatile output of the left ventricle, thereby reducing the pulse pressure. If the aorta were a rigid tube, the pulse pressure would be very high with each ven-

tricular ejection. However, as blood is ejected into the aorta, the walls of the aorta expand to accommodate the increase in blood volume contained within the aorta because the aorta is compliant. As the aorta expands, the increase in pressure is determined by the change in aortic volume divided by the compliance of the aorta at that particular range of volumes (Fig. 5.5, panel A). The less compliant the aorta, the greater the pressure change (i.e., pulse pressure) at any given change in aortic volume (Fig. 5.5, panel B). Age and arteriosclerotic disease decrease aortic compliance, which increases aortic pulse pressure. It is not uncommon for elderly people to have aortic pulse pressures of 60 mm Hg or more, whereas younger adults have aortic pulse pressures of about 40 to 45 mm Hg at resting heart rates.

A change in compliance affects only pulse pressure and not the mean pressure, which remains unchanged as long as cardiac output and systemic vascular resistance do not change. In contrast, a change in stroke volume normally changes mean aortic pressure in addition to pulse pressure because the cardiac output changes. For example, if stroke volume and cardiac output are increased by an increase in inotropy, both pulse pressure and mean arterial pressure

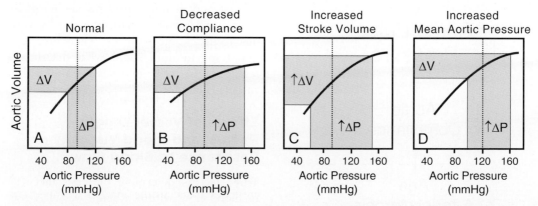

■ **FIGURE 5.5** Effects of stroke volume, aortic compliance, and mean aortic pressure on aortic pulse pressure. **Panel A**. At a given stroke volume (*ΔV*), the pulse pressure (*ΔP*) is determined by the aortic compliance (*red line*). **Panel B**. Decreasing the aortic compliance (slope of *red line*) increases the pulse pressure at a given stroke volume. **Panel C**. Increasing the stroke volume into the aorta increases the pulse pressure. **Panel D**. At higher mean aortic pressures (*dotted line*), a given stroke volume produces a greater pulse pressure because the aortic compliance is less at higher pressures and volumes. **Panels A–C** assume a constant mean aortic pressure.

increase. If, however, cardiac output is not changed when stroke volume changes (e.g., if a decrease in heart rate accompanies the increase in stroke volume), then only the pulse pressure changes—the mean aortic pressure does not change (Fig. 5.5, panel C).

No single value for aortic compliance exists because the relationship between volume and pressure (compliance curve; red line in Fig. 5.5) is not linear. At higher aortic volumes and pressures, the slope of the relationship decreases and compliance decreases (see Fig. 5.5, panel D). Therefore, at elevated mean arterial pressures, the reduced compliance results in an increase in pulse pressure at a given stroke volume.

In summary, aortic pulse pressure is determined by ventricular stroke volume and aortic compliance (Fig. 5.6). Any factor that

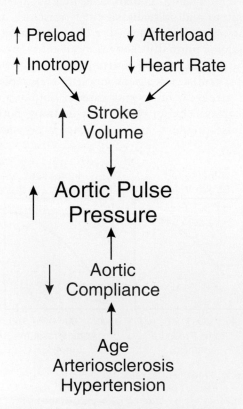

■ **FIGURE 5.6** Factors affecting aortic pulse pressure. Pulse pressure is increased by those factors that increase stroke volume or decrease aortic compliance.

changes stroke volume (e.g., ventricular preload, afterload, and inotropy; heart rate) or aortic compliance (e.g., age, arteriosclerosis, hypertension) alters aortic pulse pressure. Beat–to–beat changes in pulse pressure occur owing to changes in stroke volume. In contrast, chronic, long–term increases in pulse pressure are commonly due to decreased aortic compliance.

## HEMODYNAMICS (PRESSURE, FLOW, AND RESISTANCE)

The term **hemodynamics** describes the physical factors governing blood flow within the circulatory system. Blood flow through an organ is determined by the pressure gradient ($\Delta P$) driving the flow divided by the resistance (R) to flow (Equation 5–5), which is a rearrangement of Equation 5–1. The pressure gradient (or perfusion pressure) driving flow through an organ is the arterial minus the venous pressure. For an individual blood vessel, the pressure gradient is the pressure difference between two defined points along the vessel.

Eq. 5-5
$$F = \frac{\Delta P}{R}$$

Blood flow through organs is determined largely by changes in resistance because arterial and venous pressures are normally maintained within a narrow range by various feedback mechanisms. Therefore, it is important to understand what determines resistance in individual vessels and within vascular networks.

### Effects of Vessel Length, Radius, and Blood Viscosity on Resistance to Blood Flow

Three factors determine the resistance (R) to blood flow within a single vessel: vessel length (L), blood viscosity ($\eta$), and diameter (or radius, r) of the vessel. These are described by Equation 5–6 as follows:

Eq. 5-6
$$R \propto \frac{\eta \cdot L}{r^4}$$

Resistance is directly proportional to vessel length. Therefore, a vessel that is twice as long as another vessel with the same radius will have twice the resistance to flow. In the body, individual vessel lengths do not change appreciably; therefore, changes in vessel length have only a minimal effect on resistance.

Resistance to flow is directly related to the viscosity of the blood. Viscosity is related to friction generated by interactions between fluid molecules in the plasma and suspended formed substances (e.g., red blood cells) as the blood is flowing. Viscosity also takes into account the friction generated between the blood and the lining of the vessel. Therefore, viscosity can be thought of as a force that opposes blood flow. If viscosity increases twofold, the resistance to flow increases twofold, thereby decreasing flow by one–half at constant $\Delta P$. At normal body temperatures, the viscosity of plasma is about 1.8 times the viscosity of water. The viscosity of whole blood is about three to four times the viscosity of water owing to the presence of red cells and proteins. Blood viscosity normally does not change much; however, it can be significantly altered by changes in hematocrit and temperature and by low flow states. Hematocrit is the volume of red blood cells expressed as a percentage of a given volume of whole blood. If hematocrit increases from a normal value of 40% to an elevated value of 60% (this is termed polycythemia), the blood viscosity approximately doubles. Decreasing blood temperature increases viscosity by about 2% per degree centigrade. The flow rate of blood also affects viscosity. At very low flow states in the microcirculation—as occurs during circulatory shock—the blood viscosity can increase severalfold. This occurs because at low flow states, cell–to–cell and protein–to–cell adhesive interactions increase, which can cause erythrocytes to adhere to one another and increase the blood viscosity.

Of the three independent variables in Equation 5–6, vessel radius is the most important quantitatively for determining resistance to flow. Because radius and resistance are inversely related, an increase in radius reduces resistance. Furthermore, *a change in radius alters resistance inversely to the fourth power of the radius.* For example, a twofold increase in radius decreases resistance 16–fold! Therefore, vessel resistance is exquisitely sensitive to changes in radius. Because changes in radius and diameter are directly proportional, diameter can be substituted for radius in Equation 5–6.

If the expression for resistance (Equation 5–6) is combined with the equation describing the relationship between flow, pressure, and resistance (F = $\Delta P$/R; Equation 5–5), the following relationship is obtained:

**Eq. 5-7**
$$F \propto \frac{\Delta P \cdot r^4}{\eta \cdot L}$$

This relationship (**Poiseuille's equation**) was first described by the French physician Poiseuille (1846). The full equation contains $\pi$ in the numerator, and the number 8 in the denominator (a constant of integration). Equation 5–7 describes how flow is related to perfusion pressure, radius, length, and viscosity. In the body, however, flow does not conform precisely to this relationship because the equation assumes the following: (1) the vessels are long, straight, rigid tubes; (2) the blood behaves as a Newtonian fluid in which viscosity is constant and independent of flow; and (3) the blood is flowing under steady laminar flow (nonturbulent) conditions. Despite these assumptions, which clearly are not always achieved in vivo, the relationship is important because it describes the dominant influence of vessel radius on resistance and flow, and therefore provides a conceptual framework to understand how physiologic and pathologic changes in blood vessels and blood viscosity affect pressure and flow.

The relationship between flow and radius (Equation 5–7) for a single vessel is shown graphically in Figure 5.7. In this analysis, laminar flow conditions are assumed, and driving pressure, viscosity, and vessel length are held constant. As vessel radius decreases from a relative value of 1.0, a dramatic fall in flow occurs because flow is directly related to radius to the fourth power. For example,

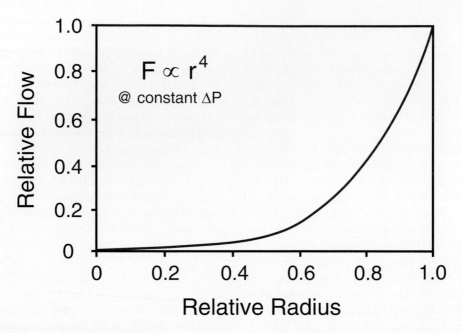

$$F \propto r^4$$

@ constant ΔP

Relative Flow (y-axis)

Relative Radius (x-axis)

■ **FIGURE 5.7** The effects of changes of vessel radius on flow through a single vessel. This quantitative relationship is derived from Poiseuille's equation (Equation 5–7). Decreasing vessel radius (*r*) dramatically increases resistance and decreases flow (*F*) at constant perfusion pressure (ΔP) because flow is proportional to radius to the fourth power.

when radius is one–half normal (0.5 relative radius), flow is decreased 16–fold. Therefore, the new flow is only about 6% of the original flow. This figure dramatically illustrates how very small changes in vessel radius can have profound effects on flow (and on perfusion pressure if this were the dependent variable and flow were held constant).

### PROBLEM 5-1

An isolated, cannulated arteriole is perfused with an oxygenated physiologic salt solution at a constant flow, and the pressure gradient across the two ends of the arteriole is initially 2 mm Hg. If the application of a drug constricts the vessel diameter by 50%, what will be the new pressure gradient across the arteriole?

## Laminar versus Turbulent Flow

Poiseuille's equation (Equation 5–7) and the simplified equations for the relationship between pressure, flow, and resistance (Equations 5–1 and 5–5) assume laminar, nonturbulent conditions for flow. Laminar flow is the normal condition for blood flow in most blood vessels. It is characterized by concentric layers of blood moving down the length of a blood vessel (see Fig. 5.8, top panel). The orderly movement of adjacent layers of blood moving through a vessel helps to minimize energy losses in the flowing blood caused by viscous interactions between the adjacent layers and the wall of the blood vessel. Turbulence occurs when laminar flow becomes disrupted (see Fig. 5.8, bottom panel). Turbulence is found distal to stenotic (narrowed) heart valves or arterial vessels, at large artery branch points, and in the ascending aorta at high cardiac ejection velocities (e.g., during exercise). Turbulence in large arteries results in characteristic sounds (e.g., carotid bruits) that can be heard with a stethoscope. Because higher velocities enhance turbulence, murmurs resulting from turbulence become louder whenever blood flow increases across narrowed valves or vessels.

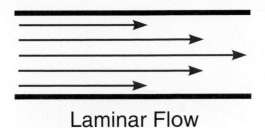

## Laminar Flow

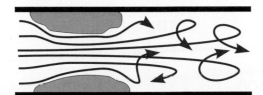

## Turbulent Flow

■ **FIGURE 5.8** Laminar versus turbulent flow. In laminar flow, blood flows smoothly in concentric layers parallel with the axis of the blood vessel, with the highest velocity in the center of the vessel and the lowest velocity next to the endothelial lining of the vessel. When laminar flow becomes disrupted (e.g., by a atherosclerotic plaque), it becomes turbulent; blood no longer flows in concentric, parallel layers, but rather moves in different paths, often forming vortices.

## Normal Flow

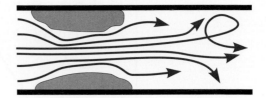

## $\Delta P = 10$ mmHg

## 2-Times Normal Flow

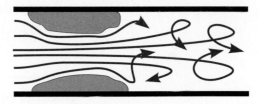

## $\Delta P = 35$ mmHg

■ **FIGURE 5.9** Effects of flow on turbulence. A twofold increase in flow across a stenotic lesion causes a disproportionate increase in the pressure drop ($\Delta P$) across the lesion due to increased turbulence. In this illustration, $\Delta P$ may increase threefold or fourfold instead of twofold as predicted by Poiseuille relationship when flow is doubled.

Turbulence causes increased energy loss and a greater pressure drop along a vessel length than predicted by the Poiseuille relationship (Equation 5–7). For example, as illustrated in Figure 5.9, if blood flow is increased twofold across a stenotic arterial segment that already has mild turbulence, the pressure drop across the stenosis may increase threefold or fourfold, and the turbulence enhanced. The Poiseuille relationship predicts a twofold increase in the pressure drop across the lesion because the pressure drop is proportionate to flow under laminar flow conditions (see Fig. 5.10). Turbulence, however, alters the relationship between flow and perfusion pressure so that the relationship is no longer linear and proportionate as described by the Poiseuille relationship. Instead, a greater perfusion pressure is required to propel the blood at a given flow rate when turbulence is present. Alternatively, a given flow causes a greater pressure drop

across a resistance than predicted simply by the radius and length of the resistance element because of increased energy losses associated with turbulence.

## Series and Parallel Arrangement of the Vasculature

It is crucial that Poiseuille's equation should be applied only to single vessels. If, for example, a single arteriole within the kidney were constricted by 50%, although the resistance of that single vessel would increase 16–fold, the vascular resistance for the *entire* renal circulation would not increase 16–fold. The change in overall renal resistance would be so small that it would be immeasurable. This is because the single arteriole is one of many resistance vessels within a complex network of vessels, and therefore, it constitutes

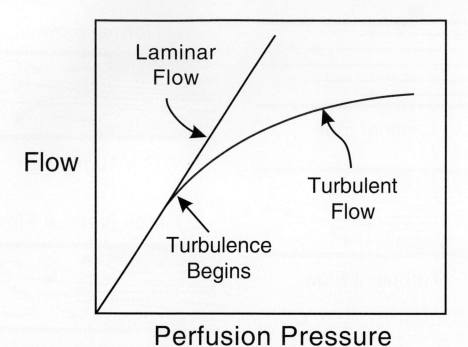

■ **FIGURE 5.10** Effects of turbulence on the pressure–flow relationship. Turbulence decreases flow at any given perfusion pressure, or requires a greater perfusion pressure to drive a given flow.

only a small fraction of the resistance for the whole organ. To help understand this complex arrangement of vessel architecture, it is necessary to examine the vascular components in terms of series and parallel elements.

The parallel arrangement of organs and their circulations (see Fig. 1.2) is important because *parallel vessels decrease total vascular resistance*. When there is a parallel arrangement of resistances, the reciprocal of the total resistance is equal to the sum of the reciprocals of the individual resistances. For example, the total resistance ($R_T$) of three parallel resistances ($R_1$, $R_2$, $R_3$) would be

$$\frac{1}{R_T} = \frac{1}{R_1} + \frac{1}{R_2} + \frac{1}{R_3}$$

*or,* solving for $R_T$,

**Eq. 5-8**
$$R_T = \frac{1}{\dfrac{1}{R_1} + \dfrac{1}{R_2} + \dfrac{1}{R_3}}$$

Two important principles emerge from Equation 5–8. First, *the total resistance of*

*a network of parallel resistances is less than the resistance of the single lowest resistance;* therefore, parallel vessels greatly reduce resistance. For example, assume that $R_1 = 5$, $R_2 = 10$, and $R_3 = 20$. When the equation is solved, $R_T = 2.86$, a value that is less than the lowest individual resistance. The resistance calculation for parallel networks explains why capillaries constitute a relatively small fraction of the total vascular resistance of an organ or microvascular network. Although capillaries have the highest resistance of individual vessels because of their small diameter, they also form a large network of parallel vessels. This reduces their resistance as a group of vessels. The second principle is that *when many parallel vessels exist, changing the resistance of a small number of these vessels will have little effect on total resistance.*

Within an organ, the vascular arrangement is a combination of series and parallel elements. In Figure 5.11, the artery, arterioles, capillaries, venules, and vein as groups of vessels are in series with each other. All of the blood that flows through the artery

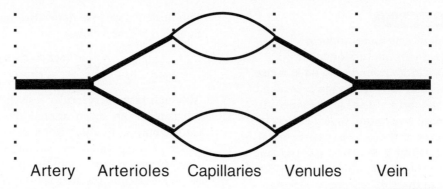

Artery    Arterioles    Capillaries    Venules    Vein

■ **FIGURE 5.11** Model of the circulation within an organ showing the series arrangement of multiple segments of parallel vessels.

likewise flows through each of the other vascular segments. Within each of the series elements, many parallel components may exist (e.g., several parallel capillaries may arise from a single arteriole). Each vascular element (e.g., the arterioles) will have a resistance value that is determined by vessel length, radius, and number of parallel vessels.

For an in–series resistance network, the total resistance ($R_T$) equals the sum of the individual segmental resistances. The total resistance for the model depicted in Figure 5.11 is

**Eq. 5-9**    $R_T = R_A + R_a + R_c + R_v + R_V$

(A = artery; a = arterioles; c = capillary;
v = venules; V = vein)

The resistance of each segment relative to the total resistance of all the segments determines how changing the resistance of one segment affects total resistance. To illustrate this principle, assign a relative resistance value to each of the five resistance segments in this model. The relative resistances are similar to what is observed in a typical vascular bed.

**Assume $R_A = 1$, $R_a = 70$, $R_c = 20$,**

**$R_v = 8$, $R_V = 1$;**

Therefore, $R_T = 1 + 70 + 20 + 8 + 1 = 100$
If $R_A$ were to increase fourfold (to a value of 4), $R_T$ would increase to 103, a 3% increase. In contrast, if $R_a$ were to increase fourfold (to a value of 280), the $R_T$ would increase to 310, a 210% increase. In this model, $R_A$ represents a large artery distributing blood flow to an organ

(e.g., renal artery), and $R_a$ represents the small arteries and arterioles within the organ, which are the primary site of vascular resistance. Therefore, this empirical example demonstrates that *changes in large artery resistance have relatively little effect on total resistance, compared to changes in small artery and arteriolar resistances that have a large affect on total resistance.* This is why small arteries and arterioles are the principal vessels regulating organ blood flow and systemic vascular resistance.

The above analysis explains why the radius of a large, distributing artery must be decreased by more than 60% or 70% to have a significant effect on organ blood flow. This is referred to as a **critical stenosis**. The concept of a critical stenosis can be confusing because Poiseuille equation indicates that resistance to flow is inversely related to radius to the fourth power. Therefore, a 50% reduction in radius should increase resistance 16–fold (a 1500% increase). Indeed, within that single vessel segment, resistance will increase 16–fold; however, total resistance will increase only by about 15% if the large artery resistance is normally 1% of the total resistance.

---

**PROBLEM 5-2**

A parent arteriole branches into two smaller arterioles. In relative terms, the resistance of the parent arteriole is 1, and the resistance of each daughter vessel is 4. What is the combined resistance of the parent vessel and its branches?

## REGULATION OF SYSTEMIC VASCULAR RESISTANCE

**Systemic vascular resistance**, which is sometimes called total peripheral resistance (TPR), is the resistance to blood flow offered by all of the systemic vasculature, excluding the pulmonary vasculature. Systemic vascular resistance primarily is determined by changes in vascular diameters, although changes in blood viscosity also affect systemic vascular resistance. Mechanisms that cause generalized vasoconstriction will increase systemic vascular resistance, and mechanisms that cause vasodilation will decrease systemic vascular resistance. The increase in systemic vascular resistance in response to sympathetic stimulation, for example, depends on the degree of sympathetic activation, the responsiveness of the vasculature, and the number of vascular beds involved.

### Calculation of Systemic Vascular Resistance

Systemic vascular resistance (SVR) can be calculated if cardiac output (CO), mean arterial pressure (MAP), and CVP are known.

This calculation is done by rearranging Equation 5–3 as follows:

Eq. 5-10
$$SVR = \frac{(MAP - CVP)}{CO}$$

Although systemic vascular resistance can be calculated from mean arterial pressure and cardiac output, its value is not determined by either of these variables (although its value changes depending upon the pressure—see below). Systemic vascular resistance is determined by vascular diameters, length, anatomical arrangement of vessels, and blood viscosity. Because vessels are compliant, increasing intravascular pressure expands the vessels, thereby causing a small reduction in resistance. Nonetheless, the decrease in systemic vascular resistance that occurs when pressure increases is not owing to the pressure directly but rather is caused by passive increases in vessel diameter. Mathematically, systemic vascular resistance is the dependent (calculated) variable in Equation 5–10; however, physiologically, systemic vascular resistance and cardiac output are the independent variables normally, and mean arterial pressure is the dependent variable; that is, mean arterial pressure changes in response to changes in cardiac output and systemic vascular resistance.

When calculating systemic vascular resistance, it is customary to use the units of mm Hg/mL·min$^{-1}$ (peripheral resistance units, PRU) or the units of dynes·s/cm$^5$ (in which pressure is expressed in dynes/cm$^2$ instead of mm Hg; 1 mm Hg = 1330 dynes/cm$^2$) and flow is expressed in cm$^3$/s. When calculating resistance in PRU, pressure has the units of mm Hg and cardiac output is expressed in mL/min.

## Vascular Tone

Under normal physiologic conditions, changes in the diameter of precapillary resistance vessels (small arteries and arterioles) represent the most important mechanism for regulating systemic vascular resistance. Resistance vessels are normally in a partially constricted state that is referred to as the **vascular tone** of the vessel. This tone is generated by smooth muscle contraction within the wall of the blood vessel. From this partially constricted state, a vessel can constrict further and thereby increase resistance, or it can dilate by smooth muscle relaxation and thereby decrease resistance. Venous vessels likewise possess a level of vascular tone.

Extrinsic and intrinsic mechanisms determine the degree of smooth muscle activation (Fig. 5.12). Extrinsic mechanisms, such as sympathetic nerves and circulating hormones, originate outside of the organ or tissue. Intrinsic mechanisms originate from within the blood vessel or the tissue surrounding the vessel. Examples of intrinsic mechanisms include endothelial–derived factors, smooth muscle myogenic tone, locally produced hormones, and tissue metabolites. Some of these extrinsic and intrinsic factors promote vasoconstriction (e.g., sympathetic nerves, angiotensin II, and endothelin–1), whereas others promote smooth muscle relaxation and vascular dilation (e.g., endothelial–derived nitric oxide and tissue metabolites such as adenosine and hydrogen ion). Therefore, at any given time, vasoconstrictor and vasodilator influences are competing to determine the vascular tone. The extrinsic and intrinsic mechanisms regulating vascular tone are described in more detail in Chapters 6 and 7.

In general, the vasoconstrictor mechanisms are important for maintaining systemic vascular resistance and arterial pressure, whereas vasodilator mechanisms regulate blood flow within organs. For example, if the body needs to maintain arterial blood pressure when a person stands up, vasoconstrictor mechanisms (primarily sympathetic adrenergic) are activated to constrict resistance vessels and increase systemic vascular resistance. If an organ requires more blood flow and oxygen delivery (e.g., exercising muscle), vasodilator mechanisms will predominate and override vasoconstrictor influences. Therefore, the competition between vasoconstrictor and vasodilator influences can be thought of as competition between maintenance of arterial blood pressure and organ perfusion.

## VENOUS BLOOD PRESSURE

Venous pressure is a general term that represents the average blood pressure within the venous compartment. A more specific term, **central venous pressure** (CVP), describes the blood pressure in the thoracic vena cava near the right atrium. This pressure is important because it determines the filling pressure of the right ventricle, and thereby determines ventricular stroke volume through the Frank–Starling mechanism as discussed in Chapter 4.

## Venous Blood Volume and Compliance

Several factors influence CVP: cardiac output, respiratory activity, contraction of skeletal muscles (particularly leg and abdominal muscles), sympathetic vasoconstrictor tone, and gravitational forces. All of these factors ultimately

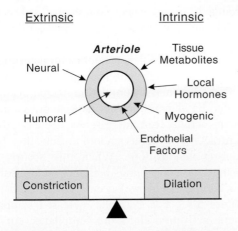

■ **FIGURE 5.12** Vascular tone. The state of vessel tone is determined by the balance between constrictor and dilator influences. Extrinsic influences originate outside of the tissue, whereas intrinsic influences originate from the vessel or surrounding tissue.

change CVP ($\Delta P_v$) by changing either venous blood volume ($\Delta V_v$) or venous compliance ($C_v$) as described by Equation 5–11.

**Eq. 5-11**      $$\Delta P_v \propto \frac{\Delta V_v}{C_v}$$

Equation 5–11 is a rearrangement of the equation used to define compliance (Equation 5–4), in which compliance (in this case venous compliance) equals a change in venous volume divided by a change in venous pressure. Therefore, an increase in venous volume increases venous pressure by an amount determined by the compliance of the veins. Furthermore, a decrease in venous compliance, as occurs during sympathetic activation of veins, increases venous pressure.

The relationship described by Equation 5–11 can be depicted graphically as shown in Figure 5.13, in which venous blood volume is plotted against venous blood pressure. The different curves represent different states

of venous tone, and the slope of a tangent line at any point on the curve represents the compliance. Looking at a single curve, it is evident that an increase in venous volume will increase venous pressure (point A to B). The amount by which the pressure increases for a given change in volume depends on the slope of the relationship between the volume and pressure (i.e., the compliance). As with arterial vessels (see Fig. 5.5), the relationship between venous volume and pressure is not linear (see Fig. 5.13). The slope of the compliance curve ($\Delta V/\Delta P$) is greater at low pressures and volumes than at higher pressures and volumes. The reason for this is that at very low pressures, a large vein collapses. As the pressure increases, the collapsed vein assumes a more cylindrical shape with a circular cross–section. Until a cylindrical shape is attained, the walls of the vein are not stretched appreciably. Therefore, small changes in pressure can result in a large change in volume by changes in vessel geometry rather than by stretching the vessel wall. At higher pressures, when the vein is cylindrical in shape, increased pressure can increase the volume only by stretching the vessel wall, which is resisted by the structure and composition of the wall (particularly by collagen, smooth muscle, and elastin components). Therefore, at higher volumes and pressures, the change in volume for a given change in pressure (i.e., compliance) is less.

The smooth muscle within veins is ordinarily under some degree of tonic contraction. Like arteries and arterioles, a major factor determining venous smooth muscle contraction is sympathetic adrenergic stimulation, which occurs under basal conditions. Changes in sympathetic activity can increase or decrease the contraction of venous smooth muscle, thereby altering venous tone. When this occurs, a change in the volume–pressure relationship (or compliance curve) occurs, as depicted in Figure 5.13. For example, increased sympathetic activation shifts the compliance curve down and to the right, decreasing its slope (compliance) at any given volume (from point A to C in Fig. 5.13). This rightward diagonal shift in the venous compliance curve results in a decrease in venous volume and an increase

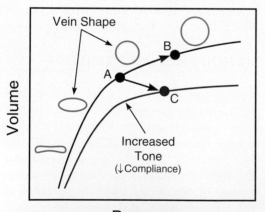

■ **FIGURE 5.13** Compliance curves for a vein. Venous compliance (the slope of line tangent to a point on the curve) is very high at low pressures because veins collapse. As pressure increases, the vein assumes a more circular cross–section and its walls become stretched; this reduces compliance (decreases slope). Point A is the control pressure and volume. Point B shows how pressure increases along the compliance curves as volume increases. Point C shows how pressure increases as volume decreases when venous tone is increased (decreased compliance) by sympathetic stimulation of the vein, for example.

in venous pressure. Drugs that reduce venous tone (e.g., nitrodilators) will decrease venous pressure while increasing venous volume by shifting the compliance curve to the left.

## Mechanical Factors Affecting Central Venous Pressure and Venous Return

Several of the factors affecting CVP can be classified as mechanical (or physical) factors. These include gravitational effects, respiratory activity, and skeletal muscle contraction. Gravity passively alters CVP and volume, and respiratory activity and muscle contraction actively promote or impede the return of blood into the central venous compartment, thereby altering CVP and volume.

### GRAVITY

Gravity exerts significant effects on CVP and venous return. When a person is reclining (supine position), systemic blood vessels are positioned near the hydrostatic level of the heart, which causes a generally uniform distribution of the blood volume between the head, thorax, abdomen, and legs. When supine, CVP averages about 2 mm Hg, and venous pressure in the legs is only a few mm Hg above CVP. When a person changes from supine to a standing posture, gravity acts on the vascular volume, causing blood to accumulate in the lower extremities (Fig. 5.14). Because venous compliance is much higher than arterial compliance, the shift in blood volume to the legs increases their venous pressure and volume. In fact, venous pressures in the feet when a person is standing still may reach 90 mm Hg because of the increased hydrostatic pressure owing to the influence of gravity. The shift in blood volume from the thorax to the dependent limbs causes thoracic venous volume and CVP to fall. This reduces right ventricular filling pressure (preload)

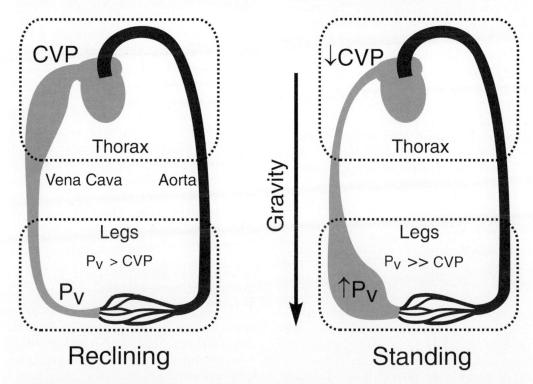

■ **FIGURE 5.14** Effects of gravity on central venous pressure (*CVP*) and venous pressure ($P_v$) in the lower leg. When horizontal (reclining), thoracic blood volume and CVP are relatively high, and $P_v$ is only a few mm Hg above CVP. When standing upright, the force of gravity causes a large increase in venous pressure in the legs, expanding the compliant veins and increasing their volume. This translocation of blood volume to the veins in the legs reduces thoracic volume and pressure.

and stroke volume by the Frank–Starling mechanism. Left ventricular stroke volume subsequently falls because of reduced pulmonary venous return to the left ventricle; the reduced stroke volume causes cardiac output and arterial blood pressure to decrease. If systemic arterial pressure falls by more than 20 mm Hg upon standing, this is termed **orthostatic** or **postural hypotension**. When this occurs, cerebral perfusion may fall and a person may become "light headed" and experience a transient loss of consciousness (syncope). Normally, baroreceptor reflexes (see Chapter 6) are activated to restore arterial pressure by causing peripheral vasoconstriction and cardiac stimulation (increased heart rate and inotropy). Furthermore, as seen in the next section, limb movement (e.g., walking) in the upright position facilitates venous return, thereby lowering venous pressures in the leg and partially restoring CVP.

The influence of gravity on venous volume can be visualized by looking at the veins on the back of the hand when below the level of the heart and then raising the hand above the head. When this is done, the veins collapse because they are above the level of the heart and the negative hydrostatic pressure caused by gravity acting on the column of blood reduces the pressure within the veins. If the hand is suddenly brought down below the heart, the veins will refill with blood as the positive hydrostatic pressure increases the venous pressure and distends the veins.

### SKELETAL MUSCLE PUMP

Veins, particularly in extremities, contain one–way valves that permit blood flow toward the heart and prevent retrograde flow. Deep veins in the lower limbs are surrounded by large groups of muscle that compress the veins when the muscles contract. This compression increases the pressure within the veins, which closes upstream valves and opens downstream valves, thereby functioning as a pumping mechanism (Fig. 5.15). This pumping mechanism plays a significant role in facilitating venous return during exercise. Rhythmical contraction of leg muscles also

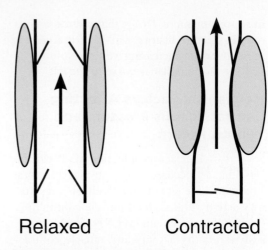

## Relaxed        Contracted

■ **FIGURE 5.15** Rhythmic contraction of skeletal muscle compresses veins, particularly in the lower limbs, and propels blood toward the heart through a system of one–way valves.

helps to counteract gravitational forces when a person stands up by facilitating venous return and lowering venous and capillary pressures in the feet and lower limbs. For example, human experiments have shown that when a person is standing still, the venous pressure measured at the ankle is about 90 mm Hg. When the person begins to walk, the venous pressure falls to 30 to 40 mm Hg after several steps. When the venous valves become incompetent, as occurs when veins become enlarged (varicose veins), muscle pumping becomes ineffective. Besides the loss of muscle pumping in aiding venous return, blood volume and pressure increase in the veins of the dependent limbs, which increases capillary pressure and may cause edema (see Chapter 8).

### RESPIRATORY ACTIVITY (ABDOMINOTHORACIC OR RESPIRATORY PUMP)

Venous return to the right atrium from the abdominal vena cava is determined by the pressure difference between the abdominal vena cava and the right atrial pressure, as well as by the resistance to flow, which is primarily determined by the diameter of the thoracic vena cava. Therefore, increasing right atrial pressure impedes venous return, whereas lowering right atrial pressure facilitates venous return. These changes in venous return significantly influence stroke volume through the Frank–Starling mechanism.

Pressures and volumes in the right atrium and thoracic vena cava depend on the surrounding **intrapleural pressure**. This pressure is measured in the space between the thoracic wall and the lungs and is generally negative (subatmospheric). During inspiration, the chest wall expands and the diaphragm descends (red arrows on chest wall and diaphragm in Fig. 5.16). This causes the intrapleural pressure ($P_{pl}$) to become more negative, causing expansion of the lungs, atrial and ventricular chambers, and vena cava (smaller red arrows). This expansion decreases the pressures within the vessels and cardiac chambers. As right atrial pressure falls during inspiration, the pressure gradient for venous return to the heart is increased. During expiration the opposite occurs, although the net effect of respiration is that the increased rate and depth of ventilation facilitates venous return and ventricular stroke volume.

Although it may appear paradoxical, the fall in right atrial pressure during inspiration is associated with an *increase* in right atrial and ventricular preloads and right ventricular stroke volume. This occurs because the fall in intrapleural pressure causes the **transmural pressure** to increase across the chamber walls. The transmural pressure is the difference between the pressure within the chamber and the pressure outside the chamber ($P_{pl}$). When transmural pressure increases, the chamber volume increases, which increases sarcomere length and myocyte preload. For example, if intrapleural pressure is normally –4 mm Hg at end–expiration and right atrial pressure is 0 mm Hg, the transmural pressure (the pressure that distends the atrial chamber) is 4 mm Hg. During inspiration, if intrapleural pressure decreases to –8 mm Hg and atrial pressure decreases to –2 mm Hg, the transmural pressure across the atrial chamber increases from 4 to 6 mm Hg, thereby expanding the chamber. At the same time, because blood pressure within the atrium is diminished, this leads to an increase in venous return to the right atrium from the abdominal vena cava. Similar increases in right ventricular transmural pressure and preload occur during inspiration. The increase in sarcomere length during inspiration augments right ventricular stroke volume by the Frank–Starling mechanism. In addition, changes in intrapleural pressure during inspiration influence the left atrium and ventricle; however, the expanding lungs and pulmonary vasculature act as a capacitance reservoir (pulmonary blood volume increases) so that

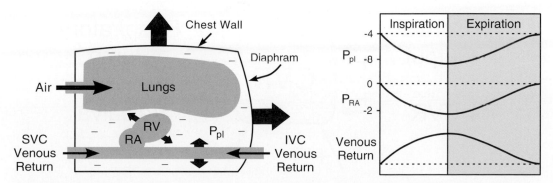

■ **FIGURE 5.16** Effects of respiration on venous return. **Left panel**. During inspiration, intrapleural pressure ($P_{pl}$) decreases as the chest wall expands and the diaphragm descends (large red arrows). This increases the transmural pressure across the superior and inferior vena cava (*SVC* and *IVC*), right atrium (*RA*), and right ventricle (*RV*), which causes them to expand. This facilitates venous return and leads to an increase in atrial and ventricular preloads. **Right panel**. During inspiration, $P_{pl}$ and right atrial pressure ($P_{RA}$) become more negative, which increases venous return. During expiration, $P_{pl}$ and $P_{RA}$ become less negative and venous return falls. Numeric values for $P_{pl}$ and $P_{RA}$ are expressed as mm Hg.

the left ventricular filling is not enhanced during inspiration. During expiration, however, blood is forced from the pulmonary vasculature into the left atrium and ventricle, thereby increasing left ventricular filling and stroke volume. *The net effect of respiration is that increasing the rate and depth of respiration increases venous return and cardiac output.*

If a person exhales forcefully against a closed glottis (**Valsalva maneuver**), intrapleural pressure becomes very positive, which causes the transmural pressure to become negative, thereby collapsing the thoracic vena cava. This dramatically increases resistance to venous return and reduces venous return. Because of the accompanying decrease in transmural pressure across the ventricular chamber walls, ventricular volume decreases (particularly the more compliant right ventricle) despite the large increase in the pressure within the chamber. Decreased chamber volume (i.e., decreased preload) leads to a fall in ventricular stroke volume by the Frank–Starling mechanism. Similar changes can occur when a person strains while having a bowel movement or when a person lifts a heavy weight while holding his or her breath.

## Summary of Factors Affecting Central Venous Pressure

As previously discussed, CVP plays a very important role in cardiac filling and ventricular stroke volume (via the Frank–Starling mechanism). Conditions that elevate CVP increase cardiac output, whereas conditions that decrease CVP decrease cardiac output. Furthermore, as described in Chapter 8, elevation in CVP can lead to peripheral edema. Therefore, it is important to understand how the following different conditions influence CVP (see Fig. 5.17):

1. An increase in total blood volume (hypervolemia), as occurs in renal failure or with activation of the renin–angiotensin–aldosterone system (see Chapter 6), increases thoracic blood volume and therefore CVP.
2. A decrease in cardiac output, caused by decreased heart rate (e.g., bradycardia) or stroke volume (e.g., ventricular failure), causes blood to back up into the venous circulation (increased venous volume) as less blood is pumped into the arterial circulation. The resultant increase in thoracic blood volume elevates CVP.

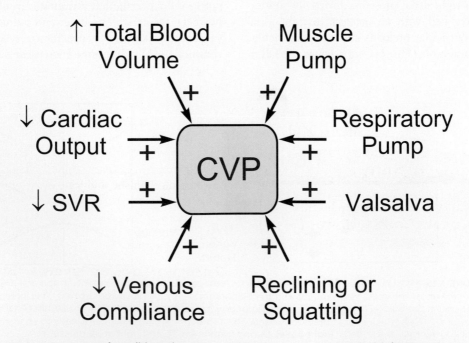

■ **FIGURE 5.17** Summary of conditions that alter central venous pressure (*CVP*). (+), increase CVP; (−), decrease CVP.

3. A decrease in systemic vascular resistance by selective arterial dilation increases blood flow from the arterial into the venous compartments, thereby increasing venous volume and CVP, while at the same time reducing arterial volume and pressure (discussed later in this chapter).

4. Constriction of peripheral veins (reduced venous compliance) elicited by sympathetic activation or circulating vasoconstrictor substances (e.g., catecholamines, angiotensin II) causes blood volume to be translocated from peripheral veins into the thoracic compartment, thereby increasing CVP.

5. Postural changes such as moving from a standing to a reclining or squatting position diminishes venous pooling in the legs caused by gravity, which increases thoracic volume and CVP.

6. A forceful expiration against a high resistance (Valsalva maneuver) causes external compression of the thoracic vena cava (decrease in functional compliance), which increases CVP.

7. Increased respiratory activity (abdominothoracic pump) facilitates venous return into the thorax, thereby helping to maintain CVP when cardiac output is elevated during exercise.

8. Rhythmic muscular contraction (muscle pump), particularly of the limbs during exercise, compresses the veins and facilitates venous return into the thoracic compartment, which increases CVP.

## VENOUS RETURN AND CARDIAC OUTPUT

### The Balance between Venous Return and Cardiac Output

Venous return is the flow of blood back to the heart. It was previously described how the venous return to the right atrium from the abdominal vena cava is determined by the pressure gradient between the abdominal vena cava and the right atrium, divided by the resistance of the vena cava. However, that analysis looks at only a short segment of the venous system and does not show what factors determine venous return from the capillaries. Venous return from capillaries is determined by the difference between the mean capillary and right atrial pressures divided by the resistance of all the postcapillary vessels. If we consider venous return as being all the systemic flow returning to the heart, venous return is determined by the difference between the mean aortic and right atrial pressures divided by the systemic vascular resistance. Therefore, the pressures and resistances that are used as the hemodynamic variables for determining venous return depend on whether one is defining venous return from specific locations in the systemic vasculature, or if one is viewing venous return as the flow of blood throughout all the systemic circulation as it travels back to the heart.

An important concept to note is the following: *under steady-state conditions, venous return equals cardiac output when averaged over time.* The reason for this is that the cardiovascular system is essentially a closed system. Strictly speaking, the cardiovascular system is not a closed system because fluid is lost through the kidneys and by evaporation through the skin, and fluid enters the circulation through the gastrointestinal tract. Nevertheless, a balance is maintained between fluid entering and leaving the circulation during steady–state conditions. Therefore, it is appropriate to view the system as closed, and therefore cardiac output and venous return as being equal. There may occur transient imbalances, such as when a person suddenly starts to run and venous return is augmented by the muscle and abdominothoracic pumps; however, this augmentation leads to an increase in cardiac output by the Frank–Starling mechanism and cardiac stimulation so that shortly after starting to run the cardiac output once again equals the venous return, although at a higher level of cardiac output.

### Systemic Vascular Function Curves

Blood flow through the entire systemic circulation, whether viewed as the flow leaving the heart (cardiac output) or returning to the heart (venous return), depends on both cardiac and systemic vascular function.

As described in more detail below, cardiac output under normal physiologic conditions depends on systemic vascular function. Cardiac output is limited to a large extent by the prevailing state of systemic vascular function. Therefore, it is important to understand how changes in systemic vascular function affect cardiac output and venous return (or total systemic blood flow because cardiac output and venous return are equal under steady–state conditions).

The best way to show how systemic vascular function affects systemic blood flow is by use of systemic vascular and cardiac function curves. Credit for the conceptual understanding of the relationship between cardiac output and systemic vascular function goes to Arthur Guyton and colleagues, who conducted extensive experiments in the 1950s and 1960s. To develop the concept of systemic vascular function curves, we must understand the relationship between cardiac output, mean aortic pressure, and right atrial pressure. Figure 5.18 shows that at a cardiac output of 5 L/min, the right atrial pressure is near zero and mean aortic pressure is about 95 mm Hg. If cardiac output is reduced experimentally, right atrial pressure increases and mean aortic pressure decreases. The fall in aortic pressure reflects the relationship between mean aortic pres-

sure, cardiac output, and systemic vascular resistance (see Equation 5–3). As cardiac output is reduced to zero, right atrial pressure continues to rise and mean aortic pressure continues to fall, until both pressures are equivalent, which occurs when systemic blood flow ceases. When all flow ceases, pressures throughout all the systemic circulation are equal. The pressure at zero systemic flow, which is called the **mean circulatory filling pressure**, is about 7 mm Hg. This value is found experimentally when baroreceptor reflexes are blocked; otherwise the value for mean circulatory filling pressure is higher because of vascular smooth muscle contraction and decreased vascular compliance owing to sympathetic activation.

The reason right atrial pressure increases in response to a decrease in cardiac output is that less blood per unit time is translocated by the heart from the venous to the arterial vascular compartment. This leads to a reduction in arterial blood volume and pressure, and to an increase in venous blood volume and pressure, which increases right atrial pressure. When the heart is completely stopped and there is no flow in the systemic circulation, the intravascular pressure found throughout the entire vasculature is a function of total blood volume and vascular compliance.

Finally, it is important to note in Figure 5.18 that if one attempts to increase cardiac output above 5 L/min by increasing heart rate, for example, cardiac output will not increase much above 5 L/min. The reason is that right atrial pressure falls below zero, which collapses the vena cava at the level of the diaphragm where it enters the thorax from the abdomen. This increases the resistance of the vena cava, thereby limiting venous return into the thorax, which limits the cardiac output.

The magnitude of the relative changes in aortic and right atrial pressures from a normal cardiac output to zero cardiac output is determined by the ratio of venous to arterial compliances. If venous compliance ($C_V$) equals the change in venous volume ($\Delta V_V$) divided by the change in venous pressure ($\Delta P_V$), and arterial compliance ($C_A$) equals the change in arterial volume ($\Delta V_A$) divided by the change in

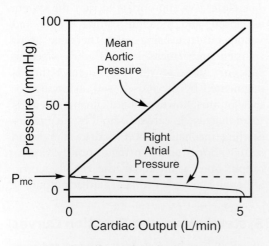

■ **FIGURE 5.18** Effects of cardiac output on mean aortic and right atrial pressures. Decreasing cardiac output results in a rise in right atrial pressure and a fall in aortic pressure. When cardiac output is zero, both pressures equilibrate at the mean circulatory filling pressure ($P_{mc}$).

arterial pressure ($\Delta P_A$), the ratio of venous to arterial compliance ($C_V/C_A$) can be expressed by the following equation:

**Eq. 5-12**
$$\frac{C_V}{C_A} = \frac{\Delta V_V / \Delta P_V}{\Delta V_A / \Delta P_A}$$

When the heart is stopped, the decrease in arterial blood volume ($\Delta V_A$) equals the increase in venous blood volume ($\Delta V_V$). Because $\Delta V_A$ equals $\Delta V_V$, Equation 5–12 can be simplified to the following relationship:

**Eq. 5-13**
$$\frac{C_V}{C_A} \propto \frac{\Delta P_A}{\Delta P_V}$$

Equation 5–13 shows that the ratio of venous to arterial compliance is proportional to the ratio of the changes in arterial to venous pressures when the heart is stopped. This ratio is usually in the range of 10 to 20. If, for example, the ratio of venous to arterial compliance is 15, there is a 1 mm Hg increase in right atrial pressure for every 15 mm Hg decrease in mean aortic pressure.

If the right atrial pressure curve from Figure 5.18 is plotted as cardiac output versus right atrial pressure (i.e., reversing the axis), the relationship shown in Figure 5.19 (black curve in both panels) is observed. This curve is called the **systemic vascular function curve.** This relationship can be thought of as either the effect of cardiac output on right atrial pressure (cardiac output being the independent variable) or the effect of right atrial pressure on venous return (right atrial pressure being the independent variable). When viewed from the latter perspective, systemic vascular function curves are sometimes called venous return curves.

The value of the x–intercept in Figure 5.19 is the mean circulatory filling pressure, which is the pressure throughout the vascular system when there is no blood flow. This value depends on the vascular compliance and blood volume (Fig. 5.19, panel A). Increased blood volume or decreased venous compliance causes a parallel shift of the vascular function curve to the right, which increases mean circulatory filling pressure. Decreased blood volume or increased venous compliance causes a parallel shift to the left and a decrease in the mean circulatory filling pressure. Therefore, at a given cardiac output, an increase in total blood volume (or decreased venous compliance) is associated with an increase in right atrial pressure.

Decreased systemic vascular resistance increases the slope without appreciably changing mean circulatory filling pressure (Fig. 5.19,

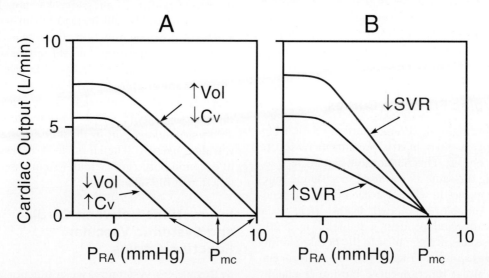

■ **FIGURE 5.19** Systemic function curves. **Panel A** shows the effects of changes in cardiac output on right atrial pressure ($P_{RA}$) and mean circulatory filling pressures ($P_{mc}$). Changes in blood volume (*Vol*) and venous compliance ($C_v$) cause parallel shifts in the curves and changing $P_{mc}$. **Panel B** shows how changes in systemic vascular resistance (*SVR*) alter the slope of the systemic function curves without changing $P_{mc}$.

panel B). Increased systemic vascular resistance decreases the slope while keeping the same mean circulatory filling pressure. Therefore, at a given cardiac output, a decrease in systemic vascular resistance increases right atrial pressure, whereas an increase in systemic vascular resistance decreases right atrial pressure. These changes can be difficult to conceptualize, but the following explanation might help to clarify. When small resistance vessels dilate at a constant cardiac output, the rate of blood flow from the arteries into the capillaries and veins increases. This causes a transient imbalance between the rate of flow into the arterial system (cardiac output) and the rate of flow out of the arterial system (more blood leaves than enters the arterial system per unit time). The increase in venous volume causes venous pressure and right atrial pressure to increase. This reduces the pressure gradient for venous return from the capillaries and will lead to a new steady state where there is once again a balance between the flow that enters and leaves the arteries. This steady state will be characterized by increased venous volume and pressure, and decreased arterial volume and pressure. If the heart were suddenly stopped, the mean circulatory filling pressure would not be appreciably different from before the systemic vascular resistance was reduced because the decrease in arterial diameter (which increases arterial compliance) has little affect on overall vascular compliance, which is overwhelmingly determined by venous compliance.

## Cardiac Function Curves

According to the Frank–Starling relationship, an increase in right atrial pressure increases cardiac output. This relationship can be depicted using the same axis as used in systemic function curves in which cardiac output (dependent variable) is plotted against right atrial pressure (independent variable) (Fig. 5.20). These curves are similar to the Frank–Starling curves shown in Figure 4.21. There is no single cardiac function curve, but rather a family of curves that depends on the inotropic state and afterload (see Chapter 4). Changes in heart rate also shift the cardiac function curve

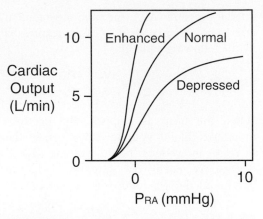

■ **FIGURE 5.20** Cardiac function curves. Cardiac output is plotted as a function of right atrial pressure ($P_{RA}$); normal (*solid black*), enhanced (*red*), and depressed curves (*red*) are shown. Cardiac performance, measured as cardiac output, is enhanced (curves shift up and to the left) by an increase in heart rate and inotropy and a decrease in afterload.

because cardiac output, not stroke volume as in Figure 4.21, is the dependent variable. With a "normal" function curve, the cardiac output is about 5 L/min at a right atrial pressure of about 0 mm Hg. If cardiac performance is enhanced by increasing heart rate or inotropy or by decreasing afterload, it shifts the cardiac function curve up and to the left. At the same right atrial pressure of 0 mm Hg, the cardiac output will increase. Conversely, a depressed cardiac function curve, as occurs with decreased heart rate or inotropy or with increased afterload, will decrease the cardiac output at any given right atrial pressure. However, *the magnitude by which cardiac output changes when cardiac performance is altered is determined in large part by the state of systemic vascular function.* Therefore, it is necessary to examine both cardiac and system vascular function at the same time.

## Interactions between Cardiac and Systemic Vascular Function Curves

By themselves, systemic vascular function and cardiac function curves provide an incomplete picture of overall cardiovascular dynamics; however, when coupled together, these curves

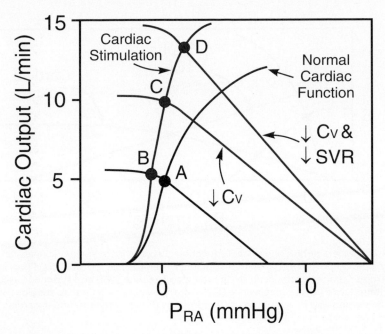

■ **FIGURE 5.21** Combined cardiac and systemic function curves: effects of exercise. Cardiac output is plotted against right atrial pressure ($P_{RA}$) to show the effects of altering both cardiac and systemic function. Point *A* represents the normal operating point described by the intercept between the normal cardiac and systemic function curves. Cardiac stimulation alone changes the intercept from point *A* to *B*. Cardiac stimulation coupled with decreased venous compliance ($C_V$) shifts the operating intercept to point *C*. If systemic vascular resistance (*SVR*) also decreases, which is similar to what occurs during exercise, the new intercept becomes point *D*.

can offer new understanding as to the way cardiac and vascular function are coupled.

When the cardiac function and vascular function curves are superimposed (Fig. 5.21), a unique intercept between a given cardiac and a given vascular function curve (point *A*) exists. This intercept is the equilibrium point that defines the relationship between cardiac and vascular function. The heart functions at this equilibrium until one or both curves shift. For example, if the sympathetic nerves to the heart are stimulated to increase heart rate and inotropy, only a small increase in cardiac output will occur, accompanied by a small decrease in right atrial pressure (point *B*). As previously discussed, cardiac stimulation alone will not increase cardiac output appreciably if right atrial pressure becomes negative. If at the same time, however, the venous compliance is decreased by sympathetic activation of venous vasculature, cardiac output will be greatly augmented (point *C*). If the decrease in venous compliance is accompanied by a

decrease in systemic vascular resistance, cardiac output would be further enhanced (point *D*). These changes in venous compliance and systemic vascular resistance, which occur during exercise, permit the cardiac output to increase. This example shows that for cardiac output to increase significantly during cardiac stimulation, there must be some alteration in vascular function so that venous return is augmented and right atrial pressure (ventricular filling) is maintained. Therefore, *in the normal heart, cardiac output is limited by factors that determine vascular function.*

In pathologic conditions such as heart failure, cardiac function limits venous return. In heart failure, ventricular inotropy is diminished, total blood volume is increased, and systemic vascular resistance is increased (see Chapter 9). The former two lead to an increase in atrial and ventricular pressures and volumes (increased preload), which enables the Frank–Starling mechanism to partially compensate for the loss of inotropy. These

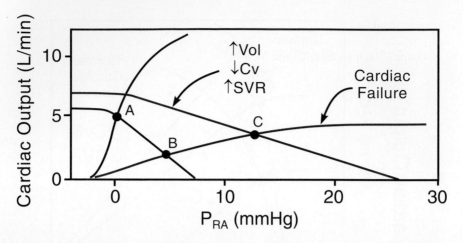

■ **FIGURE 5.22** Combined cardiac and systemic function curves: effects of chronic heart failure. The normal operating intercept (point *A*) is shifted to point *B* when cardiac function alone is depressed by diminished inotropy. Compensatory increases in total blood volume (*Vol*) and systemic vascular resistance (*SVR*), along with reduced venous compliance (*C$_v$*), shift the systemic function to the right and decrease the slope. The new combined intercept (point *C*) represents partial compensation in cardiac output at the expense of a large increase in right atrial pressure (*P$_{RA}$*).

changes during heart failure can be depicted using cardiac and systemic function curves as shown in Figure 5.22. In this figure, point *A* represents the operating point in a normal heart, and point *B* indicates where a heart might operate when it is in failure in the absence of systemic compensation—cardiac output would be greatly reduced and right atrial pressure would be elevated. Compensatory increases in blood volume and systemic vascular resistance, along with reduced venous compliance, shift the systemic function curve to the right and decrease the slope. The new, combined intercept (point *C*) represents a partial compensation in the cardiac output at the expense of a large increase in right atrial pressure. The increased atrial pressure helps to support ventricular preload and stroke volume through the Frank–Starling mechanism.

In summary, total blood flow through the systemic circulation depends on both cardiac and systemic vascular function. Cardiac stimulation in a normal heart has only a modest effect on cardiac output; however, if systemic function is additionally altered by decreasing venous compliance and systemic vascular resistance, the cardiac output is able to increase. Without changes in systemic function, cardiac output is limited by the return of blood to the heart and ventricular filling.

## SUMMARY OF IMPORTANT CONCEPTS

- Regulation of arterial pressure and organ blood flow is primarily the function of the small resistance vessels—arteries and arterioles. Capillaries are the principal site for exchange and most of the blood volume is found in the venous capacitance vessels.

- Mean arterial pressure is determined by the product of cardiac output and systemic vascular resistance, plus CVP.

- Aortic pulse pressure is primarily determined by ventricular stroke volume and aortic compliance.

- Vascular resistance is inversely related to the vessel radius to the fourth power, and it is directly related to vessel length and blood viscosity. Vessel radius is the most important factor for regulating resistance.

- The parallel arrangement of vascular beds in the body reduces overall resistance. Furthermore, because of this arrangement, a resistance change in one vascular bed has minimal influence on pressure and flow in other vascular beds.

- Changes in large artery resistance have little effect on total resistance of a vascular bed because these vessels normally comprise only a small percentage of the total resistance of a vascular bed. In contrast, changes in small artery and arteriolar resistances greatly affect total resistance.

- Arteries and veins are normally in a partially constricted state (i.e., they possess vascular tone), which is determined by the net effect of vasoconstrictor and vasodilator influences acting upon the vessel.

- CVP is altered by changes in thoracic blood volume and venous compliance. Gravity, respiratory activity, and the pumping action of rhythmically contracting skeletal muscle have important influences on CVP.

- Cardiac output is strongly influenced by changes in systemic vascular function as described by cardiac and systemic vascular function curves. In the normal heart, cardiac output is limited by factors that determine vascular function.

## REVIEW QUESTIONS

For each question, choose the one best answer:

1. Concerning different types of blood vessels in a vascular network,

    a. Arterioles have the highest individual resistance and, therefore, as a group of vessels, have the greatest pressure drop.
    b. Capillaries as a group of vessels constitute the greatest resistance to flow within an organ.
    c. Capillaries and venules are the primary site for fluid exchange.
    d. Large arteries are the most important vessels for blood flow and pressure regulation.

2. A 17–year–old male patient who runs on the high school cross–country team is found to have an arterial pressure of 115/60 and a resting heart rate of 55 beats/minute. The most likely explanation for his elevated arterial pulse pressure is

    a. Decreased mean arterial pressure.
    b. Elevated ventricular stroke volume.
    c. Increased aortic compliance.
    d. Reduced systemic vascular resistance.

3. A patient who has coronary artery disease is treated with a drug that reduces heart rate by 10% without changing stroke volume. Furthermore, the drug is found to decrease mean arterial pressure by 10%. Assume that central venous pressure remains at 0 mm Hg. This drug

   a. Decreases systemic vascular resistance by 10%.
   b. Does not alter cardiac output.
   c. Does not alter systemic vascular resistance.
   d. Reduces pressure by dilating the systemic vasculature.

4. Which of the following will increase blood flow to the greatest extent in a single isolated blood vessel that is perfused with blood in vitro at a constant perfusion pressure?

   a. Decreasing the blood temperature by 10°C
   b. Increasing perfusion pressure by 100%
   c. Increasing blood viscosity by 100%
   d. Increasing the vessel diameter by 50%

5. If cardiac output is 4500 mL/min, mean arterial pressure is 94 mm Hg, and right atrial pressure is 4 mm Hg, systemic vascular resistance (in peripheral resistance units, PRU; mm Hg/mL · min$^{-1}$) is

   a. 0.02
   b. 20
   c. 50
   d. $4.05 \times 10^5$

6. A patient recently diagnosed with hypertension is found to have a stenotic (narrowed) right renal artery. The internal diameter is reduced by 50%. Assuming that renal artery resistance is 1% of total renal resistance and that vascular resistance in the kidney is unchanged, blood flow to the right kidney will decrease by what amount?

   a. 50%
   b. <20%
   c. 8–fold
   d. 16–fold

7. A patient in the Emergency Department with traumatic injuries from an automobile accident suddenly shows a fall in arterial pressure accompanied by an increase in central venous pressure. These hemodynamic changes could be explained by

   a. A sudden fall in cardiac output.
   b. Increased systemic venous compliance.
   c. Loss of blood volume.
   d. Sympathetic activation.

8. Venous return to the right atrium is

   a. Decreased as cardiac output increases.
   b. Decreased by sympathetic activation of veins.
   c. Increased during a forced expiration against a closed glottis.
   d. Increased during inspiration.

9. Mean circulatory filling pressure is increased by

   a. Decreased venous compliance.
   b. Increased systemic vascular resistance.
   c. Decreased blood volume.
   d. Increased cardiac output.

10. In a normal heart, cardiac output and right atrial pressure are both increased by

    a. Decreased blood volume.
    b. Decreased systemic vascular resistance.
    c. Increased heart rate.
    d. Increased venous compliance.

1. The correct answer is "c" because these vessels are the most permeable to fluid. Choice "a" is incorrect because capillaries, not arterioles, have the highest individual resistance because of their small diameter. Choice "b" is incorrect because the large number of parallel capillaries reduces their overall resistance as a group of vessels. Choice "d" is incorrect because the small arteries and arterioles are the primary sites for pressure and flow regulation.

2. A pathological decrease in aortic compliance, which would increase pulse pressure, is very unlikely in this young, healthy adult. Therefore, the correct answer most likely involves increased stroke volume, and for this reason choice "b" is correct. Stroke volume would be elevated because of the low resting heart rate and perhaps more forceful ventricular contractions because of exercise conditioning. Choice "a" is incorrect because aortic compliance increases at lower aortic pressures and volumes; therefore, this would decrease pulse pressure. Choice "c" is incorrect because increased aortic compliance decreases pulse pressure. Choice "d" is incorrect because reduced systemic vascular resistance has no effect on pulse pressure except if mean arterial pressure is reduced, which would then decrease pulse pressure.

3. The correct answer is "c." Choices "a" and "b" are incorrect because reducing heart rate by 10% without changing stroke volume decreases cardiac output by 10%. Because mean arterial pressure is also reduced by 10% and mean arterial pressure equals cardiac output times systemic vascular resistance (when central venous pressure is zero), systemic vascular resistance is not changed. Choice "d" is incorrect because systemic vascular resistance changes if the systemic vasculature dilates.

4. The correct answer is "d" because a 50% increase in diameter will increase flow by about fivefold because flow is proportional to radius (or diameter) to the fourth power in a single vessel segment (assuming that the pressure gradient does not change appreciably). Choice "a" is incorrect because decreasing temperature increases blood viscosity, which decreases flow. Choice "b" is incorrect because increasing perfusion pressure by 100% increases flow by twofold. Choice "c" is incorrect because flow is inversely related to blood viscosity.

5. The correct answer is "a" because systemic vascular resistance equals arterial minus venous pressure (mm Hg) divided by cardiac output (mL/min).

6. The correct answer is "b" because the renal artery is the distributing artery to the kidney, and therefore is in series with the kidney. Although decreasing the renal artery diameter by 50% increases its resistance 16–fold, the total renal resistance increases only about 15% because the renal artery resistance is about 1% of total renal resistance. Therefore, flow will decrease (assuming no change in perfusion pressure) about 13% because $F = \Delta P/R$ and R is increased by a factor of 1.15. With increased perfusion pressure because of the hypertension, the reduction in flow would be <13%.

7. The correct answer is "a" because a fall in cardiac output causes arterial pressure to fall and blood to back up into the venous circulation, which increases central venous pressure. Choices "b" and "c" are incorrect because increased systemic venous compliance and decreased blood volume reduce central venous pressure, cardiac output, and arterial pressure. Choice "d" is incorrect because generalized sympathetic activation would raise arterial pressure by increasing systemic vascular resistance and cardiac output.

8. Choice "d" is correct because inspiration reduces intrapleural pressure, which expands the right atrium, lowers its pressure, and thereby enhances venous return. Choice "a" is incorrect because an increase in cardiac output must increase venous return because the circulatory system is closed. Choice "b" is incorrect because decreased sympathetic activation of the veins causes them to relax, which increases their compliance. This reduces preload on the heart, which leads to a reduction in cardiac output and venous return. Choice "c" is incorrect because a Valsalva maneuver increases intrapleural pressure, compresses the vena cava, and reduces venous return.

9. Choice "a" is correct because decreased venous compliance shifts the systemic function curve to the right, which increases the mean circulatory filling pressure (value of the x–intercept). Choice "b" is incorrect because changes in systemic vascular resistance alter the slope of the systemic function curve, but not its x–intercept. Choice "c" is incorrect because a decrease in blood volume causes a parallel shift in the systemic function curve to the left, which decreases mean circulatory filling pressure. Choice "d" is incorrect because mean circulatory filling pressure, by definition, is the intravascular pressure when cardiac output is zero, and therefore it is independent of cardiac output.

10. The correct answer is "b" because a decrease in systemic vascular resistance increases the slope of the systemic function curve, which increases cardiac output and right atrial pressure. Choices "a" and "d" are incorrect because decreased blood volume and increased venous compliance decrease right atrial pressure and cardiac output by causing a leftward parallel shift in the systemic function curve. Choice "c" is incorrect because increased heart rate increases cardiac output a small amount and decreases right atrial pressure.

## ANSWERS TO PROBLEMS AND CASES

### PROBLEM 5-1
Under constant flow conditions, $\Delta P \propto \Delta R$ (from Equation 5–1). Furthermore, $R \propto 1/r^4$ (from Equation 5–6). Therefore, $\Delta P \propto 1/r^4$. Using this relationship, we find that decreasing diameter (or radius, which is proportional to diameter) by 50% (to 1/2 its original radius) increases $\Delta P$ by a factor of 16 (reciprocal of 1/2 to the fourth power). Therefore, the new pressure gradient along the length of vessel will be 32 mm Hg (2 mm Hg × 16).

### PROBLEM 5-2
In this problem, the two smaller daughter arterioles ($R_D$) are parallel with each other and in series with the parent arteriole ($R_P$). Therefore, the total resistance ($R_T$) can be found by the following equation:

$$R_T = R_P + \cfrac{1}{\cfrac{1}{R_D} + \cfrac{1}{R_D}}$$

Substituting the relative resistances given in this problem, we obtain

$$R_T = 1 + \cfrac{1}{\cfrac{1}{4} + \cfrac{1}{4}} = 3$$

### PROBLEM 5-3
From Equation 5–10, we know that

$$SVR = \frac{(MAP - CVP)}{CO}$$

Because CVP is zero, this equation simplifies to

$$SVR = \frac{MAP}{CO}$$

In this problem, CO is increased by 30% and MAP is decreased by 10%:

$$SVR = \frac{0.9\,MAP}{1.3\,CO} = 0.69$$

Therefore, SVR is decreased by 31% (0.69 SVR is the equivalent of a 31% decrease), and the drug is a vasodilator. Note: In solving this problem, MAP and CO cannot be multiplied by their percentage change.

### CASE 5-1

The total coronary resistance ($R_T$) equals the sum of the series resistance elements. Therefore, the left main coronary artery resistance ($R_L$) would be in series with the remainder of the resistance elements ($R_X$), so that $R_T = R_L + R_X$. Normally, $R_L = 0.01(R_T)$ and $R_X = 0.99(R_T)$ because $R_L$ is 1% of $R_T$, and therefore $R_T = 0.01(R_T) + 0.99(R_T) = 1(R_T)$. Decreasing the vessel diameter by 50% increases $R_L$ by a factor of 16 because $R \propto 1/r^4$. Therefore, the resistance of the stenotic vessel will be 16 times its normal resistance, so that $R_L = 16(0.01)R_T$, or $R_L = 0.16(R_T)$. We can now say that $R_T = 0.16(R_T) + 0.99(R_T)$. Therefore, $R_T = 1.15(R_T)$, which means that total coronary resistance increases by only 15% (1.15 - 1.00) × 100] when the resistance of the left main coronary artery increases 1500% (16–fold increase).

**SUGGESTED RESOURCES**

Belloni FL. Teaching the principles of hemodynamics. Am J Physiol 1999;277 (Adv Physiol Educ 1999;22:S187–S202.

Berne RM, Levy MN. Cardiovascular Physiology. 8th Ed. Philadelphia: Mosby, 2001.

Burton, AC. Physiology and Biophysics of the Circulation. 2nd Ed. Chicago: Year Book Medical Publishers, 1972.

Folkow B, Neil E. Circulation. New York: Oxford University Press, 1971.

Guyton AC, Jones CE, Coleman TG. Circulatory Physiology: Cardiac Output and its Regulation. 2nd Ed. Philadelphia: W.B. Saunders, 1973.

Rhoades RA, Bell DR. Medical Physiology: Principles for Clinical Medicine. 3rd Ed. Philadelphia: Lippincott Williams & Wilkins, 2009.

# NEUROHUMORAL CONTROL OF THE HEART AND CIRCULATION

# 6

## LEARNING OBJECTIVES

Understanding the concepts presented in this chapter will enable the student to:

1. Describe the origin and distribution of sympathetic and parasympathetic nerves to the heart and circulation.

2. Know the location and function of alpha- and beta-adrenoceptors and muscarinic receptors in the heart and blood vessels.

3. Describe the location and afferent connections from the carotid sinus, aortic arch, and cardiopulmonary baroreceptors to the medulla oblongata.

4. Describe how carotid sinus baroreceptors respond to changes in arterial pressure (mean pressure and pulse pressure), and explain how changes in baroreceptor activity affect sympathetic and parasympathetic outflow to the heart and circulation.

5. Describe (a) the location of peripheral and central chemoreceptors; (b) the way they respond to hypoxemia, hypercapnia, and acidosis; and (c) the effects of their stimulation on autonomic control of the heart and circulation.

6. List the factors that stimulate the release of catecholamines, renin, aldosterone, atrial natriuretic peptide, and vasopressin.

7. Describe how sympathetic nerves, circulating catecholamines, angiotensin II, aldosterone, atrial natriuretic peptide, and vasopressin interact to regulate arterial blood pressure.

## INTRODUCTION

Autonomic nerves and circulating hormones serve as important mechanisms for regulating cardiac and vascular function. These mechanisms are controlled by sensors that monitor blood pressure (baroreceptors), blood volume (volume receptors), blood chemistry (chemoreceptors), and plasma osmolarity (osmoreceptors). Peripheral sensors such as baroreceptors are found in arteries, veins, and cardiac chambers. They have afferent nerve fibers that travel to the central nervous system, where their activity is monitored and compared against a "set point" for arterial pressure. Deviations from the set point result in selective activation or deactivation of neurohumoral efferent control systems. Sensors located within the central nervous system (e.g., central

chemoreceptors and osmoreceptors) also interact with regions within the brain that control neurohumoral status. The sensors work together with the neurohumoral mechanisms to ensure that arterial blood pressure is adequate for perfusing organs. Although the following sections describe several individual neurohumoral mechanisms, note that these mechanisms interact together to ensure cardiovascular homeostasis.

## AUTONOMIC NEURAL CONTROL

### Autonomic Innervation of the Heart and Vasculature

Autonomic regulation of cardiovascular function is controlled by the central nervous system. The medulla oblongata located within the brainstem, the hypothalamus, and the cortical regions work together to regulate autonomic function (Fig. 6.1). Regions within the **medulla** contain the cell bodies for the parasympathetic (vagal) and sympathetic efferent nerves that control the heart and vasculature. The **hypothalamus** (in particular, the paraventricular nucleus and dorsal medial nucleus) plays an integrative role by modulating medullary neuronal activity, for example, during exercise or when the body needs to adjust blood flow to the skin to regulate body temperature. Higher centers, including the **cortex** and limbic and midbrain structures, connect with the hypothalamus and medulla. The higher centers can alter cardiovascular function during times of emotional stress (e.g., caused by fear and anxiety).

The central nervous system receives sensory (afferent) input from peripheral sensors and from sensors within the brain. Afferent fibers from peripheral baroreceptors and chemoreceptors, as well as respiratory stretch receptors, enter the medulla at the **nucleus tractus solitarius (NTS)** (see Fig. 6.2). Inhibitory interneurons from cells within the NTS project to other medullary regions containing cell bodies of sympathetic nerves. In addition, excitatory interneurons from

the NTS project to medullary regions containing cell bodies of parasympathetic (vagal) nerves. Therefore, increased activity of the NTS enhances vagal efferent nerve activity and inhibits sympathetic nerve efferent activity. The NTS also sends fibers to the hypothalamus and receives input from the hypothalamus. Sensors within the hypothalamus that monitor blood temperature (thermoreceptors) send fibers to medullary regions to modulate sympathetic outflow to the cutaneous circulation.

## PARASYMPATHETIC INNERVATION

The parasympathetic vagal fibers innervating the heart originate from cell bodies located within the medulla of the brainstem (see Figs. 6.1 and 6.2). These cell bodies are found in collections of neurons called the **dorsal vagal nucleus (DVN)** and **nucleus ambiguus (NA)**. Increased activity of these nuclei reduces sinoatrial (SA) nodal firing (negative chronotropy) and slows AV nodal conduction (negative dromotropy). It is important to note that under normal resting conditions, these neurons are tonically active, thereby producing what is termed "**vagal tone**" on the heart, resulting in resting heart rates significantly below the intrinsic firing rate of the SA nodal pacemaker. Afferent nerves, particularly from peripheral baroreceptors that enter the medulla through the NTS, modulate the activity of these vagal neurons. Excitatory interneurons from the NTS, which normally are excited by tonic baroreceptor activity, stimulate vagal activity.

Efferent vagal fibers (also referred to as **preganglionic fibers**) exit the medulla as the tenth cranial nerve (see Fig. 6.3) and travel to the heart within the left and right vagus nerves. Branches from these nerves innervate specific regions within the heart such as the SA and atrioventricular (AV) nodes, conduction pathways, atrial myocytes, and the coronary vasculature. The preganglionic efferent fibers synapse within or near the target tissue and form small ganglia, from which short **postganglionic fibers** innervate specific tissue sites. The right vagus is usually the primary vagal branch that innervates the SA

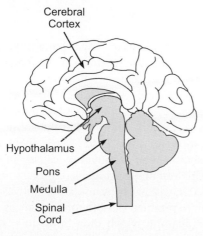

Cerebral
Cortex

Hypothalamus

Pons

Medulla

Spinal
Cord

■ **FIGURE 6.1** Regions of the central nervous system involved in cardiovascular regulation. The primary site of cardiovascular regulation resides in the medulla; the hypothalamus serves as an integrative region for coordinating cardiovascular responses. Higher centers such as the cortex influence cardiovascular function.

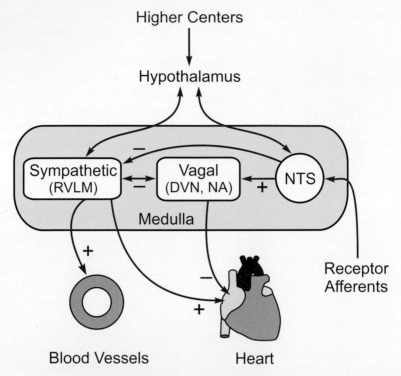

**■ FIGURE 6.2** Schematic representation of autonomic sympathetic and vagal interconnections within the central nervous system. Receptor afferent nerve fibers (e.g., from baroreceptors) enter the medulla at the nucleus tractus solitarius (*NTS*), which projects inhibitory interneurons to the sympathetic neurons in the rostral ventrolateral medulla (*RVLM*) and excitatory fibers to the vagal neurons in the dorsal vagal nucleus (*DVN*) and nucleus ambiguus (*NA*). The medulla receives input from the hypothalamus and higher brain centers. Sympathetic activation (+) of blood vessels and the heart causes smooth muscle contraction (vasoconstriction), increased heart rate (positive chronotropy), increased conduction velocity within the heart (positive dromotropy), and increased contractility (positive inotropy). Vagal activation of the heart decreases (−) chronotropy, dromotropy, and inotropy.

node, whereas the left vagus primarily innervates the AV node. This can be demonstrated experimentally by electrically stimulating the right vagus nerve, which causes bradycardia (or SA nodal arrest) with little change in AV nodal conduction, as evidenced by a relatively small increase in the P-R interval of the electrocardiogram. Left vagal stimulation, in contrast, usually results in a pronounced AV nodal block (see Chapter 2), with relatively little decrease in heart rate. However, these responses to vagal stimulation can be markedly different between individuals because of crossover of the left and right vagal efferent nerves.

Some efferent parasympathetic fibers innervate blood vessels in specific organs in which they directly or indirectly cause vasodilation.

Direct vasodilation by parasympathetic activation in some tissues (e.g., genitalia erectile tissue) is achieved through the release of acetylcholine (Ach), which binds to muscarinic receptors on the vascular endothelium to cause vasodilation through the subsequent formation of nitric oxide (see Chapter 3). Parasympathetic stimulation causes indirect vasodilation in some organs (e.g., gastrointestinal circulation) by stimulating nonvascular tissue to produce vasodilator substances such as bradykinin, which then binds to vascular receptors to cause vasodilation. Note that *any existing parasympathetic nerves primarily serve to regulate blood flow within specific organs and do not play a significant role in the regulation of systemic vascular resistance and arterial blood pressure.*

## SYMPATHETIC INNERVATION

The sympathetic adrenergic control of the heart and vasculature originates from neurons found within the medulla, the most important of which are located in the **rostral ventrolateral medulla** (RVLM). Increased activity of these neurons produces cardiac stimulation and systemic vasoconstriction. Sympathetic neurons within the RVLM have spontaneous action potential activity, which results in tonic stimulation of the heart and vasculature. Therefore, acute sympathetic denervation of the heart and systemic blood vessels usually results in cardiac slowing and systemic vasodilation. At low resting heart rates, the effects of sympathetic denervation on the heart rate are relatively small because the heart is under a high level of vagal tone and relatively weak sympathetic tone. In contrast, sympathetic vascular tone is relatively high in most organ circulations; therefore, sudden removal of sympathetic tone produces significant vasodilation and hypotension.

Axons from sympathetic neurons leave the medulla, travel down the spinal cord and synapse within the intermediolateral cell column of the spinal cord, and then exit at specific thoracolumbar levels (T1-L2) (Fig. 6.3). These preganglionic fibers (short compared to preganglionic parasympathetic fibers) then

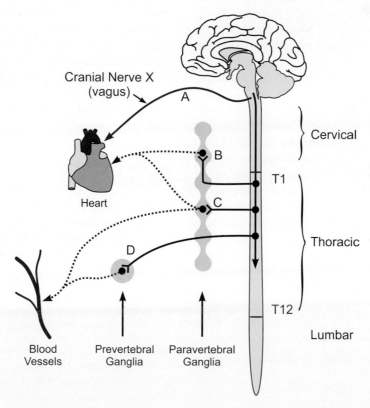

■ **FIGURE 6.3** Organization of sympathetic and vagal innervation of the heart and circulation. The tenth cranial nerve (vagus; parasympathetic) arises from the brainstem. Preganglionic fibers (*solid red line, A*) travel to the heart, where they synapse with cell bodies of short postganglionic fibers that innervate the heart. Preganglionic sympathetic nerves (*solid black lines*) arise from thoracic (T1–T12) and lumbar segments of the spinal cord. Some of these fibers (*B*) enter the paravertebral ganglia (sympathetic chain) on both sides of the spinal cord, and travel within the ganglia to synapse above (B) or below their entry level, or at their level of entry (*C*). Postganglionic fibers (*dotted black lines*) from the cervical ganglia primarily innervate the heart, whereas those from thoracic ganglia travel to blood vessels and to the heart. Preganglionic fibers from lower thoracic and upper lumbar segments generally synapse in prevertebral ganglia (*D*), from which postganglionic fibers travel to blood vessels.

synapse within sympathetic **paravertebral ganglia** (cervical, stellate, and thoracolumbar sympathetic chain) located on either side of the spinal cord, or they synapse within **prevertebral ganglia** located within the abdomen (celiac, superior mesenteric, and inferior mesenteric ganglia) (Fig. 6.3). Some fibers also travel to the adrenal glands where they synapse. Postganglionic sympathetic fibers (long compared to postganglionic parasympathetic fibers) travel to target organs where they innervate arteries and veins; capillaries are not innervated. Small branches of these efferent nerves are found in the adventitia (outer) layer of blood vessels. **Varicosities**, which are small enlargements along the sympathetic nerve fibers, provide the site of neurotransmitter release.

Postganglionic sympathetic fibers traveling to the heart innervate the SA and AV nodes, the conduction system, and cardiac myocytes, as well as the coronary vasculature. Sympathetic activation increases chronotropy, dromotropy, and inotropy (see Table 6-1). In blood vessels, sympathetic activation directly constricts both resistance and capacitance vessels, thereby increasing systemic vascular resistance (and arterial blood pressure) and decreasing venous capacitance (which increases venous pressure) (see Table 6-1). As described in Chapter 7, sympathetic activation of the heart leads to paradoxical coronary vasodilation because increased cardiac activity produces metabolic coronary vasodilation that overrides the direct sympathetic vasoconstrictor effects on the coronary vessels.

Sympathetic activation of resistance vessels significantly contributes to the vascular tone in many organs. This can be demonstrated by abruptly removing sympathetic influences (e.g., by blocking α-adrenoceptors with drugs). When this is done, blood flow increases, the amount of which depends upon the degree of sympathetic tone and the strength of local autoregulatory mechanisms that will attempt to maintain constant blood flow (see Chapter 7). For example, if α-adrenoceptors in the forearm circulation are blocked pharmacologically, blood flow increases two- or threefold. Over time, however, intrinsic autoregulatory mechanisms restore normal tone and blood flow.

As described further in Chapter 7, the vascular response to sympathetic activation differs among organs. Nevertheless, generalized sympathetic activation of the circulation increases arterial pressure and reduces organ perfusion throughout the body except in the heart and brain.

## RECIPROCAL SYMPATHETIC AND VAGAL ACTIVITY

Normally, there is reciprocal activation of the medullary sympathetic RVLM and the nuclei controlling vagal outflow. An example of this reciprocity occurs when a person stands up

| **TABLE 6-1 EFFECTS OF SYMPATHETIC AND PARASYMPATHETIC STIMULATION ON CARDIAC AND VASCULAR FUNCTION** | | |
|---|---|---|
| | SYMPATHETIC | PARASYMPATHETIC |
| Heart | | |
| Chronotropy (rate) | + + + | – – – |
| Inotropy (contractility) | + + + | –1 |
| Dromotropy (conduction velocity) | + + | – – – |
| Vessels (Vasoconstriction) | | |
| Resistance (arteries, arterioles) | + + + | –2 |
| Capacitance (veins, venules) | + + + | 0 |

Relative magnitude of responses (+, increase; –, decrease; 0, no response) indicated by number of + or – signs.
[1]More pronounced in atria than ventricles.
[2]Vasodilator effects only in specific organs such as genitalia.

and arterial blood pressure falls. Baroreceptor reflexes (discussed later in this chapter) cause the RVLM to increase sympathetic outflow to stimulate the heart (increase heart rate and inotropy) and to constrict the systemic vasculature. These cardiac and vascular responses help to restore normal arterial pressure. As sympathetic neurons in the RVLM are being activated, parasympathetic vagal activity originating from the DVN and nucleus ambiguus is decreased. This is important because without removal of vagal influences on the heart, the ability of enhanced sympathetic activity to increase heart rate is impaired. The reason for this is that *vagal influences are dominant over sympathetic influences in the heart.*

Regions within the hypothalamus can integrate and coordinate cardiovascular responses by providing input to medullary centers. Studies have shown that electrical stimulation of dorsomedial hypothalamus produces autonomic responses that mimic those that occur during exercise, or the **flight-or-fight response**. These coordinated responses include sympathetic-mediated tachycardia, increased inotropy, catecholamine release, and systemic vasoconstriction. These are brought about by hypothalamic activation of sympathetic neurons within the RVLM and inhibition of vagal nuclei.

Input from higher cortical regions can alter autonomic function as well. For example, sudden fear or emotion can sometimes cause vagal activation leading to bradycardia, withdrawal of sympathetic vascular tone, and fainting (**vasovagal syncope**). Fear and anxiety can lead to sympathetic activation that causes tachycardia, increased inotropy, and hypertension. Chronic sympathetic activation induced by long-term emotional stress can result in sustained hypertension, cardiac hypertrophy, and arrhythmias.

### CARDIAC AND VASCULAR AUTONOMIC RECEPTORS

Activation of sympathetic efferent nerves to the heart releases the neurotransmitter norepinephrine that binds primarily to $\beta_1$-adrenoceptors located in nodal tissue, conducting tissues, and myocardium (see Fig. 6.4). There are also postjunctional $\beta_2$-adrenoceptors in the heart;

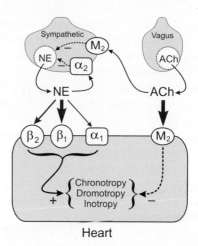

Heart

■ **FIGURE 6.4** Adrenergic and muscarinic receptors in the heart. Norepinephrine (NE) released from sympathetic nerve terminals binds to postjunctional adrenoceptors (order of functional importance: $\beta_1 > \beta_2 > \alpha_1$) to increase (+) inotropy, chronotropy, and dromotropy. Prejunctional $\alpha_2$–adrenoceptors serve as a feedback mechanism to inhibit NE release. Parasympathetic (vagal) nerves release acetylcholine (ACh), which binds to postjunctional $M_2$ receptors to decrease (−) inotropy, chronotropy, and dromotropy. ACh also binds to prejunctional muscarinic receptors ($M_2$) on sympathetic nerve terminals to inhibit NE release.

however, they are normally less important than $\beta_1$-adrenoceptors. Beta-adrenoceptors are coupled to the Gs-protein/cAMP signal transduction pathway as described in Chapter 3. There are also postjunctional $\alpha_1$-adrenoceptors located in cardiac tissue that bind to norepinephrine, which activates the Gq-protein/IP$_3$ pathway to stimulate the heart (see Chapter 3). Released norepinephrine can also bind to prejunctional $\alpha_2$-adrenoceptors located on the sympathetic nerve terminal. These receptors inhibit norepinephrine release through a negative feedback mechanism.

Activation of postganglionic vagal fibers causes the release of the neurotransmitter ACh. In the heart, this neurotransmitter binds to muscarinic receptors ($M_2$) principally in nodal tissue, and in atrial myocardium (Fig. 6.4). These receptors are coupled to the Gi-protein/cAMP signal transduction pathway (see Chapter 3), which decreases chronotropy, dromotropy, and inotropy (more so in the atria than in the ventricles). Released ACh can also bind to prejunctional $M_2$ muscarinic receptors found on nearby sympathetic adrenergic nerve terminals, which inhibits their release of norepinephrine.

In blood vessels, norepinephrine released by sympathetic adrenergic nerves preferentially binds to postjunctional $\alpha_1$-adrenoceptors to cause smooth muscle contraction and vasoconstriction (see Fig. 6.5). Similar responses occur when norepinephrine binds to postjunctional $\alpha_2$-adrenoreceptors located primarily on small arteries and arterioles, although postjunctional $\alpha_1$-adrenoceptors are generally the more important $\alpha$-adrenoceptor subtype in most vessels. These $\alpha$-adrenoceptors are coupled to the Gq-protein/$IP_3$ signal transduction pathway as described in Chapter 3. In addition, norepinephrine can bind to prejunctional $\alpha_2$-adrenoreceptors, which acts as a negative feedback mechanism for modulating norepinephrine release.

Blood vessels possess postjunctional $\beta_2$-adrenoceptors in addition to $\alpha$-adrenoceptors. Activation of postjunctional $\beta_2$-adrenoceptors by norepinephrine (and, more importantly, by circulating epinephrine) causes vasodilation in the absence of opposing $\alpha$-adrenoceptor-mediated

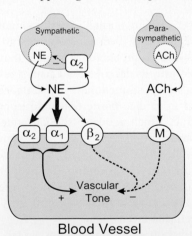

**■ FIGURE 6.5** Adrenergic and muscarinic receptors in blood vessels. Norepinephrine (NE) released from sympathetic nerve terminals binds to postjunctional adrenoceptors (order of functional importance: $\alpha_1 > \alpha_2 > \beta_2$). NE binding to postjunctional $\alpha$-adrenoceptors causes increased (+) vascular tone (vasoconstriction), whereas binding to $\beta_2$-adrenoceptors causes decreased (−) vascular tone (vasodilation). In a few specific organs (e.g., genitalia), ACh released by parasympathetic nerves binds to muscarinic (M) receptors to produce endothelial-dependent vasodilation.

vasoconstriction. To observe this $\beta_2$-adrenoceptor-induced vasodilation experimentally, one can stimulate vascular sympathetic nerves in the presence of complete $\alpha$-adrenoceptor blockade. Normally, this small $\beta_2$-receptor-mediated vasodilator effect of norepinephrine is completely overwhelmed by simultaneous $\alpha$-adrenoceptor activation, leading to vasoconstriction.

Although there is relatively little or no parasympathetic innervation of most blood vessels in the body, muscarinic receptors on coronary arteries can respond to vagal activation in the heart by dilating, and similar receptors in genital erectile tissue respond by dilating to ACh release by parasympathetic nerves (Fig. 6.5).

## Baroreceptor Feedback Regulation of Arterial Pressure

As described above, sympathetic nerves play an important role in regulating systemic vascular resistance and cardiac function, and therefore arterial blood pressure. But, how does the body control the systemic vascular resistance and cardiac output to establish and maintain an arterial blood pressure to ensure adequate organ perfusion?

Arterial blood pressure is regulated through negative feedback systems incorporating pressure sensors (i.e., baroreceptors) found in strategic locations within the cardiovascular system. **Arterial baroreceptors** are found in the carotid sinus (at the bifurcation of external and internal carotids) and in the aortic arch (Fig. 6.6). The sinus nerve (nerve of Hering), a branch of the glossopharyngeal nerve (cranial nerve IX), innervates the carotid sinus. Afferent fibers from the carotid sinus travel in the glossopharyngeal nerve up to the brainstem, where they synapse at the NTS. As already described, the NTS modulates the activity of sympathetic neurons within the RVLM and medullary vagal nuclei. The aortic arch baroreceptors are innervated by the aortic nerve, which then combines with the vagus nerve (cranial nerve X) before traveling to the NTS.

The arterial baroreceptors respond to the stretching of the vessel walls produced by increases in arterial blood pressure (Fig. 6.7). Increased arterial pressure increases the firing

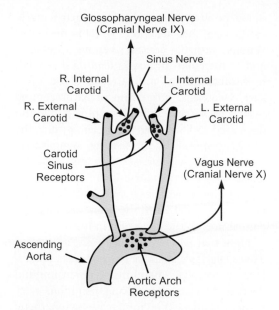

**■ FIGURE 6.6** Location and innervation of arterial baroreceptors. Carotid sinus receptors are located on the internal carotid artery just above the junction with the external carotid artery. These receptors are innervated by the sinus nerve of Hering, which joins the glossopharyngeal nerve (cranial nerve IX) before traveling up to the medulla. Afferent nerves from the aortic arch receptors join the vagus nerve (cranial nerve X), which then travel to the medulla. *R*, right; *L*, left.

rate of individual receptors and nerves. Each individual receptor has its own threshold and sensitivity to changes in pressure; therefore, additional receptors are recruited as pressure increases. Overall, the receptors of the carotid

sinus respond to pressures ranging from about 60 to 180 mm Hg. Therefore, if arterial blood pressure decreases from normal, it lowers the firing rate of the carotid sinus baroreceptors; conversely, increased arterial pressure increases receptor firing.

Baroreceptors are sensitive to the rate of pressure change and to a steady or mean pressure. At a given mean arterial pressure, decreasing the arterial pulse pressure decreases firing rate. This is important during conditions such as hemorrhagic shock in which pulse pressure (as well as mean pressure) decreases because of the decline in stroke volume caused by decreased ventricular preload and increased heart rate. Therefore, reduced pulse pressure reinforces the baroreceptor reflex when mean arterial pressure falls. The curve representing the frequency of baroreceptor firing in Figure 6.7 is the integrated receptor firing at a given pulse pressure. At reduced pulse pressures, the curve shifts to the right, thereby decreasing the firing at any given mean arterial pressure.

Maximal carotid sinus sensitivity (the point of greatest slope of the response curve in Fig. 6.7) occurs near the "set point" of normal mean arterial pressures (~95 mm Hg in adults). Therefore, small deviations from this set point elicit large changes in baroreceptor firing frequency. This set point, and the entire receptor response curve, is not fixed. Chronic shifts in this curve can occur during hypertension, heart failure, and other disease

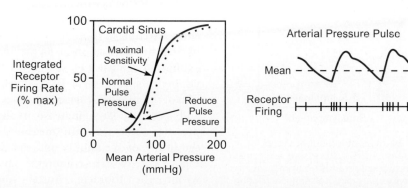

**■ FIGURE 6.7** Effects of arterial pressure on integrated carotid sinus firing rate. **Left panel:** The threshold for receptor activation occurs at mean arterial pressures of about 60 mm Hg; maximal firing occurs at about 180 mm Hg. Maximal receptor sensitivity occurs at normal mean arterial pressures. The receptor firing–response curve shifts to the right with decreased pulse pressures; therefore, a decrease in pulse pressure at a given mean pressure decreases firing. **Right panel:** Single receptor firing in response to pulsatile pressure. Receptors fire more rapidly when arterial pressure is rapidly increasing during cardiac systole.

states. In hypertension, for example, the curve shifts to the right, thereby reducing the firing rate at any given mean arterial pressure. This resetting of the baroreceptor response can occur at the level of the receptors themselves as well as in the brainstem. In arteriosclerosis, the carotid arteries at the region of the carotid sinus become less compliant, and therefore they stretch less in response to changes in arterial blood pressure—this decreases their sensitivity. During exercise, medullary and hypothalamic control centers can modulate autonomic efferent responses at a given level of baroreceptor firing, thereby resetting arterial pressure to a higher level.

Receptors located within the aortic arch function similarly to carotid sinus receptors; however, they have a higher threshold pressure for firing and are less sensitive than the carotid sinus receptors. Therefore, the aortic arch baroreceptors serve as secondary baroreceptors, with the carotid sinus receptors normally being the dominant arterial baroreceptor.

To understand how the baroreceptor reflex operates, consider the events that occur in response to a decrease in arterial pressure (mean, pulse, or both) when a person suddenly stands up (Fig. 6.8). When upright posture is suddenly assumed from the supine position, gravity causes venous blood pooling below the heart, particularly in the legs (see Chapter 5). This decreases venous return, central venous pressure, and ventricular preload, leading to a fall in cardiac output and arterial blood pressure. Decreased stretching of baroreceptors results in decreased baroreceptor firing and decreased NTS activity. Nuclei within the RVLM respond by increasing sympathetic outflow, which increases systemic vascular resistance (vasoconstriction) and cardiac output (increased heart rate and inotropy). Decreased vagal outflow from the medulla contributes to the elevation in heart rate.

Note that *baroreceptor firing normally exerts a tonic inhibitory influence on sympathetic outflow from the medulla.* Therefore, hypotension and decreased baroreceptor firing disinhibits sympathetic outflow (i.e., it increases sympathetic activity) from the medulla. The combined effects on systemic vascular resistance and cardiac output increases arterial blood pressure back toward its set point.

The carotid sinus reflex can be activated by rubbing the neck over the carotid sinus (i.e., **carotid sinus massage**). This mechanical stimulation of the receptors increases their firing, which leads to decreased sympathetic and increased parasympathetic outflow from the medulla. This action is sometimes used to abort certain types of arrhythmias by activating the vagus efferents to the heart.

Another example of the operation of the baroreceptor reflex is when a **Valsalva maneuver** is performed, which is sometimes used to assess autonomic reflex control of cardiovascular function in humans. It is performed by having the subject conduct a maximal, forced expiration against a closed glottis and maintaining this for at least 10 seconds. Contraction of the thoracic cage compresses the lungs and causes a large increase in intrapleural pressure (the pressure measured between the lining of the thorax and the lungs—see Fig. 5.16), which compresses the vessels within the thoracic. Aortic compression results in a transient rise in aortic pressure (Phase I of Fig. 6.9). This results in a reflex bradycardia caused by baroreceptor activation. Because the thoracic vena cava also

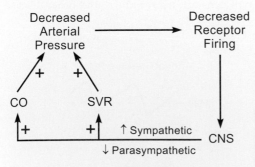

■ **FIGURE 6.8** Baroreceptor feedback loop. A sudden decrease in arterial pressure, as occurs when a person suddenly stands up from a supine position, decreases baroreceptor firing, activating sympathetic nerves and inhibiting parasympathetic (vagal) nerves. This change in autonomic balance increases (+) cardiac output (*CO*) and systemic vascular resistance (*SVR*), which helps to restore normal arterial pressure. *CNS*, central nervous system.

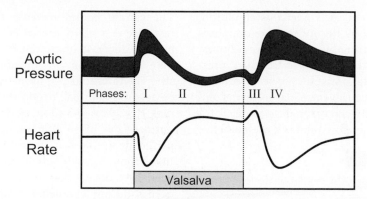

■ **FIGURE 6.9** Baroreceptors responses during a Valsalva maneuver. During Phase I, which occurs at the beginning of the forced expiration, aortic pressure increases (due to aortic compression) and heart rate decreases reflexively. Aortic pressure falls during Phase II because compression of thoracic veins reduces venous return and cardiac output; reflex tachycardia occurs. Phase III begins when normal respiration resumes, and is characterized by a small transient fall in aortic pressure (because of removal of aortic compression) and a small increase in heart rate. Aortic pressure increases (and heart rate reflexively decreases) during Phase IV because resumption of normal cardiac output occurs while systemic vascular resistance is elevated from sympathetic activation that occurred during Phase II.

becomes compressed, venous return to the heart is compromised, causing cardiac output and aortic pressure to fall (Phase II). As aortic pressure falls, the baroreceptor reflex increases heart rate. A decrease in stroke volume accounts for the fall in pulse pressure. After several seconds, arterial pressure (both mean and pulse pressure) is reduced, and heart rate is elevated. When the subject begins breathing again, the sudden loss of compression on the aorta causes a small, transient dip in arterial pressure and a further reflex increase in heart rate (Phase III). When compression of the vena cava is removed, venous return suddenly increases, causing a rapid rise in cardiac output several seconds later, which leads to a transient increase in arterial pressure (Phase IV). Arterial pressure overshoots during Phase IV because the systemic vascular resistance is increased by sympathetic activation that occurred during Phase II owing to the baroreceptor reflex. Heart rate reflexively decreases during Phase IV in response to the transient elevation in arterial pressure.

In addition to arterial baroreceptors, stretch receptors are located at the venoatrial junctions of the heart (**cardiopulmonary receptors**) and respond to atrial filling and contraction. These tonically active receptors are innervated by myelinated vagal afferents. Increased stretch

caused by an increase in venous return can under some conditions increase heart rate via medullary activation of sympathetic efferent activity to the SA node. This response, which is called the **Bainbridge reflex**, increases heart rate when the initial heart rate is low.

An increase in blood volume and venous pressure stimulates other types of cardiopulmonary receptors to decrease antidiuretic hormone (ADH, vasopressin) release by the posterior pituitary. Decreased circulating ADH causes diuresis, which leads to a fall in blood volume and venous pressure. If blood volume is lost as a result of dehydration or hemorrhage, these receptors will increase ADH release so that the kidneys excrete less water.

Unmyelinated vagal afferents are found throughout the atria and ventricles. Receptors associated with these vagal afferents respond to stretch such that the firing rate of these receptors is enhanced with increased atrial and ventricular pressures. The effects of these receptors on sympathetic and vagal outflow are similar to those on the arterial baroreceptors. Depending upon the circumstances, however, these receptors can either oppose or reinforce arterial baroreceptor function. In heart failure, atrial and ventricular filling pressures are increased, whereas arterial pressure is decreased. Under this condition, increased firing by the AV receptors opposes the decreased firing by arterial baroreceptors. During hemorrhage, cardiac chamber pressures and arterial pressures are both reduced. This causes the atrioventricular receptors and the arterial baroreceptors to decrease their firing rates and therefore reinforce each other.

---

**PROBLEM 6-1**

How do the carotid sinus baroreceptors respond to occlusion of both common carotid arteries? What are the cardiovascular responses to bilateral carotid occlusion? How would these responses be altered by bilateral vagotomy?
How would these responses be altered by the pharmacologic blockade of β-adrenoceptors?

---

## Chemoreceptors

Chemoreceptors are specialized cells located on arteries (peripheral chemoreceptors) and within the medulla (central chemoreceptors) that monitor blood $PO_2$ (partial pressure of oxygen), $PCO_2$ (partial pressure of carbon dioxide), or pH (log $H^+$ concentration). Their primary function is to regulate respiratory activity to maintain arterial blood $PO_2$, $PCO_2$, and pH within a narrow physiologic range. Chemoreceptor activity, however, affects cardiovascular function either directly by influencing medullary cardiovascular centers or indirectly through altered pulmonary stretch receptor activity. Impaired respiratory gas exchange, hypoxic environments, cerebral ischemia, and circulatory shock, for example, increase chemoreceptor activity, leading to enhanced sympathetic outflow to the heart and vasculature by activating neurons in the RVLM.

The **peripheral chemoreceptors** are found in two locations. Small **carotid bodies** are associated with the external carotid arteries near their bifurcation with the internal carotids. Afferent nerve fibers from the carotid body receptors join with the sinus nerve before entering the glossopharyngeal nerve to synapse in the RTS in the medulla.

The carotid bodies increase their firing in response to a fall in arterial $PO_2$ (hypoxemia) or to an increase in arterial $PCO_2$ (hypercapnia) and hydrogen ion concentration (acidosis). The threshold $PO_2$ for activation is about 80 mm Hg (normal arterial $PO_2$ is about 95 mm Hg). Any elevation of $PCO_2$ above its normal value of 40 mm Hg, or a decrease in pH below 7.4, also increases receptor firing. In addition, carotid body firing can be stimulated by reduced carotid body perfusion, as occurs during hypotension associated with circulatory shock. This response to reduced perfusion can occur without changes in arterial $PO_2$, $PCO_2$, and pH. The mechanism may involve cellular hypoxia resulting from inadequate oxygen delivery to the carotid bodies (i.e., "stagnant hypoxia"). Another set of peripheral chemoreceptors, the **aortic bodies**, are located on the aortic arch, and they function similarly to the carotid bodies. Their afferent connections to the NTS travel with vagal afferent fibers.

**Central chemoreceptors** are found in medullary regions that control cardiovascular and respiratory activity. These receptors increase their firing in response to hypercapnia and acidosis but not directly in response to hypoxia. Carbon dioxide diffusing from the blood into the cerebrospinal fluid forms hydrogen ion by the bicarbonate buffer system, and it is the hydrogen ion rather than the carbon dioxide that stimulates receptor firing.

If a subject breathes a gas mixture containing 10% instead of 21% oxygen, chemoreceptor activation (primarily peripheral) increases respiratory activity and stimulates sympathetic activity to the heart and systemic vasculature, causing arterial blood pressure to increase. If, however, respiratory rate and depth are not allowed to change, the sympathetic-mediated pressor response is accompanied by bradycardia resulting from vagal activation of the heart. This demonstrates that the tachycardia normally found during hypoxemia is secondary to respiratory stimulation and activation of pulmonary stretch receptors. Cardiovascular responses to hypercapnia and acidosis likewise depend in part upon respiratory responses.

## Other Autonomic Reflexes Affecting the Heart and Circulation

In addition to the baroreceptor and chemoreceptor reflexes already described, several other reflexes affect cardiovascular function.

1. **Ischemic brain reflexes.** Insufficient blood flow to the brain (cerebral ischemia), which occurs during severe hypotension (a mean arterial pressure <60 mm Hg), or when there is cerebral vascular occlusion, causes intense sympathetic activation and constriction of the systemic circulation. Mean arterial pressure can rise to well over 200 mm Hg during severe cerebral ischemia. This can be thought of as a final effort by the body to restore perfusion to the brain. An increase in intracranial pressure, which can occur following hemorrhagic stroke or brain trauma, can cause ischemia within the brainstem. This elicits a strong, sympathetic-mediated pressor response (**Cushing reflex**), often accompanied by baroreceptor-mediated bradycardia.

2. **Pain reflexes.** Chest pain associated with myocardial ischemia (insufficient coronary blood flow) or myocardial infarction can cause generalized sympathetic activation, leading to elevated arterial pressure, tachycardia, and increased sweating (diaphoresis). If cardiac output decreases significantly because of the ischemic injury, arterial pressure may fall despite the enhanced sympathetic activity. Deep pain produced by trauma or visceral distension can produce hypotension (i.e., circulatory shock) caused by enhanced parasympathetic and decreased sympathetic activity. Another example of a pain reflex is the **cold pressor response.** If a person's hand or foot is submerged into ice-cold water, arterial pressure increases as a result of sympathetic activation. This test is sometimes used clinically to evaluate autonomic function and vascular reactivity in patients.

3. **Bezold-Jarisch reflex.** This reflex is triggered by stimulation of specific types of chemoreceptors within the heart and coronary arteries and produces bradycardia and hypotension mediated by vagus nerve afferents and efferents. This reflex is sometimes stimulated when dye or other chemical agents are injected into coronary arteries during coronary arteriography. Ventricular ischemia, particularly caused by right coronary artery occlusion, can also trigger this reflex.

4. **Pulmonary and muscle stretch receptors.** Lung inflation activates stretch receptors located in the airways and respiratory muscles that inhibit medullary sympathetic centers and cause arterial pressure to fall; heart rate increases reflexively. These receptors contribute to the normal cyclical changes in heart rate and arterial pressure associated with respiratory activity. Limb muscles and tendons also possess receptors that sense tension and length changes. Passive or active movement of joints can stimulate sympathetic activity to the heart and circulation and help to reinforce cardiovascular responses to exercise.

5. **Temperature reflexes.** Changes in environmental temperature sensed by cold and warm thermoreceptors in the skin can lead to reflex changes in cutaneous blood flow and sweating. Similarly, changes in core temperature, sensed by thermoreceptors located in the hypothalamus, produce changes in sympathetic activity to the skin circulation. For example, a decrease in either skin surface temperature or hypothalamic blood temperature leads to cutaneous vasoconstriction.

## HUMORAL CONTROL

In addition to autonomic nerves, many circulating factors (humoral substances) affect cardiac and vascular function. Some of these humoral factors directly influence the heart and blood vessels, whereas others indirectly alter cardiovascular function through changes in blood volume. Major humoral factors include circulating catecholamines, the renin-angiotensin-aldosterone system, atrial natriuretic peptide, and antidiuretic hormone (vasopressin). Although not addressed in this chapter, note that many other hormones and circulating substances (e.g., thyroxin, estrogen, insulin, and growth hormone) have direct or indirect cardiovascular effects.

## Circulating Catecholamines

Circulating catecholamines originate from two sources. The adrenal medulla releases catecholamines (80% epinephrine, 20% norepinephrine) when preganglionic sympathetic nerves innervating this tissue are activated. This occurs during times of stress (e.g., exercise, heart failure, blood loss, emotional stress, excitement, or pain). Sympathetic nerves innervating blood vessels are another source of circulating catecholamines, principally norepinephrine. Normally, most of the norepinephrine released by sympathetic nerves is taken back up by the nerves and metabolized (some is taken up by extraneuronal tissues). A small amount of released norepinephrine, however, diffuses into the blood and circulates throughout the body. At times of high levels of sympathetic nerve activation, the amount of norepinephrine spilling over into the blood can increase dramatically.

Circulating **epinephrine** has several direct cardiovascular actions that depend upon the relative distribution of adrenergic receptors in different organs and the relative affinities of the different receptors for epinephrine. Epinephrine binds to $\beta_1$-, $\beta_2$-, $\alpha_1$-, and $\alpha_2$-adrenoceptors; however, the affinity of epinephrine for $\beta$-adrenoceptors is much greater than for $\alpha$-adrenoceptors. The relative receptor affinities explain why, at low plasma concentrations, epinephrine binds preferentially to $\beta$-adrenoceptors. Therefore, at low to moderate circulating levels of epinephrine, heart rate, inotropy, and dromotropy are stimulated (primarily $\beta_1$-adrenoceptor mediated). Epinephrine at low concentrations binds to $\beta_2$-adrenoceptors located on small arteries and arterioles (particularly in skeletal muscle) and causes vasodilation.

If a low dose of epinephrine is injected intravenously while systemic hemodynamics are monitored, heart rate (and cardiac output) will increase, systemic vascular resistance will fall, but mean arterial pressure will change very little (Fig. 6.10). At high plasma concentrations, the cardiovascular actions of epinephrine are different because epinephrine binds to $\alpha$-adrenoceptors as well as to $\beta$-adrenoceptors. Increasing concentrations of epinephrine result in further cardiac stimulation along with $\alpha$-adrenoceptor-mediated activation of vascular smooth muscle leading to vasoconstriction. This increases arterial blood pressure (pressor response) owing

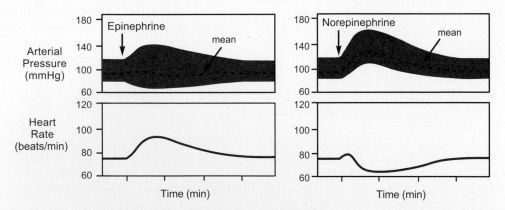

■ **FIGURE 6.10** Effects of intravenous administration of epinephrine and norepinephrine on arterial pressure and heart rate. A low dose of epinephrine (**left panel**) increases heart rate and arterial pulse pressure (it increases systolic and decreases diastolic pressure) with little change in mean arterial pressure. These changes occur because low concentrations of epinephrine preferentially bind to cardiac $\beta_1$-adrenoceptors (produces cardiac stimulation) and vascular $\beta_2$-adrenoceptors (produces systemic vasodilation). Mean pressure does not change very much because the increase in cardiac output is offset by the decrease in systemic vascular resistance. Norepinephrine (**right panel**) increases mean arterial pressure and arterial pulse pressure; heart rate transiently increases ($\beta_1$-adrenoceptor stimulation) and then decreases owing to baroreceptor reflex activation of vagal efferents to the heart. Mean arterial pressure rises because norepinephrine binds to vascular $\alpha_1$-adrenoceptors, which increases systemic vascular resistance.

to both an increase in cardiac output and an increase in systemic vascular resistance. However, even at very high circulating concentrations of epinephrine, the systemic vascular resistance does not increase very much above normal, or may still be reduced, because the vasoconstrictor actions epinephrine acting through the $\alpha$-adrenoceptors is attenuated by the epinephrine that is still bound to the $\beta_2$-adrenoceptors. If the $\beta_2$-adrenoceptors are blocked pharmacologically, then high concentrations of epinephrine produce very large increases in systemic vascular resistance because of the removal of the $\beta_2$-adrenoceptor vasodilator influence.

Circulating **norepinephrine** affects the heart and systemic vasculature by binding to $\beta_1$-, $\beta_2$-, $\alpha_1$-, and $\alpha_2$-adrenoceptors; however, the affinity of norepinephrine for $\beta_2$- and $\alpha_2$-adrenoceptors is relatively weak. Therefore, the predominant affects of norepinephrine are mediated through $\beta_1$- and $\alpha_1$-adrenoceptors. If norepinephrine is injected intravenously, it causes an increase in mean arterial blood pressure (systemic vasoconstriction) and pulse pressure (owing to increased stroke volume) and a paradoxical decrease in heart rate after an initial transient increase in heart rate (Fig. 6.10). The transient increase in heart rate is due to norepinephrine binding to $\beta_1$-adrenoceptors in the SA node, whereas the secondary bradycardia is due to a baroreceptor reflex (vagal mediated), which is in response to the increase in arterial pressure.

High levels of circulating catecholamines, caused by a catecholamine-secreting adrenal tumor (**pheochromocytoma**), causes tachycardia, arrhythmias, and severe hypertension (systolic arterial pressures can exceed 200 mm Hg).

Other actions of circulating catecholamines include (1) stimulation of renin release with subsequent elevation of angiotensin II (AII) and aldosterone, and (2) cardiac and vascular smooth muscle hypertrophy and remodeling. These actions of catecholamines, in addition to the hemodynamic and cardiac actions already described, make them a frequent therapeutic target for the treatment of hypertension, heart failure, coronary artery disease, and arrhythmias. This has led to

the development and use of many different types of $\alpha$- and $\beta$-adrenoceptor antagonists to modulate the effects of circulating catecholamines as well as the norepinephrine released by sympathetic nerves.

> ### PROBLEM 6-2
>
> How would the changes in arterial pressure and heart rate shown in Figure 6.10 be different if $\beta_1$-adrenoceptors were blocked before the administration of low-dose epinephrine?

> ### PROBLEM 6-3
>
> How would the norepinephrine-induced changes in arterial pressure and heart rate shown in Figure 6.10 be different in the presence of bilateral cervical vagotomy?

## Renin-Angiotensin-Aldosterone System

The renin-angiotensin-aldosterone system plays an important role in regulating blood volume, cardiac and vascular function, and arterial blood pressure. Although the pathways for renin and angiotensin formation have been found in a number of tissues, the most important site for renin formation and subsequent formation of circulating angiotensin is the kidney. Sympathetic stimulation of the kidneys (via $\beta_1$-adrenoceptors), renal artery hypotension, and decreased sodium delivery to the distal tubules (usually caused by reduced glomerular filtration rate secondary to reduced renal perfusion) stimulate the release of **renin** into the circulation. The renin is formed within, and released from, **juxtaglomerular cells** associated with afferent and efferent arterioles of renal glomeruli (see Chapter 7 for details), which are adjacent to the macula densa cells of distal tubule segments that sense sodium chloride concentrations in the distal tubule. Together, these components are referred to as the juxtaglomerular apparatus.

Renin is an enzyme that acts upon **angiotensinogen**, a circulating substrate synthesized and released by the liver, which undergoes proteolytic cleavage to form the decapeptide angiotensin I. Vascular endothelium, particularly in the lungs, has an enzyme, **angiotensin-converting enzyme (ACE)**, that cleaves off two amino acids to form the octapeptide, **angiotensin II.**

Angiotensin II has several important functions that are mediated by specific angiotensin II receptors $(AT_1)$ (Fig. 6.11). Angiotensin II

1. Constricts resistance vessels, thereby increasing systemic vascular resistance and arterial pressure.
2. Enhances sympathetic adrenergic activity by facilitating norepinephrine release from sympathetic nerve endings, inhibiting norepinephrine reuptake by nerve endings, and by binding to $AT_1$ receptors in the RVLM, which increases sympathetic efferent activity.
3. Acts upon the adrenal cortex to release aldosterone, which in turn acts upon the kidneys to increase sodium and fluid retention, thereby increasing blood volume.
4. Stimulates the release of vasopressin from the posterior pituitary, which acts upon the kidneys to increase fluid retention and blood volume.
5. Stimulates thirst centers within the brain, which can lead to an increase in blood volume.
6. Stimulates cardiac and vascular hypertrophy.

Angiotensin II is continuously produced under basal conditions, and this production can change under different physiologic conditions. For example, when a person exercises, circulating levels of angiotensin II increase. An increase in renin release during exercise probably results from sympathetic stimulation of the kidneys. Changes in body posture likewise alter circulating AII levels, which are increased when a person stands. As with exercise, this results from sympathetic activation. Dehydration and loss of blood volume (hypovolemia) stimulate renin release and angiotensin II formation in response to renal artery hypotension, decreased glomerular filtration rate, and sympathetic activation.

Several cardiovascular disease states are associated with changes in circulating angiotensin II and aldosterone. For example, secondary hypertension caused by renal artery stenosis is associated with increased renin release and

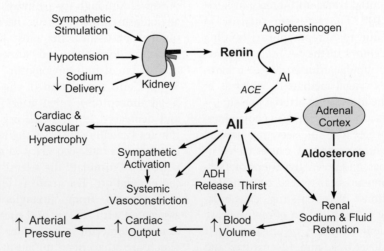

■ **FIGURE 6.11** Formation of angiotensin II and its effects on renal, vascular, and cardiac function. Renin is released by the kidneys in response to sympathetic stimulation, hypotension, and decreased sodium delivery to distal tubules. Renin acts upon angiotensinogen to form angiotensin I (*AI*), which is converted to angiotensin II (*AII*) by angiotensin–converting enzyme (*ACE*). AII has several important actions: stimulates aldosterone release, which increases renal sodium reabsorption; directly stimulates renal sodium reabsorption; stimulates thirst; stimulates release of antidiuretic hormone (*ADH*); produces systemic vasoconstriction; activates the sympathetic nervous system; and causes cardiac and vascular smooth muscle hypertrophy. The overall systemic effect of increased AII is increased blood volume, venous pressure, and arterial pressure.

circulating angiotensin II. **Primary hyperaldosteronism**, caused by an adrenal tumor that secretes large amounts of aldosterone, increases arterial pressure through its effects on renal sodium retention. This increases blood volume, cardiac output, and arterial pressure. In this condition, renin release and circulating angiotensin II levels are usually depressed because of the hypertension. In heart failure, circulating angiotensin II increases in response to sympathetic activation and decreased renal perfusion.

Therapeutic manipulation of the renin-angiotensin-aldosterone system has become important in treating hypertension and heart failure. ACE inhibitors and $AT_1$ receptor blockers effectively decrease arterial pressure, ventricular afterload, blood volume, and hence ventricular preload, and they inhibit and reverse cardiac and vascular remodeling that occurs during chronic hypertension and heart failure.

Note that local, tissue-produced angiotensin may play a significant role in cardiovascular pathophysiology. Many tissues and organs, including the heart and blood vessels, can produce renin and angiotensin II, which have actions directly within the tissue. This may explain why ACE inhibitors can reduce arterial pressure and reverse cardiac and vascular remodeling (e.g., diminish hypertrophy) even in individuals who do not have elevated circulating levels of angiotensin II. In hypertension and heart failure, for example, tissue ACE activity is often elevated, and this may be an important target for the pharmacologic actions of ACE inhibitors.

**CASE 6-1**

A 56-year-old male patient is found to have an arterial pressure of 190/115 mm Hg. Two years earlier, he was normotensive. Diagnostic tests reveal bilateral renal artery stenosis. Describe the mechanisms by which this condition elevates arterial pressure.

## Atrial Natriuretic Peptide

Atrial natriuretic peptide (ANP) is a 28-amino acid peptide that is synthesized, stored, and released by atrial myocytes in response to atrial distension, angiotensin II stimulation, endothelin, and sympathetic stimulation (β-adrenoceptor mediated). Therefore, elevated levels of ANP are found during conditions such as hypervolemia and congestive heart failure, both of which cause atrial distension.

ANP is involved in the long-term regulation of sodium and water balance, blood volume, and arterial pressure (Fig. 6.12). Most of its actions are the opposite of angiotensin II, and therefore *ANP is a counterregulatory system*

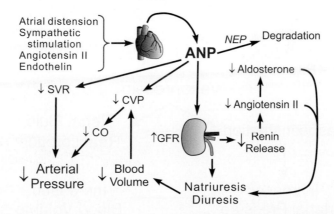

■ **FIGURE 6.12** Formation and cardiovascular/renal actions of atrial natriuretic peptide (*ANP*). ANP, which is released from cardiac atrial tissue in response to atrial distension, sympathetic stimulation, increased angiotensin II, and endothelin, functions as a counterregulatory mechanism for the renin–angiotensin–aldosterone system. ANP decreases renin release, angiotensin II and aldosterone formation, blood volume, central venous pressure, and arterial pressure. *NEP*, neutral endopeptidase; *GFR*, glomerular filtration rate; *CVP*, central venous pressure; *CO*, cardiac output; *SVR*, systemic vascular resistance.

*for the renin-angiotensin-aldosterone system.* ANP decreases aldosterone release by the adrenal cortex; increases glomerular filtration rate; produces natriuresis and diuresis (potassium sparing); and decreases renin release, thereby decreasing angiotensin II. These actions reduce blood volume, which leads to a fall in central venous pressure, cardiac output, and arterial blood pressure. Chronic elevations of ANP appear to decrease arterial blood pressure primarily by decreasing systemic vascular resistance.

The mechanism of systemic vasodilation may involve ANP receptor-mediated elevations in vascular smooth muscle cGMP (ANP activates particulate guanylyl cyclase). ANP also attenuates sympathetic vascular tone. This latter mechanism may involve ANP acting upon sites within the central nervous system as well as through inhibition of norepinephrine release by sympathetic nerve terminals.

A new class of drugs that are neutral endopeptidase (NEP) inhibitors is useful in treating acute heart failure. By inhibiting NEP, the enzyme responsible for the degradation of ANP, these drugs elevate plasma levels of ANP. NEP inhibition is particularly effective in some forms of heart failure when combined with an ACE inhibitor. The reason for this is that NEP inhibition, by elevating ANP, reinforces the effects of ACE inhibition.

Brain-type natriuretic peptide (BNP), a 32-amino acid peptide hormone related to ANP, is synthesized and released by the ventricles in response to pressure and volume overload, particularly during heart failure. BNP appears to have actions that are similar to those of ANP. Circulating BNP is now used clinically as a sensitive biomarker for heart failure.

## Vasopressin (Antidiuretic Hormone)

Vasopressin (arginine vasopressin, AVP; antidiuretic hormone, ADH) is a nonapeptide hormone released from the posterior pituitary (Fig. 6.13). AVP has two principal sites of action: the kidneys and blood vessels. The most important physiologic action of AVP is that it increases water reabsorption by the kidneys by increasing water permeability in the collecting duct, thereby permitting the formation of concentrated urine. This antidiuretic property of AVP, which acts through renal $V_2$ receptors, increases blood volume and arterial blood pressure. This hormone also constricts arterial blood vessels through $V_1$ vascular receptors; however, the normal

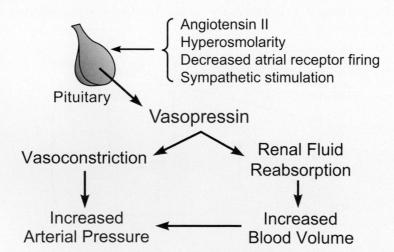

■ **FIGURE 6.13** Cardiovascular and renal effects of arginine vasopressin (AVP). AVP release from the posterior pituitary is stimulated by angiotensin II, hyperosmolarity, decreased atrial receptor firing (usually in response to hypovolemia), and sympathetic activation. The primary action of AVP is on the kidney to increase water reabsorption (antidiuretic effect), which increases blood volume. AVP also has direct vasoconstrictor actions at high concentrations. Increased arterial pressure is the overall effect of increased AVP.

physiologic concentrations of AVP are below its vasoactive range. Studies have shown, nevertheless, that in severe hypovolemic shock, when AVP release is very high, AVP contributes to the compensatory increase in systemic vascular resistance. This vasoconstrictor property of AVP is sometimes utilized in the treatment of circulatory shock; AVP is administered to increase systemic vascular resistance and therefore arterial pressure.

Several mechanisms regulate the release of AVP. Specialized stretch receptors within the atrial walls and large veins (cardiopulmonary baroreceptors) entering the atria decrease their firing rate when atrial pressure falls (as occurs with hypovolemia). Afferents from these receptors synapse within the hypothalamus, which is the site of AVP synthesis. AVP is transported from the hypothalamus via axons to the posterior pituitary, from where it is secreted into the circulation. Atrial receptor firing normally inhibits the release of AVP. With hypovolemia and decreased central venous pressure, the decreased firing of atrial stretch receptors leads to an increase in AVP release. AVP release is also stimulated by enhanced sympathetic activity accompanying decreased arterial baroreceptor activity during hypotension. An important mechanism regulating AVP release involves hypothalamic osmoreceptors, which sense extracellular osmolarity. When osmolarity rises, as occurs during dehydration, AVP release is stimulated, which increases water retention by the kidneys. Finally, angiotensin II receptors ($AT_1$) located within the hypothalamus regulate AVP release; an increase in angiotensin II stimulates AVP release.

Heart failure causes a paradoxical increase in AVP. The increased blood volume and atrial pressure associated with heart failure suggest that AVP secretion should be inhibited, but it is not. It may be that sympathetic and renin–angiotensin system activation in heart failure override the volume and low-pressure cardiovascular receptors (as well as the osmoregulation of AVP) and cause the increase in AVP secretion. This increase in AVP during heart failure may contribute to the increased systemic vascular resistance and to renal retention of fluid.

In summary, the importance of AVP in cardiovascular regulation is primarily through its effects on volume regulation, which in turn affects ventricular preload and cardiac output through the Frank-Starling relationship. Increased AVP, by increasing blood volume, increases cardiac output and arterial pressure. The vasoconstrictor effects of AVP are probably important only when AVP levels are very high, as occurs during severe hypovolemia.

## INTEGRATION OF NEUROHUMORAL MECHANISMS

Autonomic and humoral influences are necessary to maintain a normal arterial blood pressure under the different conditions in which the human body functions. Neurohumoral mechanisms enable the body to adjust to changes in body posture, physical activity, or environmental conditions. The neurohumoral mechanisms act through changes in systemic vascular resistance, venous compliance, blood volume, and cardiac function, and through these actions, they can effectively regulate arterial blood pressure (Table 6-2). Although each mechanism has independent cardiovascular actions, it is important to understand that each mechanism also has complex interactions with other control mechanisms that serve to reinforce or inhibit the actions of the other control mechanisms. For example, activation of sympathetic nerves either directly or indirectly increases circulating angiotensin II, aldosterone, adrenal catecholamines, and arginine vasopressin, which act together to increase blood volume, cardiac output, and arterial pressure. These humoral changes are accompanied by an increase in ANP, which acts as a counter-regulatory system to limit the effects of the other neurohumoral mechanisms.

Finally, it is important to note that some neurohumoral effects are rapid (e.g., autonomic nerves and catecholamine effects on cardiac output and arterial pressure), whereas others may take several hours or days because changes in blood volume must occur before alterations in cardiac output and arterial pressure can be fully expressed.

**TABLE 6-2 EFFECTS OF NEUROHUMORAL ACTIVATION ON BLOOD VOLUME, CARDIAC OUTPUT, AND ARTERIAL PRESSURE**

| INCREASED | BLOOD VOLUME | CARDIAC OUTPUT | ARTERIAL PRESSURE |
|---|---|---|---|
| Sympathetic activity | ↑ | ↑ | ↑ |
| Vagal activity | — | ↓ | ↓ |
| Circulating epinephrine | ↑ | ↑ | ↓↑[1] |
| Angiotensin II | ↑ | ↑ | ↑ |
| Aldosterone | ↑ | ↑ | ↑ |
| Atrial natriuretic peptide | ↓ | ↓ | ↓ |
| Arginine vasopressin | ↑ | ↑ | ↑ |

↑ = increase; ↓ = decrease.
[1]Dependent upon plasma epinephrine concentration.

## SUMMARY OF IMPORTANT CONCEPTS

- Autonomic regulation of the heart and vasculature is primarily controlled by special regions within the medulla oblongata of the brainstem that contain the cell bodies of sympathetic and parasympathetic (vagal) efferent nerves.

- The hypothalamus plays an integrative role by modulating medullary neuronal activity (e.g., during exercise).

- Sensory nerves from peripheral baroreceptors (e.g., carotid sinus baroreceptors) synapse within the medulla at the NTS, which modulates the activity of the sympathetic and vagal neurons within the medulla.

- Preganglionic parasympathetic efferent nerves exit the medulla as the tenth cranial nerve and travel to the heart within the left and right vagus nerves. Preganglionic fibers synapse within ganglia located within the heart; short postganglionic fibers innervate the myocardial tissue. Preganglionic sympathetic efferent nerves exit from the spinal cord and synapse within paravertebral or prevertebral ganglia before sending out postganglionic

fibers to target tissues in the heart and blood vessels.

- Sympathetic activation increases heart rate, inotropy, and dromotropy through the release of norepinephrine, which binds primarily to postjunctional cardiac $\beta_1$-adrenoceptors. Norepinephrine released by sympathetic nerves constricts blood vessels by binding primarily to postjunctional $\alpha_1$-adrenoceptors.

- Parasympathetic activation decreases heart rate, inotropy, and dromotropy, and it produces vasodilation in specific organs through the release of ACh, which binds to postjunctional muscarinic ($M_2$) receptors.

- Baroreceptors respond to stretch induced by an increase in pressure or volume. Arterial baroreceptor activity (e.g., carotid sinus and aortic arch receptors) tonically inhibits sympathetic outflow to the heart and blood vessels, and it tonically stimulates vagal outflow to the heart. Decreased arterial pressure, therefore, decreases the firing of arterial baroreceptors, which leads to reflex activation of sympathetic influences acting on the heart and blood vessels and withdrawal of the vagal activity to the heart.

- Peripheral chemoreceptors (e.g., carotid bodies) and central chemoreceptors (e.g., medullary chemoreceptors) respond to decreased $PO_2$ and pH or increased $PCO_2$ of the blood. Their primary function is to regulate respiratory activity, although chemoreceptor activation generally leads to activation of the sympathetic nervous system to the vasculature, which increases arterial pressure.

- Reflexes triggered by changes in blood volume, cerebral and myocardial ischemia, pain, pulmonary activity, muscle and joint movement, and temperature alter cardiac and vascular function.

- Sympathetic activation of the adrenal medulla stimulates the release of catecholamines, principally epinephrine. This hormone produces cardiac stimulation (via $\beta_1$-adrenoceptors), and it either decreases (via vascular $\beta_2$-adrenoceptors) or increases (via vascular $\alpha_1$- and $\alpha_2$-adrenoceptors) systemic vascular resistance, depending upon the plasma concentration.

- The renin-angiotensin-aldosterone system plays a major role in regulating renal excretion of sodium and water. The overall systemic effect of increased angiotensin II is increased blood volume, venous pressure, and arterial pressure.

- Atrial natriuretic peptide (ANP), which is released by the atria primarily in response to atrial stretch, functions as a counterregulatory mechanism for the renin-angiotensin-aldosterone system. Therefore, increased ANP reduces blood volume, venous pressure, and arterial pressure.

- Arginine vasopressin (AVP; antidiuretic hormone), which is released by the posterior pituitary when the body needs to reduce renal loss of water, enhances blood volume and increases arterial and venous pressures. At high plasma concentrations, AVP constricts resistance vessels.

## REVIEW QUESTIONS

For each question, choose the one best answer:

1.  The cell bodies for the preganglionic vagal efferents innervating the heart are found in which region of the brain?

    a. Cortex
    b. Hypothalamus
    c. Medulla
    d. Nucleus tractus solitarius

2.  Norepinephrine released by sympathetic nerves

    a. Binds preferentially to $\beta_2$-adrenoceptors on cardiac myocytes.

    b. Constricts blood vessels by binding to $\alpha_1$-adrenoceptors.
    c. Inhibits its own release by binding to prejunctional $\beta_2$-adrenoceptors.
    d. Decreases renin release in the kidneys.

3.  Stimulating efferent fibers of the right vagus nerve

    a. Decreases systemic vascular resistance.
    b. Increases atrial inotropy.
    c. Increases heart rate.
    d. Releases acetylcholine, which binds to $M_2$ receptors.

4.  A sudden increase in carotid artery pressure

    a.  Decreases carotid sinus baroreceptor firing rate.
    b.  Increases sympathetic efferent nerve activity to systemic circulation.
    c.  Increases vagal efferent activity to the heart.
    d.  Results in reflex tachycardia.

5.  Which of the following can cause tachycardia?

    a.  Increased arterial pulse pressure
    b.  Increased blood $PCO_2$
    c.  Increased firing of carotid sinus baroreceptors
    d.  Vasovagal reflex

6.  Infusion of a high dose of epinephrine following pharmacologic blockade of β-adrenoceptors will

    a.  Decrease mean arterial pressure.
    b.  Have no significant cardiovascular effects.
    c.  Increase heart rate.
    d.  Increase systemic vascular resistance.

7.  In an experimental protocol, intravenous infusion of acetylcholine was found to decrease mean arterial pressure and increase heart rate. These results can best be explained by

    a.  Direct action of acetylcholine on muscarinic receptors at the sinoatrial node.
    b.  Increased firing of carotid sinus baroreceptors.
    c.  Reflex activation of sympathetic nerves.
    d.  Reflex systemic vasodilation.

8.  A 27-year-old female patient with severe hypertension is found to have bilateral renal artery stenosis caused by fibromuscular dysplasia of the renal arteries resulting in elevated levels of circulating renin. One mechanism contributing to her hypertension is

    a.  Increased blood volume.
    b.  Increased circulating atrial natriuretic peptide.
    c.  Increased sodium loss by the kidneys.
    d.  Inhibition of aldosterone release.

9.  A hospitalized patient with acute decompensated heart failure is given a drug that increases circulating atrial natriuretic peptide by inhibiting its metabolism. What beneficial effects would this treatment have in this patient?

    a.  Decrease blood volume by promoting sodium loss by the kidneys
    b.  Increase blood pressure by constricting the arterial and venous vasculature
    c.  Increase cardiac output by increasing preload
    d.  Stimulate the release of aldosterone from the adrenal cortex

10. Following an automobile accident that resulted in significant hemorrhage, a 48-year-old male patient is admitted to the Emergency Department in critical condition with an arterial pressure of 65/45 mm Hg and a heart rate of 140 beats/min. Fluid resuscitation was augmented by administration of arginine vasopressin. The potential benefit of adding vasopressin during resuscitation is derived from its ability to

    a.  Augment sympathetic activity.
    b.  Increase systemic vascular resistance.
    c.  Produce renal fluid loss (diuresis).
    d.  Stimulate the release of renin.

1. The correct answer is "c" because this region of the brainstem contains cell bodies for both sympathetic and parasympathetic neurons; choices "a" and "b" are therefore incorrect. Choice "d" is incorrect because the nucleus tractus solitarius is the region in the medulla that receives afferent fibers from peripheral sensors (e.g., baroreceptors) and then sends excitatory or inhibitory fibers to sympathetic and parasympathetic neurons within the medulla.

2. The correct answer is "b" because norepinephrine binds to $\alpha_1$-adrenoceptors located on vascular smooth muscle to stimulate vasoconstriction. Choice "a" is incorrect because norepinephrine preferentially binds to $\beta_1$-adrenoceptors in the heart. Choice "c" is incorrect because prejunctional $\beta_2$-adrenoceptors facilitate norepinephrine release (prejunctional $\alpha_2$-adrenoceptors inhibit release). Choice "d" is incorrect because norepinephrine stimulates renin release through $\beta_1$-adrenoceptors.

3. The correct answer is "d" because the vagus nerve is parasympathetic cholinergic and therefore releases acetylcholine. Choice "a" is incorrect because efferent right vagal stimulation primarily affects the sinoatrial node and has no significant direct effects on the systemic vasculature. Choice "b" is incorrect because vagal stimulation decreases atrial inotropy. Choice "c" is incorrect because right vagal stimulation reduces heart rate by decreasing the slope of Phase 4 of the pacemaker action potential.

4. The correct answer is "c" because increased carotid artery pressure stimulates the firing of carotid sinus baroreceptors (therefore, choice "a" is incorrect), which leads to a reflex activation of vagal efferents to slow the heart rate (therefore, choice "d" is incorrect). Choice "b" is incorrect because the baroreceptor reflex would attempt to reduce

arterial pressure by withdrawing sympathetic tone on the systemic vasculature.

5. The correct answer is "b" because increased blood $PCO_2$ stimulates chemoreceptors, which activate the sympathetic nervous system to constrict the systemic vasculature and raise arterial pressure. Choice "a" is incorrect because increased arterial pulse pressure stimulates arterial baroreceptors, which leads to vagal activation of the heart. Choice "c" is incorrect because increased carotid sinus firing (usually caused by elevated arterial pressure) causes a reflex decrease in heart rate brought about by vagal activation and sympathetic withdrawal. Choice "d" is incorrect because the vasovagal reflex causes vagal activation and bradycardia.

6. The correct answer is "d" because a high dose of epinephrine binds to both $\beta_2$- and $\alpha_1$-adrenoceptors on blood vessels. Therefore, if the $\beta_2$-adrenoceptors (which produce vasodilation) are blocked, the $\alpha_1$-adrenoceptors can produce vasoconstriction unopposed by the $\beta_2$-adrenoceptors. Choice "a" is incorrect because the unopposed $\alpha$-adrenoceptor activation increases arterial pressure. Choice "b" is incorrect because epinephrine binds to $\alpha$ as well as $\beta$-adrenoceptors. Choice "c" is incorrect because epinephrine-induced increased heart rate is mediated primarily by $\beta$-adrenoceptors (which are blocked), and systemic vasoconstriction will increase arterial pressure and cause a reflex decrease in heart rate.

7. The correct answer is "c" because acetylcholine dilates blood vessels, which lowers arterial pressure and causes a baroreceptor-mediated increase in heart rate brought about by sympathetic activation. Choice "a" is incorrect because stimulation of muscarinic receptors on the sinoatrial node induces bradycardia. Choice "b" is incorrect because the hypotension causes decreased carotid sinus firing. Choice "d" is incorrect

because reflex systemic vasodilation can occur only if arterial pressure is elevated and baroreceptor firing increases.

8. The correct answer is "a" because increased renin leads to increased angiotensin II and aldosterone (therefore, choice "d" is incorrect), both of which act on the kidney to increase sodium reabsorption and blood volume (therefore, choice "c" is incorrect). Choice "b" is incorrect because although circulating atrial natriuretic peptide is increased, this hormone counteracts the pressure-elevating mechanisms of angiotensin II.

9. The correct answer is "a" because atrial natriuretic peptide produces natriuresis and diuresis, both of which are beneficial to the acutely decompensated heart failure patient who has excessive accumulation of fluid that can cause pulmonary and systemic edema. Choices "b," "c," and "d" are incorrect because atrial natriuretic peptide dilates vessels, reduces preload and cardiac output, and decreases aldosterone release.

10. The correct answer is "b" because vasopressin constricts blood vessels directly through $V_1$ receptors, and not through augmentation of sympathetic activity which will actually decline as pressure is elevated during vasopressin administration (therefore, choice "a" is incorrect). Choice "c" is incorrect because vasopressin has an antidiuretic effect. Choice "d" is incorrect because circulating renin would decline as pressure is elevated during vasopressin administration.

---

## ANSWERS TO PROBLEMS AND CASES

### PROBLEM 6-1

The common carotid arteries are below the carotid sinus baroreceptors. Therefore, occlusion of both carotid arteries reduces pressure within the carotid sinuses. This decreases their firing, leading to increased sympathetic and decreased vagal outflow from the medulla. This results in systemic vasoconstriction, cardiac stimulation, and a rise in arterial pressure.

Bilateral vagotomy enhances the response described above because as arterial pressure rises during carotid occlusion, the aortic arch baroreceptors, which are innervated by the vagus nerve, increase their firing. This partially counteracts the effects of decreased carotid sinus firing. Bilateral vagotomy removes this influence of the aortic arch baroreceptors.

Blockade of β-adrenoceptors would prevent the sympathetic-mediated increases in heart rate and inotropy (although some withdrawal of vagal tone may still result in a small increase in heart rate). The pressor response would still occur because of systemic vasoconstriction ($α_1$-adrenoceptor mediated); however, the pressor response would be blunted significantly because cardiac stimulation would be blocked.

### PROBLEM 6-2

$β_1$-adrenoceptor activation is primarily responsible for the tachycardia and increased cardiac output produced by epinephrine. Blocking $β_1$-adrenoceptors would significantly blunt the cardiac responses. Epinephrine at low plasma concentrations also binds to vascular $β_2$-adrenoceptors to cause vasodilation; therefore, arterial pressure would fall during infusion of a low dose of epinephrine in the presence of $β_1$-adrenoceptor blockade because the large decrease in systemic vascular resistance would not be offset by an increase in cardiac output.

### PROBLEM 6-3

Bilateral cervical vagotomy would prevent vagal slowing of the heart and denervate the aortic arch baroreceptors. Heart rate (and inotropy) would increase owing to norepinephrine binding to $β_1$-adrenoceptors on the heart that is now unopposed by the vagus.

This, along with aortic arch denervation, would enhance the pressor response of norepinephrine.

## CASE 6-1

Bilateral renal artery stenosis reduces the pressure within the afferent arterioles, which causes release of renin. This, in turn, increases circulating angiotensin II, which stimulates aldosterone release. Activation of the renin-angiotensin-aldosterone system causes sodium and fluid retention by the kidneys and an increase in blood volume, which increases cardiac output. Increased vasopressin (stimulated by angiotensin II) contributes to the increase in blood volume. Increased angiotensin II increases systemic vascular resistance by binding to vascular $AT_1$ receptors and by enhancement of sympathetic activity. These changes in cardiac output and systemic vascular resistance lead to a hypertensive state.

### SUGGESTED RESOURCES

Berne RM, Levy MN. Cardiovascular Physiology. 8th Ed. Philadelphia: Mosby, 2001.

Guyenet PG. The sympathetic control of blood pressure. Nature Reviews Neuroscience 2006;7:335–346.

Melo LG, Pang SC, Ackermann U. Atrial natriuretic peptide: regulator of chronic arterial blood pressure. News Physiol Sci 2000;15:143–149.

Mendolowitz D. Advances in parasympathetic control of heart rate and cardiac function. News Physiol Sci 1999;14:155–161.

Rhoades RA, Bell, DR. Medical Physiology: Principles for Clinical Medicine. 3rd Ed. Philadelphia: Lippincott Williams & Wilkins, 2009.

Touyz CB, Dominiczak AF, Webb RC, Johns DB. Angiotensin receptors: signaling, vascular pathophysiology, and interactions with ceramide. Am J Physiol 2001;281:H2337–H2365.

# ORGAN BLOOD FLOW

Understanding the concepts presented in this chapter will enable the student to:

1. Describe the distribution of cardiac output among major organs when a person is at rest.

2. Describe how various tissue and endothelial factors influence tissue blood flow.

3. Explain how extravascular compression alters blood flow in the heart and contracting skeletal muscle.

4. Define autoregulation of blood flow, reactive hyperemia, and active (functional) hyperemia and describe their mechanisms in different organs.

5. Compare and contrast autonomic control of blood flow in major vascular beds of the body.

6. Describe the specialized vascular anatomy and function in the following organs: brain, heart, intestines and liver, skin, kidneys, and lungs.

## INTRODUCTION

This chapter describes the blood flow to different organs of the body. The first part of the chapter emphasizes local regulatory mechanisms by which organs regulate their own blood flow to meet the metabolic and functional requirements of the organ. The second part of the chapter examines blood flow in specific organs of the body.

## DISTRIBUTION OF CARDIAC OUTPUT

We have previously seen that arterial pressure is generated as the heart pumps blood into the systemic circulation. This arterial pressure serves as the driving force for blood flow to all the organ systems. The relative distribution of blood flow to the organs is regulated by the vascular resistance of the individual organs, which is influenced by extrinsic (neurohumoral) and intrinsic (local regulatory) mechanisms as summarized in Chapter 5, Figure 5.12.

Table 7–1 summarizes the distribution of cardiac output when a person is at rest. Most of the cardiac output (~80%) goes to the gastrointestinal tract, kidneys, skeletal muscle, heart, and brain, although these organs make up <50% of the body mass. This relative distribution of cardiac output, however, changes greatly depending on environmental conditions and the state of physical activity. For example, in a hot, humid environment, the relative blood flow to the skin increases substantially as the body attempts to maintain its core temperature by losing heat to the environment. When a person exercises, the increased cardiac output primarily goes to the active skeletal muscles, heart, and skin (see Chapter 9); at the same time, blood flow decreases to the gastrointestinal and renal circulations. Another example of change in cardiac output distribution occurs following a meal, when blood flow to the gastrointestinal circulation increases.

Instead of one "normal" blood flow for an organ, there is a range of blood flows. **Basal flow** refers to the flow that is measured under basal conditions (i.e., when a person is in a

| TABLE 7-1 BLOOD FLOW IN MAJOR ORGANS OF THE BODY | | | | |
|---|---|---|---|---|
| ORGAN | PERCENT BODY WEIGHT | PERCENT CARDIAC OUTPUT AT REST | NORMAL FLOW (mL/min PER 100 g) | MAXIMAL FLOW (mL/min PER 100 g) |
| Heart | 0.5 | 5 | 80 | 400 |
| Brain | 2 | 14 | 55 | 150 |
| Skeletal muscle | 40 | 18 | 3 | 60 |
| Skin | 3 | 4 | 10 | 150 |
| Stomach, intestine, liver, spleen, pancreas | 6 | 23 | 30 | 250 |
| Kidneys | 0.5 | 20 | 400 | 600 |
| Other | 48 | 16 | — | — |

Normal and maximal flows are approximate values for the whole organ. Many organs (e.g., brain, muscle, kidney, and intestine) have considerable heterogeneity of flow within the organ depending on the type of tissue or region of organ being perfused. The liver receives blood flow from the gastrointestinal venous drainage as well as from the hepatic artery (only hepatic artery flow is included in this table). "Other" includes reproductive organs, bone, fat, and connective tissue.

fasted, resting state and at normal environmental conditions of temperature and humidity). The ratio of basal flow to maximal flow is a measure of the vascular tone, which is the degree of vascular constriction (see Chapter 5). The lower the basal flow relative to the maximal flow, the higher the vascular tone. The difference between basal flow and maximal flow represents the flow capacity or **vasodilator reserve** for the organ. Most organs have a relatively large vasodilator reserve, whereas others, such as the kidneys, have a relatively small vasodilator reserve (see Table 7-1).

The changes that occur in organ blood flow under different conditions depend on the interplay between neurohumoral and local regulatory mechanisms that govern vascular resistance. The neurohumoral mechanisms were discussed in Chapter 6. The following sections focus on the local regulatory mechanisms that affect vascular resistance and organ blood flow.

## LOCAL REGULATION OF BLOOD FLOW

Tissues and organs have the ability to regulate, to a varying degree, their own blood flow. This intrinsic ability to regulate blood flow is termed "local regulation" and can occur in the complete absence of any extrinsic neurohumoral influences. For example, if a muscle is removed from the body, perfused under constant pressure from a reservoir containing oxygenated blood, and then electrically stimulated to induce muscle contractions, the blood flow increases. The increase in blood flow occurs in the absence of neurohumoral influences and therefore is a local or intrinsic mechanism.

The mechanisms responsible for local regulation originate from within the blood vessels (e.g., endothelial factors, myogenic mechanisms) and from the surrounding tissue (i.e., tissue factors), many of which are related to tissue metabolism or other biochemical pathways (e.g., arachidonic acid metabolites and bradykinin). Mechanical factors (e.g., compressive forces during muscle contraction) can also influence vascular resistance and thereby alter blood flow.

### Tissue Factors

Tissue factors are substances produced by the tissue surrounding blood vessels (Fig. 7.1). These substances act on the blood vessel to produce either relaxation or contraction of the smooth muscle, thereby altering resistance and blood flow. In some cases, these substances indirectly act on the vascular smooth muscle by affecting endothelial function or by altering the release of norepinephrine by sympathetic nerves. Some of these vasoactive substances are tissue metabolites that are products of cellular metabolism or activity (e.g., adenosine, $CO_2$, $H^+$, $K^+$, lactate). In addition,

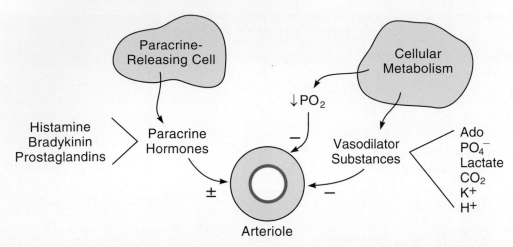

■ **FIGURE 7.1** Vasoactive substances derived from tissue cells around arterioles. Increased tissue metabolism leads to formation of metabolites that dilate (−) nearby arterioles. Increased oxygen consumption decreases the tissue partial pressure of oxygen ($PO_2$), which dilates arterioles. Some cells release locally acting, paracrine hormones (or their precursors), which can either constrict (+) or dilate (−) arterioles. *Ado*, adenosine; $PO_4^-$, inorganic phosphate; $CO_2$, carbon dioxide; $K^+$, potassium ion; $H^+$, hydrogen ion.

different cell types surrounding blood vessels can release vasoactive substances referred to as local, paracrine hormones (e.g., histamine, bradykinin, and prostaglandins). A **paracrine hormone** is a substance released by one cell that acts on another nearby cell by diffusing through the interstitial fluid. This is in contrast to **endocrine hormones** that circulate in the blood to reach distant target cells or **autocrine substances** that affect the same cell from which they are released.

Increases or decreases in metabolism alter the release of some of these vasoactive substances; thus, metabolic activity is closely coupled to blood flow in most organs of the body. For example, an increase in tissue metabolism, as occurs during muscle contraction or during changes in neuronal activity in the brain, leads to an increase in blood flow. Extensive evidence shows that the actively metabolizing cells surrounding arterioles release vasoactive substances that cause vasodilation. This is termed the **metabolic theory of blood flow regulation.** These vasoactive substances, which are linked to tissue metabolism, ensure that the tissue is adequately supplied with oxygen and that products of metabolism (e.g., $CO_2$, $H^+$, lactic acid) are removed. Several substances have been implicated in metabolic regulation of blood flow.

Their relative importance depends on the tissue in which they are formed as well as different conditions that might cause their release.

1. **Adenosine** is a potent vasodilator in most organs (although adenosine constricts renal vessels). It is formed by the action of 5′-nucleotidase, an enzyme that dephosphorylates adenosine monophosphate (AMP). The AMP is derived from hydrolysis of intracellular adenosine triphosphate (ATP) and adenosine diphosphate (ADP). Adenosine formation increases during hypoxia and increased oxygen consumption, both of which lead to increased ATP hydrolysis. Small amounts of ATP hydrolysis can lead to large increases in adenosine formation because intracellular concentrations of ATP are about a 1000-fold greater than adenosine concentrations. Experimental evidence supports the idea that adenosine formation is a particularly important mechanism for regulating coronary blood flow when myocardial oxygen consumption increases or during hypoxic conditions.

2. **Inorganic phosphate** is released by the hydrolysis of adenine nucleotides (ATP, ADP, and AMP). Inorganic phosphate may have some vasodilatory activity in

contracting skeletal muscle, but its importance is far less than that of adenosine, potassium, and nitric oxide in regulating skeletal muscle blood flow.

3. **Carbon dioxide** formation increases during states of increased oxidative metabolism. $CO_2$ concentrations in the tissue and vasculature can also increase when blood flow is reduced, which reduces the washout of $CO_2$. As a gas, $CO_2$ readily diffuses from parenchymal cells to the vascular smooth muscle of blood vessels, where it causes vasodilation. Considerable evidence indicates that $CO_2$ plays a significant role in regulating cerebral blood flow through the formation of $H^+$.

4. **Hydrogen ion** increases through the bicarbonate buffer system when $CO_2$ increases. Hydrogen ion also increases during states of increased anaerobic metabolism (e.g., during ischemia or hypoxia) when acid metabolites such as lactic acid are produced. Increased $H^+$ causes local vasodilation, particularly in the cerebral circulation.

5. **Potassium ion** is released by contracting cardiac and skeletal muscle. Muscle contraction is initiated by membrane depolarization, which results from a cellular influx of $Na^+$ and an efflux of $K^+$. Normally, the $Na^+/K^+$-ATPase pump is able to restore the ionic gradients (see Chapter 2); however, the pump does not keep up with rapid depolarizations (i.e., there is a time lag) during muscle contractions, and a small amount of $K^+$ accumulates in the extracellular space. Small increases in extracellular $K^+$ around blood vessels cause hyperpolarization of the vascular smooth muscle cells, possibly by stimulating the electrogenic $Na^+/K^+$-ATPase pump and increasing $K^+$ conductance through potassium channels. Hyperpolarization leads to smooth muscle relaxation. Potassium ion appears to play a role in causing the increase in blood flow in contracting skeletal muscle.

6. **Oxygen** levels within the blood, vessel wall, and surrounding tissue are also important in local regulation of blood flow. Decreased tissue partial pressure of oxygen ($PO_2$) resulting from reduced oxygen supply or increased oxygen utilization by tissues causes vasodilation. Hypoxia-induced vasodilation may be direct (inadequate $O_2$ to sustain smooth muscle contraction) or indirect via the production of vasodilator metabolites (e.g., adenosine, lactic acid, $H^+$). Although hypoxia causes vasodilation in nearly all vascular beds, there is a notable exception—it causes vasoconstriction in the pulmonary circulation.

7. **Osmolarity** changes in the blood and in the tissue interstitium have been implicated in local blood flow regulation. It is well known that intra-arterial infusions of hyperosmolar solutions can produce vasodilation. The molecules making up the hyperosmolar solution need not be vasoactive. Tissue ischemia and increased metabolic activity raise the osmolarity of the tissue interstitial fluid and venous blood. Therefore, it has been suggested that nonspecific changes in osmolarity may play a role in the regulation of blood flow.

Several tissue factors involved in regulating blood flow are not directly coupled to tissue metabolism. These include paracrine hormones such as histamine, bradykinin, and products of arachidonic acid (eicosanoids). **Histamine**, released by tissue mast cells in response to injury, inflammation, and allergic responses, causes arteriolar vasodilation, venous constriction in some vascular beds, and increased capillary permeability. Both $H_1$ and $H_2$ histamine receptors are involved in the vascular effects of histamine. **Bradykinin** is formed from the action of kallikrein (a proteolytic enzyme) acting on alpha2-globulin (kininogen), which is found in blood and tissues. Like histamine, bradykinin is a powerful dilator of arterioles. It acts on vascular bradykinin receptors, which stimulate nitric oxide formation by the vascular endothelium, thereby producing vasodilation. In addition, bradykinin stimulates prostacyclin formation, which produces vasodilation. One of the enzymes responsible for breaking down bradykinin is angiotensin-converting enzyme (ACE) (see Chapter 6, Fig. 6.11). Therefore, drugs that inhibit ACE not only decrease angiotensin II but also increase bradykinin, which is believed to be partly responsible for the vasodilation accompanying ACE inhibition. Some **arachidonic acid metabolites** such as prostaglandin $E_2$ ($PGE_2$) are vasodilators, whereas other eicosanoids such as $PGF_{2\alpha}$, thromboxanes, and leukotrienes are generally vasoconstrictors. Drugs that block the formation of these eicosanoids (e.g., cyclooxygenase inhibitors such as aspirin or ibuprofen) alter vascular control by these substances.

## Endothelial Factors

The vascular endothelium serves an important paracrine role in the regulation of smooth muscle tone and organ blood flow. As described in Chapter 3, the vascular endothelium produces vasoactive substances that have significant effects on vascular smooth muscle. Circulating (endocrine) and paracrine hormones, shearing forces, hypoxia, and many different drugs can stimulate the formation and release of endothelial substances (Fig. 7.2). Among their many actions, two of these substances, nitric oxide and prostacyclin, are powerful

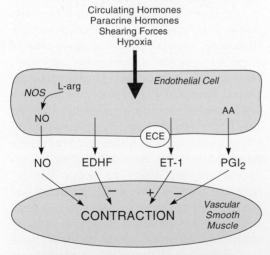

Circulating Hormones
Paracrine Hormones
Shearing Forces
Hypoxia

■ **FIGURE 7.2** Endothelial-derived vasoactive factors. Nitric oxide (NO) formed by nitric oxide synthase (*NOS*) acting on L-arginine (*L-arg*), endothelial-derived hyperpolarizing factor (*EDHF*), and prostacyclin (*PGI₂*) derived from arachidonic acid (*AA*) inhibit (−) smooth muscle contraction and cause vasodilation. Endothelin-1 (*ET-1*) formed by endothelin-converting enzyme (*ECE*) causes smooth muscle contraction (+). The formation and release of these substances are influenced by circulating and paracrine hormones, shearing forces acting on the endothelium, hypoxia, and many different drugs.

vasodilators. In contrast, endothelin-1 is a powerful vasoconstrictor.

**Nitric oxide** appears to be the most important in terms of regulating blood flow under normal physiologic conditions. Nitric oxide is synthesized in the endothelium by the action of a nitric oxide synthase (NOS) enzyme on the amino acid, L-arginine. Nitric oxide diffuses from the endothelial cell to the smooth muscle cells where it binds to and activates intracellular guanylyl cyclase to form cGMP, which leads to smooth muscle relaxation (see Chapter 3). If nitric oxide synthesis is inhibited pharmacologically using NOS inhibitors, vasoconstriction occurs in most vascular beds. This demonstrates that there normally is a basal release of nitric oxide that inhibits vascular tone; therefore, blocking nitric oxide formation leads to an increase in tone.

Nitric oxide is involved in what is termed **flow-dependent vasodilation.** Experimental studies have shown that an increase in vessel flow (actually an increase in shearing forces acting on the vascular endothelium) stimulates endothelial nitric oxide production, which causes vasodilation. Flow-dependent vasodilation is particularly important as a mechanism for increasing coronary blood flow when cardiac activity and metabolism are increased. Impaired nitric oxide synthesis or decreased bioavailability, as occurs during coronary artery disease, limits the ability of coronary blood flow to increase when cardiac activity and oxygen demand are increased. Other disorders such as hypertension, cerebrovascular disease, and diabetes are associated with impaired endothelial control of vascular function as well.

Another endothelial factor is **endothelial-derived hyperpolarizing factor (EDHF).** Some substances (e.g., acetylcholine, bradykinin) that stimulate nitric oxide production stimulate EDHF as well. The identity of this factor is not known for certain, but its release causes smooth muscle hyperpolarization and relaxation.

**Prostacyclin ($PGI_2$)** is formed from arachidonic acid and the cyclooxygenase enzyme within endothelial cells. This paracrine substance is a potent vasodilator in addition to serving as an inhibitor of platelet aggregation. $PGI_2$ synthesis is stimulated by adenosine and nitric oxide, as well as by many other substances, and therefore can play a secondary role to the vasodilation produced by other substances. It causes vasodilation by activating smooth muscle adenylyl cyclase, which increases cAMP (see Chapter 3).

**Endothelin-1** (ET-1) is a potent vasoconstrictor substance that is synthesized from an intracellular precursor by endothelin-converting enzyme (ECE) found on the endothelial cell membrane. ET-1 binds to $ET_A$ receptors on smooth muscle cells, which are coupled to Gq-proteins (see Chapter 3). ET-1 can also bind to a second type of receptor ($ET_B$) located on the vascular endothelium that stimulates nitric oxide and prostacyclin synthesis and release, which act as negative feedback mechanisms to counteract the $ET_A$-mediated vasoconstrictor effects of ET-1.

ET-1 formation and release by endothelial cells is stimulated by angiotensin II, vasopressin (antidiuretic hormone, ADH), thrombin, cytokines, reactive oxygen species, and shearing forces acting on the vascular endothelium. ET-1 release is inhibited by nitric oxide, as well as by prostacyclin and atrial natriuretic peptide. Some forms of hypertension (e.g., pulmonary artery hypertension) appear to involve ET-1 and are treated with ET-1 receptor blockers.

## Smooth Muscle (Myogenic) Mechanisms

Myogenic mechanisms originate within the smooth muscle of blood vessels, particularly in small arteries and arterioles. When the lumen of a blood vessel is suddenly expanded, as occurs when intravascular pressure is suddenly increased, the smooth muscle responds by contracting in order to restore the vessel diameter and resistance. Conversely, a reduction in intravascular pressure results in smooth muscle relaxation and vasodilation. Electrophysiologic studies have shown that vascular smooth muscle cells depolarize when stretched, leading to calcium entry into the cell (primarily through L-type calcium channels),

phosphorylation of myosin light chains, and contraction (see Chapter 3).

Myogenic behavior has been observed in many different vascular beds, although its relative functional significance differs among organs. It is difficult to evaluate myogenic mechanisms in vivo because changes in pressure are usually associated with changes in flow that trigger metabolic mechanisms, which usually dominate over myogenic mechanisms. For example, increasing venous pressure to a vascular bed should activate myogenic mechanisms to produce vasoconstriction because elevated venous pressures are transmitted back to the precapillary resistance vessels; however, the reduction in blood flow associated with the increase in venous pressure (which reduces perfusion pressure) activates tissue metabolic mechanisms that cause vasodilation. In most organs, conducting such an experiment usually results in vasodilation because the metabolic vasodilator response overrides the myogenic vasoconstrictor response, if present.

## Extravascular Compression

Mechanical compressive forces can affect vascular resistance and blood flow within organs. Sometimes this occurs during normal physiologic conditions; at other times, compressive forces can be the result of pathologic mechanisms. The pressure that distends the wall of a blood vessel is the transmural pressure (inside minus outside pressure). Therefore, if the pressure outside of the vessel increases, then the transmural pressure decreases. At very high extravascular pressures, a vessel can completely collapse. Therefore, veins, which have a relatively low intravascular pressure, are more likely to collapse when extravascular pressure is elevated; however, arteries can also become significantly compressed when extravascular pressure is elevated to very high levels.

Several examples of mechanical compression affecting organ blood flow exist. During cardiac systole or skeletal muscle contraction (particularly tetanic contractions), vascular resistance is greatly increased and blood flow is impeded by mechanical compression. Lung inflation and deflation alter pulmonary vascular transmural pressures (see Fig. 5.16) and thereby have substantial effects on pulmonary vascular resistance. Excessive distension of the gastrointestinal tract, as occurs during intestinal obstruction, can increase vascular resistance in the wall of the intestine to a point where tissues become ischemic. Blood vessels in organs such as the brain or kidneys, which are surrounded by a rigid cranium or capsule, are particularly susceptible to increases in extravascular pressure that occur with edema, vascular hemorrhage (e.g., cerebral stroke), or the growth of a tumor.

## Autoregulation of Blood Flow

*Autoregulation is the intrinsic ability of an organ to maintain a constant blood flow despite changes in perfusion pressure.* For example, if perfusion pressure is decreased to an organ by partial occlusion of the artery supplying the organ, blood flow will initially fall, then return toward normal levels over the next few minutes. This autoregulatory response occurs in isolated, perfused organs, which are not subject to neural or humoral influences. Therefore, it is a local or intrinsic response of the organ.

When perfusion pressure (arterial – venous pressure; $P_A - P_V$) initially decreases, blood flow (F) falls because of the following relationship between pressure, flow, and resistance (R):

$$F = \frac{(P_A - P_V)}{R}$$

If resistance remains unchanged, the reduction in flow will be proportionate to the reduction in perfusion pressure; however, in most organs of the body, resistance does not remain constant when perfusion pressure is decreased. The reductions in flow and perfusion pressure are thought to activate metabolic and myogenic mechanisms that cause arteriolar vasodilation and a fall in resistance (R). As resistance decreases, blood flow increases despite the presence of a reduced perfusion pressure. This autoregulatory response is shown in the left panel of Figure 7.3. For example, if perfusion pressure is reduced from 100 to 70 mm Hg, it causes flow to decrease initially by approximately 30%. Over the next few minutes, however, flow begins to increase back toward control as the organ blood flow is autoregulated (red lines). Blood flow increases because vascular resistance falls as the resistance vessels dilate.

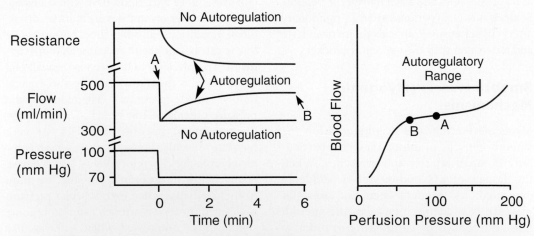

■ **FIGURE 7.3** Autoregulation of blood flow. The **left panel** shows that decreasing perfusion pressure from 100 to 70 mm Hg at point *A* results in a transient decrease in flow. If no autoregulation occurs, resistance remains unchanged and flow remains decreased. With autoregulation (*red line*), the initial fall in pressure and flow are followed by a decrease in vascular resistance, which causes flow to increase to a new steady-state level despite the reduced perfusion pressure (point *B*). The **right panel** shows steady-state, autoregulatory flows plotted against different perfusion pressures. Points *A* and *B* represent the control flow and autoregulatory steady-state flow, respectively, from the **left panel**. The autoregulatory range is the range of pressures over which flow shows little change. Below or above the autoregulatory range, flow changes are approximately proportional to the changes in perfusion pressure. The autoregulatory range as well as the flatness of the autoregulatory response curve varies among organs.

If the perfusion pressure to an organ is increased and decreased over a wide range of pressures and the steady-state autoregulatory flow response is measured, then the relationship between steady-state flow and perfusion pressure can be plotted as shown in the right panel of Figure 7.3. There is a range of pressures (autoregulatory range) over which flow changes relatively little despite a large change in perfusion pressure. The "flatness" of the autoregulation curve varies considerably among organs; the flatter the relationship, the better the autoregulation. Coronary, cerebral, and renal circulations show a high degree of autoregulation, whereas skeletal muscle and gastrointestinal circulations show only a moderate degree of autoregulation. The cutaneous circulation displays virtually no autoregulation.

Autoregulation has limits even in organs that display a high degree of autoregulation. When the perfusion pressure falls below 60 to 70 mm Hg in the cerebral and coronary circulations, the resistance vessels become maximally dilated and their ability to autoregulate is lost. Furthermore, at very high perfusion pressures (~170 mm Hg in Fig. 7.3), the upper limit of the autoregulatory range is reached and the vessels undergo no further constriction with increases in perfusion pressure; therefore, flow increases as pressure increases. The autoregulatory response can be modulated by neurohumoral influences and disease states. For example, sympathetic stimulation and chronic hypertension can shift the cerebral autoregulatory range to the right as described later in this chapter.

Autoregulation may involve both metabolic and myogenic mechanisms. If the perfusion pressure to an organ is reduced, the initial fall in blood flow leads to a fall in tissue $PO_2$ and the accumulation of vasodilator metabolites. These changes cause the resistance vessels to dilate in an attempt to restore normal flow. A reduction in perfusion pressure may also be sensed by the smooth muscle in resistance vessels, which responds by relaxing (myogenic response), leading to an increase in flow.

Under what conditions does autoregulation occur, and why is it important? In hypotension caused by blood loss, despite baroreceptor reflexes that lead to constriction of much of the systemic vasculature, blood flow to the brain and myocardium will not decline appreciably (unless the arterial pressure falls below the autoregulatory range). This is because of the strong capacity of these organs to autoregulate and their ability to escape sympathetic vasoconstrictor influences. The autoregulatory response helps to ensure that these critical organs have an adequate blood flow and oxygen delivery even in the presence of systemic hypotension.

Other situations occur in which systemic arterial pressure does not change, but in which autoregulation is very important nevertheless. Autoregulation can occur when a distributing artery to an organ (e.g., coronary artery) becomes partially occluded. This arterial stenosis increases resistance and the pressure drop along the vessel length. This reduces pressure in small distal arteries and arterioles, which are the primary vessels for regulating blood flow within an organ. These resistance vessels dilate in response to the reduced pressure and blood flow caused by the upstream stenosis. This autoregulatory response helps to maintain normal blood flow in the presence of upstream stenosis, and it is particularly important in organs such as the brain and heart that depend on a steady delivery of oxygen to maintain normal organ function.

**PROBLEM 7-1**

An experiment was conducted using an isolated perfused organ (e.g., intestinal segment) in which arterial and venous pressures were controlled while blood flow was measured. When venous pressure was suddenly raised from 0 to 15 mm Hg while arterial pressure was maintained at 100 mm Hg, flow decreased by 25%. Calculate the percentage change that occurred in vascular resistance in response to venous pressure elevation. Discuss the involvement of metabolic and myogenic mechanisms in this response.

## Reactive and Active Hyperemia

*Reactive hyperemia is the transient increase in organ blood flow that occurs following a brief period of ischemia, usually produced by temporary arterial occlusion.* Figure 7.4 shows the effects of a 2-minute arterial occlusion on blood flow. During the occlusion period, blood flow goes to zero. When the occlusion is released, blood flow rapidly increases above normal levels (hyperemia) that lasts for several minutes. In most tissues, experiments have suggested that the hyperemia occurs because during the occlusion period, tissue hypoxia and a buildup of vasoactive metabolites relax the smooth muscle of precapillary resistance vessels. When the occlusion is released and perfusion pressure is restored, flow becomes elevated because of the reduced vascular resistance. During the hyperemia, oxygen becomes replenished and vasodilator metabolites are washed out of the tissue, causing the resistance vessels to regain their normal vascular tone and thereby return flow to normal levels. The longer the period of occlusion, the greater the metabolic stimulus for vasodilation, leading to increases in peak flow and duration of hyperemia. Maximal vasodilation, as indicated by a maximal peak hyperemic flow, may occur following <1 minute of complete arterial occlusion, or it may require several minutes of occlusion depending on

the vascular bed and its metabolic activity. For example, in the beating heart (high metabolic activity), maximal reactive hyperemic responses are seen with coronary occlusions of <1 minute, whereas in resting skeletal muscle (low metabolic activity), several minutes of ischemia are necessary to elicit a maximal vasodilator response. Myogenic mechanisms may also contribute to reactive hyperemia in some tissues because arterial occlusion decreases the pressure in arterioles, which can lead to myogenic-mediated vasodilation.

Several examples of reactive hyperemia exist. The application of a tourniquet to a limb, and then its removal, results in reactive hyperemia. During surgery, arterial vessels are often clamped for a period of time; release of the arterial clamp results in reactive hyperemia. Transient coronary artery occlusions (e.g., coronary vasospasm) result in subsequent reactive hyperemia within the myocardium supplied by the coronary vessel.

*Active hyperemia is the increase in organ blood flow that is associated with increased metabolic activity of an organ or tissue.* With increased metabolic activity, vascular resistance decreases owing to vasodilation and vascular recruitment (particularly in skeletal muscle). Active hyperemia occurs during muscle contraction (also termed **exercise** or **functional hyperemia**), increased cardiac activity, increased mental activity, and increased gastrointestinal activity during food absorption.

In Figure 7.5, the left panel shows the effects of increasing tissue metabolism for 2 minutes on mean blood flow in a rhythmically contracting skeletal muscle. Within seconds of initiating contraction and the increase in metabolic activity, blood flow increases. The vasodilation is thought to be caused by a combination of tissue hypoxia and the generation of vasodilator metabolites such as potassium ion, carbon dioxide, nitric oxide, and adenosine. This increased blood flow (i.e., hyperemia) is maintained throughout the period of increased metabolic activity and then subsides after contractions cease and normal metabolism is restored. The amplitude of the active hyperemia is closely related to the increase in metabolic activity (e.g., oxygen consumption)

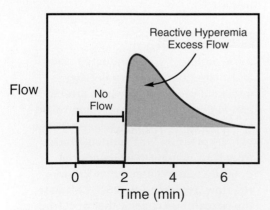

■ **FIGURE 7.4** Reactive hyperemia. Arterial occlusion (no flow) for 2 minutes followed by reperfusion results in a transient increase in blood flow (reactive hyperemia). The magnitude and duration of the reactive hyperemia are directly related to the duration of ischemia.

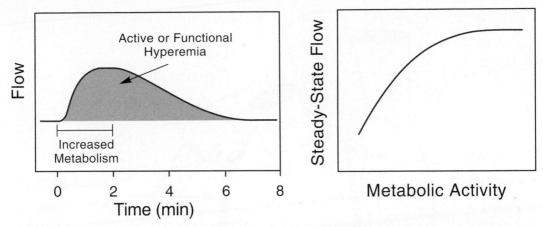

■ **FIGURE 7.5** Active hyperemia. The **left panel** shows that increasing tissue metabolism for 2 minutes transiently increases blood flow (active or functional hyperemia). The **right panel** shows that the steady-state increase in blood flow during active hyperemia is directly related to the increase in metabolic activity until the vessels become maximally dilated and flow can no longer increase.

as shown in the right panel. At high levels of metabolic activity, the vasculature becomes maximally dilated, resulting in a maximal increase in blood flow. Active hyperemia is important because it increases oxygen delivery to tissues at a time of increased oxygen demand. Furthermore, the increased blood flow enhances the removal of metabolic waste products from the tissue.

The vasodilatory capacity during active hyperemia differs considerably among organs. In skeletal muscle, blood flow can increase more than 20- to 50-fold during exercise, depending on the type of muscle. Cerebral blood flow, in contrast, increases no more than twofold at maximal metabolic activity. The reason for this difference is that resting skeletal muscle has a high degree of vascular tone in contrast to the cerebral circulation, which has a relatively low degree of vascular tone because of its higher metabolic rate under basal conditions.

## SPECIAL CIRCULATIONS

### Coronary Circulation

In order to supply sufficient oxygen to support the high oxidative metabolism of the beating heart, there must be an extensive network of vessels that provide blood flow throughout the myocardium. These vessels are the coronary arteries and veins. Regulatory mechanisms exist to ensure that adequate oxygen is delivered to the myocardium. Coronary artery disease or the failure of regulatory mechanisms can lead to insufficient oxygen delivery to the myocardium, which will impair cardiac function.

### CORONARY VASCULAR ANATOMY

The two major branches of the coronary circulation are the left main and right main coronary arteries (Fig. 7.6). These vessels arise from coronary ostia, which are small openings in the wall of the ascending aorta just distal to the aortic valve. The **left main coronary artery** is relatively short in length (~1 cm). After coursing behind the pulmonary artery trunk, it divides into the **left anterior descending artery**, which travels along the interventricular groove on the anterior surface of the heart, and the **circumflex artery**, which travels posteriorly along the groove between the left atrium and ventricle. These branches of the left coronary artery supply blood primarily to the left ventricle and atrium. The **right main coronary artery** travels between the right atrium and ventricle (left atrioventricular groove) toward the posterior regions of the heart. This vessel and its branches serve the right ventricle and atrium, and in most individuals, the inferoposterior region of the left ventricle. Significant variation is possible among

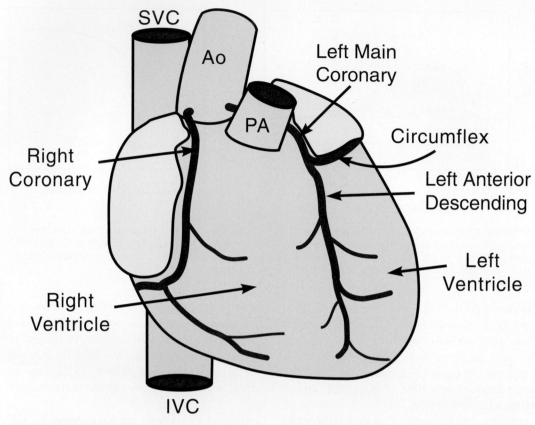

■ **FIGURE 7.6** Anterior view of the heart showing the major coronary arteries. The left main artery arises from the aorta (*Ao*) just distal to the aortic valve, travels behind the pulmonary artery (*PA*), and then branches into the circumflex artery (courses along the left atrioventricular groove) and left anterior descending artery (courses along the interventricular groove), both of which primarily supply blood to the left ventricle. The right coronary artery arises from the aorta and travels between the right atrium and ventricle toward the posterior regions of the heart to supply the right ventricle and atrium and the infero-posterior wall of the left ventricle. *SVC*, superior vena cava; *IVC*, inferior vena cava.

individuals in the anatomical arrangement and distribution of flow by the coronary vessels.

The major coronary arteries lie on the epicardial surface of the heart and serve as low-resistance distribution vessels. These epicardial arteries give off smaller branches that dive into the myocardium and become the microvascular resistance vessels that regulate coronary blood flow. The resistance vessels give rise to a dense capillary network so that each cardiac myocyte is closely associated with several capillaries. The high capillary-to-fiber density ensures short diffusion distances to maximize oxygen transport into the cells and removal of metabolic waste products (e.g., $CO_2$, $H^+$) (see Chapter 8).

Coronary veins are located adjacent to coronary arteries. These veins drain into the **coronary sinus** located on the posterior aspect of the heart. Blood flow from the coronary sinus empties into the right atrium. Some drainage also occurs directly into the cardiac chambers through the anterior cardiac veins and **thebesian vessels**.

### REGULATION OF CORONARY BLOOD FLOW

When flow is measured within an epicardial coronary artery, it is found to decrease during cardiac systole and increase during diastole (Fig. 7.7). Therefore, *most of the blood flow to the myocardium occurs during diastole*. The

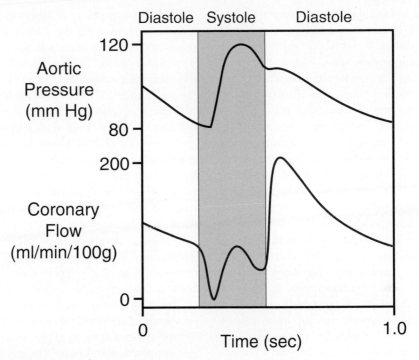

**■ FIGURE 7.7** Pulsatile nature of coronary blood flow measured in the left coronary artery. Flow is lower during systole because of mechanical compression of intramuscular coronary vessels. Flow is maximal early in diastole as the heart is relaxing, and then it falls as aortic pressure declines.

reason that coronary flow is influenced by the cardiac cycle is that during systole, the contraction of the myocardium compresses the microvasculature within the ventricular wall, thereby increasing resistance and decreasing flow. During systole, blood flow is reduced to the greatest extent within the innermost regions of the ventricular wall (i.e., in the subendocardium) because this is where the compressive forces are greatest. (This results in the subendocardial regions being more susceptible to ischemic injury when coronary artery disease or reduced aortic pressure is present.) As the ventricle begins to relax in early diastole, the compressive forces are removed and blood flow is permitted to increase. Blood flow reaches a peak in early diastole and then falls passively as the aortic pressure falls toward its diastolic value. Therefore, it is the aortic pressure during diastole that is most crucial for perfusing the coronaries. This explains why increases in heart rate can reduce coronary perfusion. At high heart rates, the length of diastole is greatly shortened, which reduces the time for coronary perfusion.

This is not a problem when the coronary arteries are normal, because they dilate with increased heart rate and metabolism; however, if the coronaries are diseased and their vasodilator reserve is limited, increases in heart rate can limit coronary flow and lead to myocardial ischemia and anginal pain.

The mechanical forces affecting coronary flow are greatest within the left ventricle because this chamber develops pressures that are severalfold greater than those developed by the right ventricle (see Chapter 4). The right ventricle and, to a lesser extent, the atria show some effects of contraction and relaxation on blood flow within their musculature, but it is much less apparent than that observed in the left ventricle.

Mean coronary blood flow (averaged over several cardiac cycles) can range from 80 mL/min per 100 g of tissue at resting heart rates to over 400 mL/min per 100 g during exercise (see Table 7-1). Therefore, the coronary vasculature normally has a relatively high vasodilator reserve capacity.

*Coronary blood flow is primarily regulated by changes in tissue metabolism.* Adenosine has been shown to be important in dilating the coronary vessels when the myocardium becomes hypoxic or when cardiac metabolism increases during increased cardiac work. Experimental studies have shown that inhibiting adenosine formation, enhancing its breakdown to inosine, or blocking vascular adenosine receptors impairs coronary vasodilation under these conditions. In addition, nitric oxide has been shown to be important in coronary vessels, particularly in producing flow-dependent vasodilation. Finally, there is also some evidence that prostaglandins play a role in regulating coronary blood flow.

Coronary vessels are innervated by both sympathetic and parasympathetic nerves. Unlike most other vascular beds, activation of sympathetic nerves to the heart causes only transient coronary vasoconstriction (α-adrenoceptor mediated) followed by vasodilation. The vasodilation occurs because sympathetic activation of the heart also increases heart rate and inotropy through β-adrenoceptors, which leads to enhanced production of vasodilator metabolites that inhibit the vasoconstrictor response and cause vasodilation. This is termed **functional sympatholysis**. If β-adrenoceptors are blocked experimentally, sympathetic stimulation of the heart causes coronary vasoconstriction. Parasympathetic stimulation of the heart (i.e., vagal nerve activation) elicits modest coronary vasodilation owing to the direct effects of released acetylcholine on the coronaries. However, if parasympathetic activation of the heart results in a significant decrease in myocardial oxygen demand, local metabolic mechanisms increase coronary vascular tone (i.e., cause vasoconstriction). Therefore, parasympathetic activation of the heart generally results in a decrease in coronary blood flow, although the direct effect of parasympathetic stimulation of the coronary vessels is vasodilation.

## INSUFFICIENT CORONARY BLOOD FLOW

Coronary blood flow is crucial for the normal function of the heart. Because of the high oxygen consumption of the beating heart (see Chapter 4) and the fact that the heart relies on oxidative metabolism (see Chapter 3), coronary blood flow (oxygen delivery) and the metabolic activity of the heart need to be tightly coupled. This is all the more important because, as discussed in Chapter 4, the beating heart extracts more than half of the oxygen from the arterial blood; therefore, there is relatively little oxygen extraction reserve. In coronary artery disease, chronic narrowing of the vessels or impaired vascular function reduces maximal coronary blood flow (i.e., there is reduced vasodilator reserve). When this occurs, coronary flow fails to increase adequately as myocardial oxygen demands increase (Fig. 7.8). This leads to cardiac hypoxia and impaired contractile function.

The relationship between coronary blood flow and the metabolic demand of the heart is often discussed in terms of the myocardial **oxygen supply/demand ratio**. The oxygen supply is the amount of oxygen delivered per minute to the myocardium in the arterial blood (mL $O_2$/min), which is the product of the coronary blood flow (mL blood/min) and arterial oxygen content (mL $O_2$/mL blood). The oxygen demand of the heart is the myocardial oxygen consumption, which is the product of coronary blood flow and the difference between the arterial and venous oxygen contents

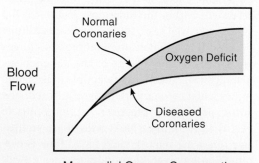

Myocardial Oxygen Consumption

■ **FIGURE 7.8** Relationship between coronary blood flow and myocardial oxygen consumption. Coronary blood flow increases as myocardial oxygen consumption increases. However, if the coronary vessels are diseased and have increased resistance owing to stenosis (*red line*), blood flow (and therefore oxygen delivery) will be limited at higher oxygen consumptions, leading to an oxygen deficit and myocardial hypoxia.

(see Equation 4-3). A decrease in the oxygen supply/demand ratio causes tissue hypoxia, which can result in chest pain (**angina pectoris**). This can occur by a decrease in oxygen supply (decreased coronary blood flow or arterial oxygen content), an increase in myocardial oxygen consumption, or a combination of the two. One of the therapeutic goals for people who have coronary artery disease and anginal pain is to increase the oxygen supply/demand ratio either by improving coronary flow (e.g., coronary bypass grafts or coronary stent placement) or by decreasing myocardial oxygen consumption by reducing heart rate, inotropy, preload, and afterload (see Chapter 4).

Both structural and functional changes occur when coronary arteries become diseased. Atherosclerotic processes decrease the lumen diameter, causing stenosis. This commonly occurs in the large epicardial arteries, although the disease also afflicts small vessels. The large coronary arteries ordinarily represent only a very small fraction of total coronary vascular resistance. Therefore, stenosis in these vessels needs to exceed a 60% to 70% reduction in lumen diameter (i.e., exceed the **critical stenosis**) to have significant effects on resting blood flow and maximal flow capacity (see Chapter 5).

In addition to narrowing the lumen and increasing resistance to flow, atherosclerosis causes endothelial damage and dysfunction. This leads to reduced nitric oxide and prostacyclin formation, which can precipitate coronary vasospasm and thrombus formation, leading to increased vascular resistance and decreased flow. Loss of these endothelial factors impairs vasodilation, which decreases the vasodilator reserve capacity. When coronary flow is compromised by coronary artery disease either at rest or during times of increased metabolic demand (e.g., during exercise), the myocardium becomes hypoxic, which can impair mechanical function, precipitate arrhythmias, and produce angina.

When coronary oxygen delivery is limited by disease, collateral vessels can play an important adjunct role in supplying oxygen to the heart. Conditions of chronic stress (e.g., chronic hypoxia or exercise training) stimulate the process of **angiogenesis**, which causes new blood vessels to form. **Collateralization** increases myocardial blood supply by increasing the number of parallel vessels, thereby reducing vascular resistance within the myocardium. This helps to supply blood flow to ischemic regions caused by vascular stenosis or thrombosis.

### CASE 7-1

A patient with known coronary artery disease (stenosis of multiple vessels) is also hypertensive. Explain why blood pressure–lowering drugs that produce reflex tachycardia should be not be used in such a patient.

## Cerebral Circulation

The brain is a highly oxidative organ that consumes almost 20% of resting total-body oxygen consumption. To deliver adequate oxygen, the cerebral blood flow needs to be relatively high, about 50 to 60 mL/min per 100 g tissue weight (see Table 7-1). Although the brain represents only about 2% of body weight, it receives approximately 14% of the cardiac output.

### MAJOR ARTERIES SUPPLYING THE BRAIN

The brain circulation is supplied by four principal arteries: the left and right **carotid arteries** and the left and right **vertebral arteries** (Fig. 7.9). The vertebral arteries join together on the ventral surface of the pons to form the **basilar artery**, which then travels up the brainstem to join the carotid arteries through interconnecting arteries, forming the **Circle of Willis**. Arterial vessels originating from the vertebral and basilar arteries as well as the Circle of Willis distribute blood flow to different regions of the brain. This interconnecting network of arterial vessels at the brainstem provides a safety mechanism for cerebral perfusion. If, for example, a carotid artery becomes partly occluded and flow is reduced through that artery, increased flow through the other interconnecting arteries can help improve perfusion of the affected portion of the brain.

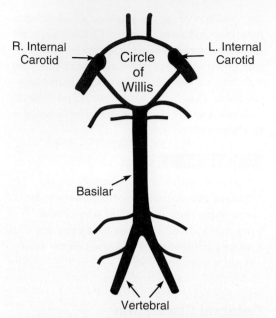

■ **FIGURE 7.9** Major cerebral arteries perfusing the brain. This view is of the ventral surface of the brain and brainstem. The carotid and vertebral arteries are the major source of cerebral blood flow and are interconnected through the Circle of Willis and basilar artery. Smaller branches from these vessels perfuse different brain regions. *L*, left; *R*, right.

## REGULATION OF CEREBRAL BLOOD FLOW

Like most other organs, cerebral blood flow is determined by its perfusion pressure (arterial–venous pressure) and its vascular resistance; however, because the cerebral circulation is located within a rigid cranium, changes in **intracranial pressure (ICP)** can have significant effects on cerebral perfusion (Fig. 7.10). ICP is the pressure found in the fluid-filled space between the rigid cranium and the brain tissue. For example, cerebral vascular hemorrhage, brain edema caused by cerebral trauma, or tumor growth can increase ICP, which can lead to vascular compression and reduced cerebral blood flow. The venous vessels are most susceptible to compression because of their low intravascular pressure, and thinner, compliant walls. Because ICP is normally greater than the venous pressure outside the cranium and the venous vessels can easily collapse, the effective perfusion pressure of the brain is not the mean arterial pressure (MAP) minus central venous pressure, but rather the MAP minus the ICP. ICP normally ranges from 0 to 10 mm Hg; however, if it becomes elevated (e.g., 20 mm Hg or greater), and especially if there is systemic hypotension, the effective cerebral perfusion pressure (CPP) and blood flow can be significantly reduced.

Like the coronary circulation, the cerebral blood flow is tightly coupled to oxygen consumption. Therefore, cerebral blood flow increases (active or functional hyperemia) when neuronal activity and oxygen

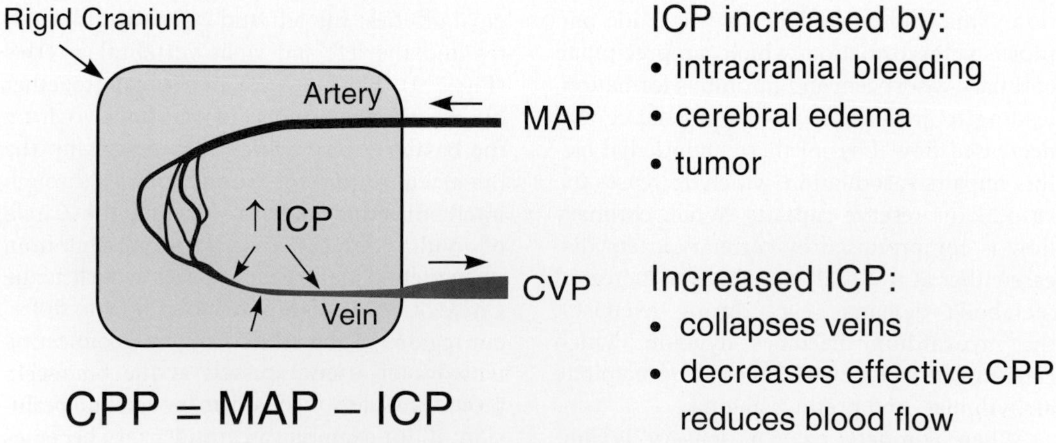

**ICP increased by:**
- intracranial bleeding
- cerebral edema
- tumor

**Increased ICP:**
- collapses veins
- decreases effective CPP reduces blood flow

$$CPP = MAP - ICP$$

■ **FIGURE 7.10** Effects of intracranial pressure (*ICP*) on cerebral blood flow. ICP is the pressure within the rigid cranium (*gray* area of figure). Increased ICP decreases transmural pressure (inside minus outside pressure) of blood vessels (particularly veins), which can cause vascular collapse, increased resistance, and decreased blood flow. Therefore, the effective cerebral perfusion pressure (*CPP*) is mean arterial pressure (*MAP*) minus ICP. *CVP*, central venous pressure.

consumption are increased. Changes in neuronal activity in specific brain regions lead to increases in blood flow to those regions.

The brain shows excellent autoregulation between MAPs of about 60 and 130 mm Hg (Fig. 7.11). This is important because cerebral function relies on a steady supply of oxygen and cannot afford to be subjected to a reduction in flow caused by a fall in arterial pressure. If MAP falls below 60 mm Hg, cerebral perfusion becomes impaired, which results in depressed neuronal function, mental confusion, and loss of consciousness. When arterial pressure is above the autoregulatory range (e.g., in a hypertensive crisis), blood flow and pressures within the cerebral microcirculation increase. This may cause endothelial and vascular damage, disruption of the blood–brain barrier, and hemorrhagic stroke. With chronic hypertension, the autoregulatory curve shifts to the right (see Fig. 7.11), which helps to protect the brain at higher arterial pressures. However, this rightward shift then makes the brain more susceptible to reduced perfusion when arterial pressure falls below the lower end of the rightward-shifted autoregulatory range.

Local metabolic mechanisms play a dominant role in the control of cerebral blood flow. Considerable evidence indicates that changes in carbon dioxide are important for coupling

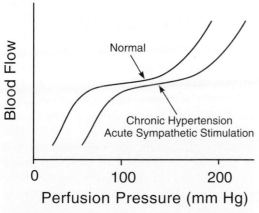

■ **FIGURE 7.11** Autoregulation of cerebral blood flow. Cerebral blood flow shows excellent autoregulation between MAPs of 60 and 130 mm Hg. The autoregulatory curve shifts to the right with chronic hypertension or acute sympathetic activation. This shift helps to protect the brain from the damaging effects of elevated pressure.

tissue metabolism and blood flow. Increased oxidative metabolism increases carbon dioxide production, which causes vasodilation. It is thought that the carbon dioxide diffuses into the cerebrospinal fluid, where hydrogen ion is formed by the action of carbonic anhydrase; the hydrogen ion then causes vasodilation. In addition, carbon dioxide and hydrogen ion increase when perfusion is reduced because of impaired washout of carbon dioxide. Adenosine, nitric oxide, potassium ion, and myogenic mechanisms have also been implicated in the local regulation of cerebral blood flow.

Cerebral blood flow is strongly influenced by the partial pressure of carbon dioxide and, to a lesser extent, oxygen in the arterial blood (Fig. 7.12). Cerebral blood flow is highly sensitive to small changes in arterial partial pressure of $CO_2$ ($PCO_2$) from its normal value of about 40 mm Hg, with increased $PCO_2$ (hypercapnia) causing pronounced vasodilation and decreased $PCO_2$ (hypocapnia) causing vasoconstriction. Hydrogen ion appears to be responsible for the changes in vascular resistance when changes occur in arterial $PCO_2$. The importance of $CO_2$ in regulating cerebral blood flow can be demonstrated when a person hyperventilates, which decreases arterial $PCO_2$. When this occurs, a person becomes "light headed" as the reduced $PCO_2$ causes cerebral blood flow to decrease. Severe arterial hypoxia (hypoxemia) increases cerebral blood flow. Arterial $PO_2$ is normally about 95 to 100 mm Hg. If the $PO_2$ falls below 50 mm Hg (severe arterial hypoxia), it elicits a strong vasodilator response in the brain, which helps to maintain oxygen delivery despite the reduction in arterial oxygen content. As described in Chapter 6, decreased arterial $PO_2$ and increased $PCO_2$ stimulate chemoreceptors, which activate sympathetic efferents to the systemic vasculature to cause vasoconstriction; however, the direct effects of hypoxia and hypercapnia override the weak effects of sympathetic activation in the brain so that cerebral vasodilation occurs and oxygen delivery is enhanced.

Although sympathetic nerves innervate larger cerebral vessels, activation of these nerves has relatively little influence on cerebral blood

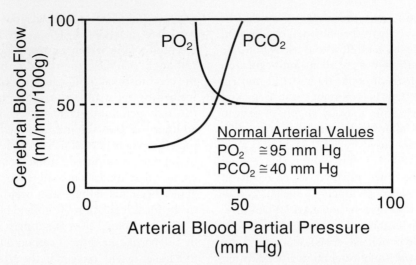

■ **FIGURE 7.12** Effects of arterial partial pressure of oxygen and carbon dioxide on cerebral blood flow. An arterial partial pressure of oxygen ($PO_2$) of <50 mm Hg (normal value is about 95 mm Hg) causes cerebral vasodilation and increased flow. A reduction in arterial partial pressure of carbon dioxide ($PCO_2$) below its normal value of 40 mm Hg decreases flow, whereas $PCO_2$ values >40 mm Hg increase flow. Therefore, cerebral blood flow is more sensitive to changes from normal arterial $PCO_2$ values than from normal arterial $PO_2$ values.

flow. Maximal sympathetic activation increases cerebral vascular resistance by no more than 20% to 30%, in contrast to an approximately 500% increase occurring in skeletal muscle. The reason, in part, for the weak sympathetic response by the cerebral vasculature is that metabolic mechanisms are dominant in regulating flow; therefore, functional sympatholysis occurs during sympathetic activation. This is crucial to preserve normal brain function; otherwise, every time a person stands up or exercises, both of which cause sympathetic activation, cerebral perfusion would decrease. Therefore, baroreceptor reflexes have little influence on cerebral blood flow. Sympathetic activation shifts the autoregulatory curve to the right, similar to what occurs with chronic hypertension.

In recent years, we have learned that neuropeptides originating in the brain significantly influence cerebral vascular tone, and they may be involved in producing headaches (e.g., migraine and cluster headaches) and cerebral vascular vasospasm during strokes. Parasympathetic cholinergic fibers innervating the cerebral vasculature release nitric oxide and **vasoactive intestinal polypeptide (VIP)**. These substances, along with acetylcholine, produce localized vasodilation. Other nerves appear to release the local vasodilators **calcitonin gene-related peptide (CGRP)** and **substance P**. Sympathetic adrenergic nerves can release **neuropeptide-Y (NPY)** in addition to norepinephrine, which causes localized vasoconstriction. Vascular and neuronal sources of endothelin-1 can also produce vasoconstriction within the brain.

## Skeletal Muscle Circulation

The primary function of skeletal muscle is to contract and generate mechanical forces to provide support to the skeleton and produce movement of joints. This mechanical activity consumes large amounts of energy and therefore requires delivery of considerable amounts of oxygen and substrates, as well as the efficient removal of metabolic waste products. Both oxygen delivery and metabolic waste removal functions are performed by the circulation.

### MICROVASCULAR ORGANIZATION IN SKELETAL MUSCLE

The circulation within skeletal muscle is highly organized (Fig. 7.13). Arterioles give

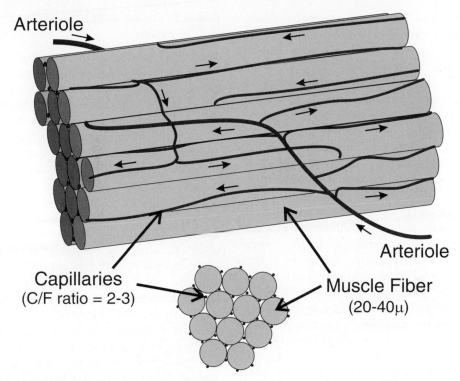

**■ FIGURE 7.13** Microvascular organization in skeletal muscle. Long, parallel muscle fibers are each surrounded by multiple, parallel capillaries that arise from arterioles. As shown in the cross section, there are typically 2 to 3 capillaries per muscle fiber (*C/F ratio*), although that varies depending on the muscle type. Arrows represent direction of flow.

rise to capillaries that generally run parallel to the muscle fibers. Because a given region of muscle may be served by multiple arterioles, the direction of flow in some capillaries may be opposite to the direction of flow in nearby capillaries. Each muscle fiber, which can be 20 to 40 µm in diameter, is surrounded by three to four capillaries. Because more than one muscle fiber may share an adjacent capillary, the overall capillary-to-fiber ratio is 2 to 3, depending on the type of muscle. Muscle fibers that have a high oxidative capacity generally have a higher capillary-to-fiber ratio than fibers that have a low oxidative capacity, but a high anaerobic (glycolytic) capacity. Muscles with a higher oxidative capacity and a greater number of capillaries generally have a higher maximal flow capacity.

When the muscle is not contracting, relatively little oxygen is required and only about one-fourth of the capillaries are perfused. In contrast, during muscle contraction and active hyperemia, all the anatomical capillaries may be perfused, which increases the number of flowing capillaries around each muscle fiber (termed **capillary recruitment**). This anatomical arrangement of capillaries and the ability to recruit capillaries decreases diffusion distances, leading to an efficient exchange of gases and molecules between the blood and the myocytes, particularly under conditions of high oxygen demand.

### MUSCLE BLOOD FLOW AT REST AND DURING CONTRACTION

In resting humans, almost 20% of cardiac output is delivered to skeletal muscle. This large cardiac output to muscle occurs not because blood flow is exceptionally high in resting muscle, but because skeletal muscle makes up about 40% of the body mass. In the resting, noncontracting state, muscle blood flow is about 3 mL/min per 100 g. This resting flow is much less than that found in organs such as the brain and kidneys, in which "resting" flows are about 55 and 400 mL/min per 100 g, respectively.

When muscles contract during exercise, blood flow can increase more than 20-fold. If muscle contraction is occurring during whole-body exercise (e.g., running), more than 80% of cardiac output can be directed to the contracting muscles. Therefore, skeletal muscle has a very large flow reserve (or capacity) relative to its blood flow at rest, indicating that the vasculature in resting muscle has a high degree of tone (see Table 7-1). This resting tone is brought about by the interplay between vasoconstrictor (e.g., sympathetic adrenergic and myogenic influences) and vasodilator influences (e.g., nitric oxide production, and tissue metabolites). In the resting state, the vasoconstrictor influences dominate, whereas during muscle contraction, vasodilator influences dominate to increase oxygen delivery to the contracting muscle fibers and remove metabolic waste products that accumulate. Vasodilation of resistance vessels, particularly the small terminal arterioles, not only increases muscle blood flow, but also increases the number of flowing capillaries. In the past, some have hypothesized that muscle capillary recruitment results from relaxation of precapillary sphincters; however, there is little or no direct evidence for their existence. Instead, capillary recruitment appears to be a consequence of altered distribution of microvascular pressures brought about by arteriolar dilation.

The blood flow response to skeletal muscle contraction depends on the type of contraction. With rhythmic or phasic contraction of muscle (Fig. 7.14, top panel), as occurs during normal locomotory activity, mean blood flow increases during the period of muscle activity. However, if blood flow is measured without filtering or averaging the flow signal, the flow is found to be phasic—flow decreases during contraction and increases during relaxation phases of the muscle activity because of mechanical compression of the vessels. In contrast, a sustained muscle contraction (e.g., lifting and holding a heavy weight) decreases mean blood flow during the period of contraction, followed by a postcontraction hyperemic response when the contraction ceases (see Fig. 7.14, bottom panel).

## REGULATION OF SKELETAL MUSCLE BLOOD FLOW

The precise mechanisms responsible for dilating skeletal muscle vasculature during contraction are not clearly understood, although many potential vasodilator candidates have been identified. These include increases in interstitial $K^+$ during muscle contraction, formation of adenosine (particularly during ischemic contractions), increased $H^+$ production, endothelial and skeletal muscle-derived nitric oxide and prostaglandins, and ATP release from red blood cells. Other candidates, although less likely, are $CO_2$, increased interstitial and blood osmolarity, and inorganic phosphate. It is very likely that multiple factors play a role and at different times during the flow response to muscle contraction. A nonchemical mechanism that is very important in facilitating blood flow during coordinated contractions of groups of muscles (as occurs during normal physical activity such as running) is the skeletal muscle pump (see Chapter 5). Regardless of the mechanisms involved in producing active hyperemia, the outcome is that there is a close correlation between the increase in oxygen consumption and the increase in blood flow during muscle contraction.

Skeletal muscle vasculature is innervated primarily by sympathetic adrenergic fibers. The norepinephrine released by these fibers binds to α-adrenoceptors and causes vasoconstriction. Under resting conditions, a significant portion of the vascular tone is generated by sympathetic activity, so that if a resting muscle is suddenly denervated or the α-adrenoceptors are blocked pharmacologically by a drug such as phentolamine, blood flow will transiently increase two- to threefold until local regulatory mechanisms reestablish a new steady-state flow. Activation of the sympathetic adrenergic nervous system (e.g., baroreceptor reflex in response to hypovolemia) can dramatically reduce blood flow in resting muscle. When this reduction in blood flow occurs, the muscle extracts more oxygen (the arterial–venous oxygen difference increases) and activates anaerobic pathways for ATP production. However,

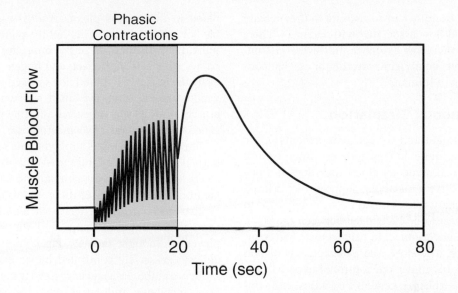

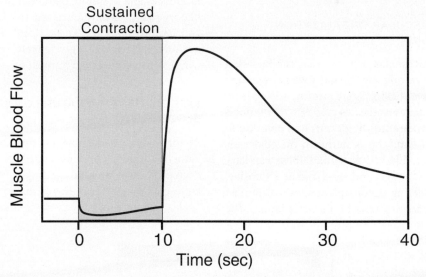

**■ FIGURE 7.14** Skeletal muscle active hyperemia following phasic and sustained (tetanic) contractions. The **top panel** shows that phasic contractions cause flow to decrease during contraction and increase during relaxation, although the net effect is an increase in flow during contraction. When contractions cease, a further increase in flow occurs because mechanical compression of the vasculature is removed. The **bottom panel** shows that sustained, tetanic contractions generate high intramuscular forces that compress the vasculature and reduce flow. When contraction ceases, a large hyperemia follows.

prolonged hypoperfusion of muscle caused by intense sympathetic activation eventually leads to vasodilator mechanisms dominating over the sympathetic vasoconstriction, leading to **sympathetic escape** and partial restoration of blood flow.

Evidence exists, at least in nonprimate species such as cats and dogs, for sympathetic cholinergic innervation of skeletal muscle resistance vessels. The neurotransmitter for these fibers is acetylcholine, which binds to muscarinic receptors to produce vasodilation. This branch of the autonomic nervous system has little or no influence on blood flow under resting conditions; however, activation of these fibers in anticipation of exercise and during exercise can contribute to the increase in blood flow associated with exercise. There is no convincing evidence, however, for similar active, neurogenic vasodilator mechanisms existing in humans.

## Cutaneous Circulation

The nutrient and oxygen requirements of the skin are quite low relative to other organs; therefore, cutaneous blood flow does not primarily serve a metabolic support role. Instead, the primary role of blood flow to the skin is to allow heat to be exchanged between the blood and the environment to help regulate body temperature. Therefore, the cutaneous circulation is primarily under the control of hypothalamic thermoregulatory centers that adjust the sympathetic outflow to the cutaneous vasculature.

### MICROVASCULAR ORGANIZATION OF THE SKIN

The microvascular network that supplies skin is unique among organs and varies depending on the type of skin. Small arteries arising from the subcutaneous tissues give rise to arterioles that penetrate into the dermis and give rise to capillaries that loop underneath the epidermis (Fig. 7.15). Blood flows from these capillary loops into venules and then into an extensive, interconnecting **venous plexus**, in which most of the cutaneous blood volume is found. The

blood in the venous plexus is also responsible for skin coloration in lightly pigmented individuals. In the skin of the nose, lips, ears, palms, toes, sole of the feet, and fingers (especially the fingertips), blood flows directly to the venous plexus from the small subcutaneous arteries through special interconnecting vessels called **arteriovenous (AV) anastomoses**.

The resistance vessels supplying the subepidermal capillary loops and the AV anastomoses are richly innervated by sympathetic adrenergic fibers. Constriction of these vessels during sympathetic activation decreases blood flow through the capillary loops and the venous plexus. Although the AV anastomoses are almost exclusively controlled by sympathetic influences, the resistance vessels respond to both metabolic influences and sympathetic influences and therefore demonstrate local regulatory phenomena such as reactive hyperemia and autoregulation. These local regulatory responses, however, are relatively weak compared to those observed in most other organs.

### EFFECTS OF TEMPERATURE ON SKIN BLOOD FLOW

At normal body and ambient temperatures, sympathetic adrenergic activity contributes to a high degree of vascular tone, and skin blood flow represents about 4% of the cardiac output (see Table 7-1). In times of severe cold stress, skin

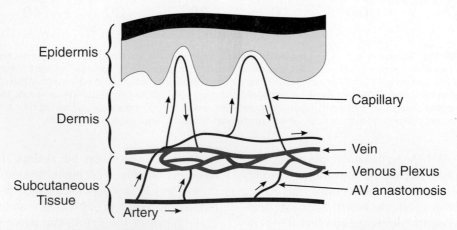

■ **FIGURE 7.15** Microvascular anatomy of the cutaneous circulation. Arteries within the subcutaneous tissue give rise to either arterioles that travel into the dermis and give rise to capillary loops or AV anastomoses that connect to a plexus of small veins in the subdermis. The venous plexus also receives blood from the capillary loops. Sympathetic stimulation constricts the resistance vessels and AV anastomoses, thereby decreasing dermal blood flow.

blood flow may be reduced to <1% of cardiac ouput, and during severe heat stress, skin blood flow can approach 60% of the cardiac output.

If core temperature decreases, heat retention mechanisms are activated by the hypothalamus, leading to increased sympathetic adrenergic outflow to the skin. This decreases cutaneous blood flow and reduces heat loss to the environment. If core temperature begins to rise (e.g., during physical exertion), heat loss mechanisms are activated by the hypothalamus, which decrease sympathetic adrenergic outflow to the skin. This reduces vasoconstrictor tone, thereby causing cutaneous vasodilation and increased blood flow. Vasodilation resulting from withdrawal of sympathetic vasoconstrictor influences is referred to as "passive vasodilation." If core temperature continues to rise, then "active vasodilation" results from sympathetic cholinergic nerve activation and the neuronal co-release of vasodilator substances such as vasoactive intestinal polypeptide (VIP). There is also evidence that substance P, histamine, prostaglandins, and nitric oxide may contribute to active vasodilation. Vasodilation enables more warm blood to circulate in the subepidermal layer of the skin so that more heat can be transferred to the environment.

Local changes in skin temperature selectively alter blood flow to the affected region. For example, if a heat source is placed on a small region of the skin on the back of the hand, blood flow will increase only to the region that is heated. This response appears to be mediated by local axon reflexes and local formation of nitric oxide instead of by changes in sympathetic discharge mediated by the hypothalamic thermoregulatory regions. Localized cooling produces vasoconstriction through local mechanisms that involve sympathetic adrenergic nerves and locally stimulated norepinephrine release. If tissue is exposed to extreme cold, a phenomenon called **cold-induced vasodilation** may occur following an initial vasoconstrictor response, especially if the exposed body region is a hand, foot, or face. This phenomenon causes light-colored skin to appear red, and it explains the rosy cheeks, ears, and nose a person may exhibit when exposed to very cold air temperatures. With continued exposure, alternating periods of dilation and constriction may occur ("**hunting response**"). The mechanism for cold-induced vasodilation is not clear, but it probably involves changes in local control of blood vessels.

## VASCULAR RESPONSES TO TISSUE INJURY

Tissue injury from mechanical trauma, heat, or chemicals releases paracrine substances such as histamine and bradykinin, which increase blood flow and cause localized edema by increasing microvascular permeability. If the skin is firmly stroked with a blunt object, the skin initially blanches owing to localized vasoconstriction. This is followed within a minute by the formation of a red line that spreads away from the site of injury (red flare); both the red line and red flare are caused by an increase in blood flow. Localized swelling (wheal formation) may then follow, caused by increased microvascular permeability and leakage of fluid into the interstitium. The red line, flare, and wheal are called the **triple response**. Both paracrine hormones and **local axon reflexes** are believed to be involved in the triple response. The vasodilator neurotransmitter involved in local axon reflexes has not been identified.

# Splanchnic Circulation

The splanchnic circulation includes blood flow to the gastrointestinal tract, spleen, pancreas, and liver. Blood flow to these combined organs represents 20% to 25% of cardiac output (see Table 7-1). Three major arteries arising from the abdominal aorta supply blood to the stomach, intestine, spleen, and liver—the celiac, superior mesenteric, and inferior mesenteric arteries. The following focuses on blood flow to the intestines and liver.

## INTESTINAL CIRCULATION

Several branches arising from the superior mesenteric artery supply blood to the intestine. These and subsequent branches travel through the mesentery that supports the intestine. Small arterial branches enter the outer muscular wall of the intestine and divide into several smaller orders of arteries and arterioles, most of which enter into the submucosa from which arterioles and capillaries arise to supply blood to the intestinal villi. Water and nutrients transported from the intestinal lumen into the villi enter the blood and are carried away by the portal venous circulation.

Intestinal blood flow is closely coupled to the primary function of the intestine, which is the absorption of water, electrolytes, and nutrients from the intestinal lumen. Therefore, intestinal blood flow increases when food is present within the intestine. In an adult human, blood flow to the intestine (superior mesenteric artery) in the fasted state is about 300 mL/min, and increases two- to threefold following a meal. This functional (absorptive) hyperemia is stimulated by gastrointestinal hormones such as gastrin and cholecystokinin, as well as by glucose, amino acids, and fatty acids that are absorbed by the intestine. Evidence exists that submucosal arteriolar vasodilation during functional hyperemia is mediated by hyperosmolarity and nitric oxide.

The intestinal circulation is strongly influenced by the activity of sympathetic adrenergic nerves. Increased sympathetic activity during exercise or in response to decreased baroreceptor firing (e.g., during hemorrhage or standing) constricts both arterial resistance vessels and venous capacitance vessels. Because the intestinal circulation receives such a large fraction of cardiac output, sympathetic stimulation of the intestine causes a substantial increase in total systemic vascular resistance. Additionally, the large blood volume contained within the venous vasculature is mobilized during sympathetic stimulation to increase central venous pressure. The spleen is also an important venous reservoir, and in some species (e.g., dogs), this organ stores hemoconcentrated blood. Stressful conditions in the dog (e.g., blood loss) can cause splenic contraction, which can substantially increase circulating blood volume and hematocrit.

Parasympathetic activation of the intestine increases motility and glandular secretions, which is associated with an increase in blood flow. This may involve metabolic mechanisms or local paracrine influences such as the formation of bradykinin and nitric oxide.

## HEPATIC CIRCULATION

Venous blood leaving the gastrointestinal tract, spleen, and pancreas drains into the hepatic portal vein, which supplies approximately 75% of the hepatic blood flow. The remainder of the hepatic blood flow is supplied by the hepatic artery, which is a branch of the celiac artery. Note that in this arrangement, most of the liver circulation is in series with the gastrointestinal, splenic, and pancreatic circulations. Therefore, changes in blood flow in these vascular beds have a significant influence on hepatic flow.

Terminal vessels from the hepatic portal vein and hepatic artery form sinusoids within the liver, which function as capillaries. The pressure within these sinusoids is very low, just a few mm Hg above central venous pressure. This is important because hepatic sinusoids are very permeable (see Chapter 8). Changes in central venous and hepatic venous pressure are almost completely transmitted to the sinusoids. Therefore, elevations in central venous pressure during right ventricular failure can cause substantial increases in sinusoid pressure and fluid filtration, leading to hepatic edema and accumulation of fluid within the abdominal cavity (ascites).

The liver circulation does not show classical autoregulation; however, decreases in hepatic portal flow result in reciprocal increases in hepatic artery flow, and vice versa. Sympathetic nerve activation constricts vessels derived from both the hepatic portal system and hepatic artery. The most important effect of sympathetic activation is on venous capacitance vessels, which contain a significant fraction (~15%) of the venous blood volume in the body. The liver, like the gastrointestinal circulation, functions as an important venous reservoir.

## Renal Circulation

Approximately 20% of the cardiac output perfuses the kidneys although the kidneys represent only about 0.4% of total body weight. Renal blood flow, therefore, is about 400 mL/min per 100 g of tissue weight, which is the highest of any major organ within the body (see Table 7-1). Only the pituitary and carotid bodies have higher blood flows per unit tissue weight. Whereas blood flow in many organs is closely coupled to tissue oxidative metabolism, this is not the case for the kidneys, in which the blood flow greatly exceeds the need for oxygen delivery. The very high blood flow results in a relatively low extraction of oxygen from the blood (about 1 to 2 mL $O_2$/mL blood) despite the fact that renal oxygen consumption is high (~5 mL $O_2$/min per 100 g). The reason for renal blood flow being so high is that the primary function of the kidneys is to filter blood and form urine. The kidney comprises three major regions: the cortex (the outer layer that contains glomeruli for filtration), the medulla (the middle region that contains renal tubules and capillaries involved in concentrating the urine), and the hilum (the inner region where the renal artery and vein, nerves, lymphatics, and ureter enter or leave the kidney). Because most of the filtering takes place within the cortex, about 90% of the total renal blood

flow supplies the cortex, with the remainder supplying the medullary regions.

## RENAL VASCULAR ORGANIZATION

The vascular organization within the kidneys is very different from most organs. The abdominal aorta gives rise to renal arteries that distribute blood flow to each kidney. The renal artery enters the kidney at the hilum and gives off several branches (**interlobar arteries**) that travel in the kidney toward the cortex. Subsequent branches (**arcuate and interlobular arteries**) then form **afferent arterioles**, which supply blood to each glomerulus (Fig. 7.16). As the afferent arteriole enters the glomerulus, it gives rise to a cluster of **glomerular capillaries**, from which fluid is filtered into Bowman capsule and into the renal proximal tubule. The glomerular capillaries then form an **efferent arteriole** from which arise **peritubular capillaries** that surround the renal tubules. Efferent arterioles associated with **juxtamedullary nephrons**

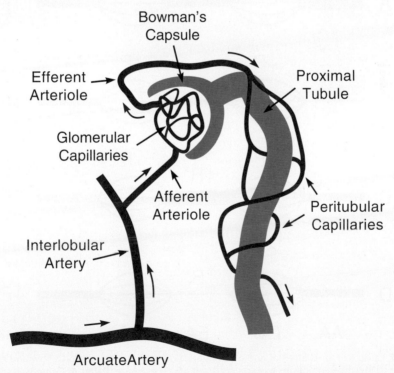

■ **FIGURE 7.16** Renal microvascular anatomy. Small vessels derived from branches of the renal artery form arcuate arteries and interlobular arteries, which then become afferent arterioles that supply blood to the glomerulus. As the afferent arteriole enters the glomerulus, it gives rise to a cluster of glomerular capillaries, from which fluid is filtered into Bowman capsule and into the renal proximal tubule. The glomerular capillaries then form an efferent arteriole from which arise peritubular capillaries that surround the renal tubules.

located in the inner cortex near the outer medulla give rise to very long capillaries (**vasa recta**) that loop down deep within the medulla. The capillaries are involved with countercurrent exchange and the maintenance of medullary osmotic gradients. Capillaries eventually form venules and then veins, which join together to exit the kidney as the renal vein. Therefore, within the kidney, a capillary bed (glomerular capillaries) is located between the two principal sites of resistance (afferent and efferent arterioles). Furthermore, a second capillary bed (peritubular capillaries) is in series with the glomerular capillaries and is separated by the efferent arteriole.

## RENAL HEMODYNAMICS

The vascular arrangement within the kidney is very important for filtration and reabsorption functions of the kidney. Changes

in afferent and efferent arteriole resistance affect not only blood flow, but also the hydrostatic pressures within the glomerular and peritubular capillaries. Glomerular capillary pressure, which is about 50 mm Hg, is much higher than that in capillaries found in other organs. This high pressure drives fluid filtration (see Chapter 8). The peritubular capillary pressure, however, is low (about 10 to 20 mm Hg). This is important because it permits fluid reabsorption to limit water loss and urine excretion. About 20% of the plasma entering the kidney is filtered. If significant reabsorption did not occur, a high rate of urine formation would rapidly lead to hypovolemia and hypotension and an excessive loss of electrolytes. Figure 7.17 shows the effects of afferent and efferent arteriole dilation and constriction on blood flow and glomerular

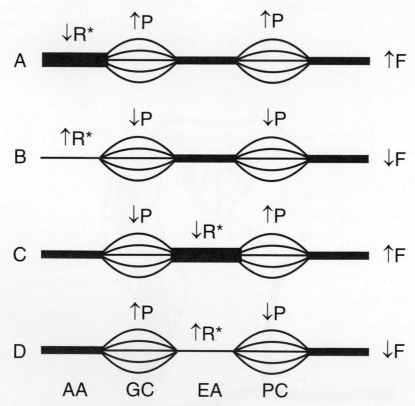

■ **FIGURE 7.17** Effects of renal afferent and efferent arteriole resistances on blood flow and renal capillary pressures. The following descriptions assume constant aortic pressure. **Panel A**. Decreased afferent arteriole (*AA*) resistance (*R*) increases glomerular capillary (*GC*) and peritubular capillary (*PC*) pressures (*P*) and increases flow (*F*). **Panel B**. Increased AA resistance decreases GC and PC pressures and decreases F. **Panel C**. Decreased efferent arteriole (*EA*) resistance decreases GC pressure, increases PC pressure, and increases F. **Panel D**. Increased EA resistance increases GC pressure, decreases PC pressure, and decreases F. *, arteriole undergoing resistance change.

capillary pressure. Dilation of the afferent arteriole (panel A) increases distal pressures (glomerular capillaries, efferent arteriole, and peritubular capillaries), while increasing total flow (assuming constant aortic pressure); this causes increased glomerular filtration. If the afferent arteriole constricts (panel B), distal pressures, glomerular filtration, and blood flow are reduced. If the efferent arteriole dilates (panel C), this increases total flow but reduces glomerular capillary pressure and filtration, while increasing peritubular capillary pressure. Efferent arteriole constriction increases glomerular capillary pressure and glomerular filtration while reducing flow and peritubular capillary pressure (panel D).

## REGULATION OF RENAL BLOOD FLOW

The renal circulation exhibits strong autoregulation between arterial pressures of about 80 to 180 mm Hg. Autoregulation of blood flow is accompanied by autoregulation of glomerular filtration so that filtration remains essentially unchanged over a wide range of arterial pressures. For this to occur, glomerular capillary pressure must remain unchanged when arterial pressure changes. This takes place because the principal site for autoregulation is the afferent arteriole. If arterial pressure falls, the afferent arteriole dilates, which helps to maintain the glomerular capillary pressure and flow despite the fall in arterial pressure.

Two mechanisms have been proposed to explain renal autoregulation: myogenic mechanisms and tubuloglomerular feedback. Myogenic mechanisms were described earlier in this chapter. Briefly, a reduction in afferent arteriole pressure is sensed by the vascular smooth muscle, which responds by relaxing; an increase in pressure induces smooth muscle contraction. The **tubuloglomerular feedback** mechanism is poorly understood, and the actual mediators have not been identified. It is believed, however, that changes in perfusion pressure alter glomerular filtration and therefore tubular flow and sodium delivery to the macula densa of the juxtaglomerular apparatus, which then signals the afferent arteriole to constrict or dilate. The macula densa of

the juxtaglomerular apparatus is a group of specialized cells of the distal tubule that lie adjacent to the afferent arteriole as the distal tubule loops up back toward the glomerulus. These cells sense solute osmolarity, particularly sodium chloride. Some investigators have proposed that adenosine (which is a vasoconstrictor in the kidney), locally produced angiotensin II (a vasoconstrictor), or vasodilators such as nitric oxide, $PGE_2$, and prostacyclin are involved in tubuloglomerular feedback and autoregulation. Locally produced angiotensin II strongly influences efferent arteriole tone. Thus, inhibition of angiotensin II formation by an ACE inhibitor dilates the efferent arteriole, which decreases glomerular capillary pressure and reduces glomerular filtration under some conditions (e.g., renal artery stenosis). Drugs that inhibit prostaglandin and prostacyclin biosynthesis (cyclooxygenase inhibitors such as aspirin or ibuprofen) alter renal hemodynamics and may impair renal function, particularly with long-term use.

The renal circulation responds strongly to sympathetic adrenergic stimulation. Under normal conditions, relatively little sympathetic tone on the renal vasculature occurs; however, with strenuous exercise or in response to severe hemorrhage, increased renal sympathetic nerve activity can virtually shut down renal blood flow. Because renal blood flow receives a relatively large fraction of cardiac output and therefore contributes significantly to systemic vascular resistance, renal vasoconstriction can serve an important role in maintaining arterial pressure under these conditions; however, intense renal vasoconstriction seriously impairs renal perfusion and function, and it can lead to renal failure.

## Pulmonary Circulation

Two separate circulations perfusing respiratory structures exist: the pulmonary circulation, which is derived from the pulmonary artery and supplies blood flow to the alveoli for gas exchange, and the bronchial circulation, which is derived from the thoracic aorta and supplies nutrient flow to the trachea and bronchial structures. The pulmonary circulation receives all of the cardiac output of the right ventricle, whereas the bronchial circulation receives about 1% of the left ventricular output. The following focuses on the pulmonary circulation.

The pulmonary circulation is a low-resistance, low-pressure, high-compliance vascular bed. Although the pulmonary circulation receives the same cardiac output as the systemic circulation, the pulmonary pressures are much lower. The pulmonary artery systolic and diastolic pressures are about 25 and 10 mm Hg, respectively. The mean pulmonary artery pressure is therefore about 15 mm Hg. If we assume that the left atrial pressure averages 8 mm Hg, the perfusion pressure for the pulmonary circulation (mean pulmonary artery pressure minus left atrial pressure) is only about 7 mm Hg. This is considerably lower than the perfusion pressure for the systemic circulation (about 90 mm Hg). Because the flow is the same, but the perfusion pressure is much lower in the pulmonary circulation, the pulmonary vascular resistance must be very low. In fact, pulmonary vascular resistance is generally 10- to 15-fold lower than systemic vascular resistance. The reason for the much lower pulmonary vascular resistance is that the vessels are larger in diameter, shorter in length, and have many more parallel elements than the systemic circulation.

Pulmonary vessels are also much more compliant than systemic vessels. Because of this, an increase in right ventricular output does not cause a proportionate increase in pulmonary artery pressure. The reason for this is that the pulmonary vessels passively distend as the pulmonary artery pressure increases, which lowers their resistance. Increased pressure also recruits additional pulmonary capillaries, which further reduces resistance. This high vascular compliance and ability to recruit capillaries are important mechanisms for preventing pulmonary vascular pressures from rising too high when cardiac output increases (e.g., during exercise). If there were no change in pulmonary vascular resistance, then increasing cardiac output five-fold during exercise would cause mean pulmonary artery pressure to increase from 15 to 43 mm Hg (assuming left atrial pressure remains at 8 mm Hg), and the pulmonary artery systolic pressure would be even higher.

Increased pulmonary vascular pressure can have two adverse consequences. First, increased pulmonary artery pressure increases the afterload on the right ventricle, which can impair ejection, and with chronic pressure elevation, cause right ventricular failure. Second, an increase in pulmonary capillary pressure increases fluid filtration (see Chapter 8), which can lead to pulmonary edema. Pulmonary capillary pressures are ordinarily about 10 mm Hg, which is less than half the value found in most other organs, and this low pressure is necessary to ensure that excessive fluid filtration from the pulmonary capillaries does not occur under normal circumstances.

Unlike other major organs, the concept of blood flow autoregulation is not applicable to the pulmonary circulation because pulmonary artery pressure is the dependent variable instead of flow. The reason for this is that the entire pulmonary blood flow is determined by the right ventricular output, and therefore, pulmonary artery pressure changes as a function of this flow and the pulmonary vascular resistance. Because other organs of the body are in parallel with each other, changes in left ventricular output do not necessarily change blood flow in a given organ except through changes in arterial pressure that may occur. Therefore, in other organs, blood flow is the dependent variable because flow depends on perfusion pressure and organ vascular resistance. Instead of autoregulating blood flow, the pulmonary circulation autoregulates pulmonary arterial pressure through passive changes in resistance of highly compliant vessels and through vessel recruitment.

Because of their low pressures and high compliance, pulmonary vascular diameters are strongly influenced by gravity and by changes in intrapleural pressure during respiration. When a person stands up, gravity increases hydrostatic pressures within vessels located in the lower regions of the lungs, which distends these vessels, decreases resistance, and increases blood flow to the lower regions. In contrast, vessels located in the upper regions of the lungs have reduced intravascular pressures; this increases resistance and reduces blood flow when a person is standing. Changes in intrapleural pressure during respiration (see Chapter 5) alter the transmural pressure that distends the vessels. For example, during normal inspiration, the fall in intrapleural pressure increases vascular transmural pressure, which distends extra-alveolar vessels (i.e., pulmonary arteries and veins), decreases resistance, and increases regional flow. The opposite occurs during a forced expiration, particularly against a high resistance (e.g., Valsalva maneuver). Vessels associated with the alveoli are compressed as the alveoli fill with air and enlarge during inspiration. With very deep inspirations, this capillary compression can cause an increase in overall pulmonary resistance.

The primary purpose of the pulmonary circulation is to perfuse alveoli for the exchange of blood gases. Gas exchange depends, in part, on diffusion distances and the surface area available for exchange. The capillary–alveolar arrangement is such that diffusion distances are minimized and surface area is maximized. Pulmonary capillaries differ from their systemic counterparts in that they form thin interconnecting sheets around and between adjacent alveoli, which greatly increase their surface area and reduce diffusion distances.

Unlike other organs, alveolar or arterial hypoxia causes pulmonary vasoconstriction. The mechanism is not known; however, evidence suggests that endothelin, reactive oxygen species, and intracellular calcium mobilization may be involved. This **hypoxic vasoconstriction**, especially in response

to regional variations in ventilation, helps to maintain normal ventilation–perfusion ratios in the lung. Maintenance of normal ventilation–perfusion ratios is important because high blood flow to hypoxic regions, for example, would decrease the overall oxygen content of the blood leaving the lungs.

Sympathetic adrenergic nerves innervate the pulmonary vasculature, although their activation has relatively weak effects on pulmonary vascular resistance and pulmonary artery pressure.

## Summary of Special Circulations

Perfusion pressure and vascular resistance determine blood flow in organs. Under normal circumstances, the perfusion pressure remains fairly constant owing to baroreceptor mechanisms. Therefore, the primary means by which blood flow changes within an organ is by changes in vascular resistance, which is influenced by extrinsic factors (e.g., sympathetic nerves and hormones) and intrinsic factors (e.g., tissue metabolites and endothelial-derived substances). Basal vascular tone is determined by the net effect of the extrinsic and intrinsic factors acting on the vasculature. Resistance can either increase or decrease from the basal state by alterations in the relative contribution of extrinsic and intrinsic factors. Table 7-2 summarizes the relative importance of sympathetic and metabolic control mechanisms and the intrinsic autoregulatory capacity of several major organ vascular beds.

**TABLE 7-2  COMPARISON OF VASCULAR CONTROL MECHANISMS IN DIFFERENT VASCULAR BEDS**

| CIRCULATORY BED | SYMPATHETIC CONTROL | METABOLIC CONTROL | AUTOREGULATION |
|---|---|---|---|
| Coronary | +[1] | +++ | +++ |
| Cerebral | + | +++ | +++ |
| Skeletal muscle | ++ | +++ | ++ |
| Cutaneous | +++ | + | + |
| Intestinal | +++ | ++ | ++ |
| Renal | ++ | + | +++ |
| Pulmonary | + | +[2] | NA |

+, weak; ++, moderate; +++, strong.
NA, not applicable because pressure is the dependent variable instead of flow as in other organs.
[1]Sympathetic vasoconstriction in the coronaries is overridden by metabolic vasodilation during sympathetic activation of the heart.
[2]Hypoxia causes vasoconstriction, the opposite of all other organs.

## SUMMARY OF IMPORTANT CONCEPTS

- The relative distribution of blood flow to organs is regulated by the vascular resistance of the individual organs, which is determined by extrinsic (neurohumoral) and intrinsic (local regulatory) mechanisms.

- Important local mechanisms regulating organ blood flow include the following: (1) tissue factors such as adenosine, $K^+$, $O_2$, $CO_2$, and $H^+$; (2) paracrine hormones such as bradykinin, histamine, and prostaglandins; (3) endothelial factors such as nitric oxide, endothelin-1, and prostacyclin; and (4) myogenic mechanisms intrinsic to the vascular smooth muscle.

- The following local factors produce vasodilation in most tissues: adenosine, $K^+$, $H^+$, $CO_2$, hypoxia, bradykinin, histamine, $PGE_2$, prostacyclin, and nitric oxide. The following local factors produce vasoconstriction: endothelin-1 and the myogenic response to vascular stretch.

- Mechanical compression of blood vessels strongly influences blood flow in the coronary circulation and in contracting skeletal muscle.

- Flow autoregulation is very important in organs such as the heart, brain, and kidneys; the gastrointestinal and skeletal muscle circulations show moderate autoregulation.

- Blood flow is tightly coupled to oxidative metabolism particularly in coronary, cerebral, skeletal muscle, and gastrointestinal circulations; therefore, an increase in tissue oxygen consumption leads to an increase in blood flow (functional or active hyperemia).

- Blood flow in the following organs is moderately to strongly influenced by sympathetic vasoconstrictor mechanisms: resting skeletal muscle, kidneys, gastrointestinal circulation, and skin (related to thermoregulation).

- Vascular control mechanisms linked to oxidative metabolism (metabolic mechanisms) are particularly strong in the heart, brain, and skeletal muscle.

## REVIEW QUESTIONS

For each question, choose the one best answer:

1. Two minutes after perfusion pressure to a kidney is suddenly reduced from 100 to 70 mm Hg, which of the following will occur?

    a. Afferent arterioles will be dilated.
    b. Renal blood flow will be reduced by 30%.
    c. Renal vascular resistance will be increased.
    d. The kidney will become hypoxic.

2. If a coronary artery is occluded for 1 minute and then the occlusion is released,

    a. A period of active hyperemia follows.
    b. Coronary flow increases because of vasoconstriction occurring during the ischemia.
    c. Endothelial release of nitric oxide will contribute to the reactive hyperemia.
    d. Interstitial adenosine concentrations will increase and constrict coronary arterioles.

3. Which one of the following organ circulations is most strongly constricted during sympathetic activation resulting from a baroreceptor reflex when a person suddenly stands up?

   a. Brain
   b. Heart
   c. Intestine
   d. Skin

Match the organs listed in questions 4 to 9 with answers "a" through "i" below. Each question may have more than one correct answer.

   a. Blood flow is primarily regulated by $CO_2$ and $H^+$.
   b. Capillary beds found between two in-series arterioles
   c. Hypoxic vasoconstriction
   d. Highest capillary pressure
   e. Highest arterial–venous oxygen difference
   f. Abundant arterial–venous anastomoses
   g. Largest organ mass
   h. Receives most of its blood supply directly from other organs
   i. Controlled primarily by hypothalamic thermoregulatory centers

4. Skin circulation _____

5. Renal circulation _____

6. Coronary arteries _____

7. Pulmonary circulation _____

8. Cerebral circulation _____

9. Skeletal muscle circulation _____

10. A hypertensive patient is diagnosed with bilateral renal artery stenosis. You consider administering an ACE inhibitor to lower the blood pressure. By what mechanism might this drug adversely affect renal glomerular filtration?

    a. Constriction of afferent arterioles
    b. Constriction of efferent arterioles
    c. Dilation of afferent arterioles
    d. Dilation of efferent arterioles

11. A patient with anginal symptoms is diagnosed with coronary artery disease and coronary vasospasm. Which of the following might be responsible for increased susceptibility to vasospasm?

    a. Diminished endothelial production of nitric oxide
    b. Diminished sympathetic tone on the coronary vessels
    c. Ischemia-induced production of adenosine
    d. Reduced coronary endothelial production of endothelin-1

12. Intracranial pressure is steadily increasing in a patient who has recently suffered a hemorrhagic stroke. You are concerned about this finding because elevated intracranial pressure can result in

    a. Decreased blood flow.
    b. Decreased cerebral vascular resistance.
    c. Increased cerebral perfusion pressure.
    d. Increased cerebral vascular transmural pressure.

## ANSWERS TO REVIEW QUESTIONS

1. The correct answer is "a" because in response to a reduction in perfusion pressure and blood flow, the kidney undergoes autoregulation through dilation of the afferent arterioles. Choice "b" is incorrect. When the pressure is first reduced, blood flow will fall by about 30%, but after 2 minutes, the blood flow will be near normal owing to the autoregulation. Choice "c" is incorrect because afferent arteriolar vasodilation reduces renal vascular resistance. Choice "d" is incorrect because autoregulation, by maintaining blood flow, protects the kidney against ischemia and hypoxia.

2. The correct answer is "c" because the increase in flow (reactive hyperemia) following release of the occlusion causes a flow-dependent release of nitric oxide by the vascular endothelium, which further contributes to the increase in blood flow. Choice "a" is incorrect because active hyperemia is associated with increased tissue metabolic activity and not with postischemic hyperemia. Choice "b" is incorrect because vasodilation occurs during ischemia. Choice "d" is incorrect because increased interstitial adenosine dilates coronary arterioles.

3. The correct answer is "c." Choice "a" is incorrect because the brain responds little to sympathetic activation. Although the coronary vasculature in the heart (choice "b") is capable of responding to sympathetic activation, concurrent stimulation of heart rate and inotropy lead to metabolic vasodilation. Choice "d" is incorrect because sympathetic control of the skin circulation is primarily related to thermoregulation; therefore, the baroreceptor reflex associated with standing has little influence on cutaneous blood flow.

4. The correct answers are "f" and "i."

5. The correct answers are "b" and "d."

6. The correct answer is "e."

7. The correct answer is "c."

8. The correct answer is "a."

9. The correct answer is "g."

10. The correct answer is "d" and the other choices are incorrect because in renal artery stenosis, increased angiotensin II, which preferentially constricts the efferent arteriole, helps to maintain glomerular capillary pressure and filtration despite the fall in renal perfusion pressure. Therefore, decreasing angiotensin II with an ACE inhibitor removes this constriction, which leads to a decrease in glomerular capillary pressure and glomerular filtration.

11. The correct answer is "a" because coronary artery disease is associated with endothelial dysfunction and decreased nitric oxide production. The vasodilator actions of nitric oxide normally oppose vasoconstrictor mechanisms, and therefore, reduced nitric oxide enhances vasoconstrictor responses and can increase susceptibility to vasospasm. Choice "b" is incorrect because diminished sympathetic tone reduces vasoconstrictor influences on the vessels. Choice "c" is incorrect because adenosine is a vasodilator and therefore opposes vasoconstriction. Choice "d" is incorrect because endothelin-1 is a vasoconstrictor and may contribute to vasospasm.

12. The correct answer is "a" because increased intracranial pressure reduces cerebral blood flow by compressing vessels and increasing their resistance (therefore, choice "b" is incorrect) and decreases the effective perfusion pressure, which can be approximated as the mean arterial pressure minus the intracranial pressure (therefore, choice "c" is incorrect). Choice "d" is incorrect because the increased intracranial pressure increases the pressure outside of the vessels so that the transmural pressure decreases.

## ANSWERS TO PROBLEMS AND CASES

### PROBLEM 7-1

The initial perfusion pressure was 100 mm Hg (mean arterial pressure minus venous pressure). Elevating the venous pressure to 15 mm Hg reduced the perfusion pressure to 85 mm Hg. According to the equation relating blood flow, perfusion pressure, and vascular resistance (F = ΔP/R), flow would decrease by 15% with a 15% decrease in perfusion pressure (assuming that resistance does not change). However, in this case, flow decreased by 25% indicating that resistance increased by 13.3% (R = ΔP/F = 0.85/0.75). The metabolic theory for autoregulation states that as perfusion pressure and flow are reduced, an accumulation of vasodilator metabolites decreases resistance in an attempt to restore flow; however, resistance did not decrease in this experiment. The myogenic theory states that increased transmural pressure causes vascular smooth muscle to contract, thereby increasing resistance and decreasing flow. Increasing venous pressure in this experiment increased the transmural pressure in arterioles, causing them to constrict and increase their resistance. Therefore, increasing venous pressure produces opposite and competing responses between these two mechanisms. Because vascular resistance increased

in this experiment, we can conclude that the myogenic (vasoconstrictor) mechanism was dominant over the metabolic (vasodilator) mechanism. These results have been observed experimentally in organs such as the intestine.

### CASE 7-1

It is important to control arterial pressure in patients with coronary artery disease because hypertension increases ventricular afterload and myocardial oxygen demand. However, it is important to lower arterial pressure using drugs that do not cause a reflex tachycardia for two reasons. First, reflex tachycardia (baroreceptor-mediated) increases myocardial oxygen demand and offsets the beneficial effects of reducing afterload (see Chapter 4). Second, tachycardia further impairs coronary perfusion because the duration of diastole relative to systole decreases at elevated heart rates. This reduces the time available for coronary perfusion during diastole, which is the time when the greatest amount of coronary perfusion occurs. It is common in clinical practice to give a drug such as a β-blocker to a patient with both coronary artery disease and hypertension because it lowers arterial pressure and prevents reflex tachycardia.

### SUGGESTED RESOURCES

Clifford PS, Hellsten Y. Vasodilatory mechanisms in contracting skeletal muscle. J Appl Physiol 2004:393–403.

Deussen A, Brand M, Pexa A, Weichsel J. Metabolic coronary flow regulation – Current concepts. Basic Res Cardio 2006;101:453–464.

Hill MA, Meininger GA, Davis MJ, Laher I. Therapeutic potential of pharmacologically targeting arteriolar myogenic tone. Trends Pharmacol Sci 2009;30:363–374.

Johnson PC. Autoregulation of blood flow. Circ Res 1986;59:483–495.

Joyner MJ, Halliwill JR. Sympathetic vasodilation in human limbs. J Physiol 2000;526:471–480.

Kellogg DL. In vivo mechanisms of cutaneous vasodilation and vasoconstriction in humans during thermoregulatory challenges. J Appl Physiol 2006;100:1709–1718.

Lassen NA: Brain. In Johnson PC, ed. Peripheral Circulation. New York: John Wiley & Sons, 1978.

Rhoades RA, Bell, DR. Medical Physiology: Principles for Clinical Medicine. 3rd Ed. Philadelphia: Lippincott Williams & Wilkins, 2009.

# EXCHANGE FUNCTION OF THE MICROCIRCULATION

**8** CHAPTER

Understanding the concepts presented in this chapter will enable the student to:

1. Describe the principal mechanisms by which gases, fluid, electrolytes, and macromolecules move across the capillary endothelium.

2. Name three different types of capillaries; know the organs in which they are found, and describe their differences in permeability to macromolecules and fluid.

3. Describe the factors that determine oxygen's rate of exchange between the microcirculation and tissue.

4. Explain the relationship between oxygen content of blood, percent saturation, and partial pressure of oxygen.

5. Describe the relationship between oxygen delivery to a tissue, oxygen extraction, and oxygen consumption.

6. Describe the mechanisms responsible for the movement of fluid across capillaries.

7. Describe the relationship between interstitial fluid volume, interstitial hydrostatic pressure, and interstitial compliance.

8. Describe how changes in capillary hydrostatic pressure, plasma oncotic pressure, capillary permeability, and lymphatic function can lead to tissue edema.

LEARNING OBJECTIVES

## INTRODUCTION

The microcirculation consists of small arteries, arterioles, capillaries, venules, small veins, and small lymphatic vessels found within organs and tissues (see Chapter 5, Fig. 5.1) and has the following important functions:

1. Small arteries and arterioles are the principal sites of resistance within the systemic circulation and therefore play a major role in the regulation of arterial blood pressure and blood flow within organs (see Chapter 5).

2. Venules and small veins have an important capacitance function and therefore determine the distribution of blood volume within the body.

3. The microcirculation allows passage of leukocytes from the blood into the extravascular space, which is important in inflammation and infection.

4. The microcirculation is where gases, circulating substances (e.g., nutrients, hormones, therapeutic drugs), metabolic wastes from the tissues, fluid, and thermal energy are exchanged between the blood and tissues.

Within the microcirculation, capillaries are quantitatively the most important site for exchange because of their physical structure (small volume-to-surface area ratio and thin walls), large number, and enormous surface area available for exchange. This chapter focuses on the exchange function of capillaries.

## MECHANISMS OF EXCHANGE

Fluid, electrolytes, gases, and small and large molecular weight substances transverse the capillary endothelium by several different mechanisms: diffusion, bulk flow, vesicular transport, and active transport (Fig. 8.1). Some substances

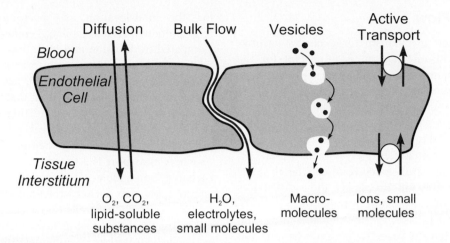

**■ FIGURE 8.1** Mechanisms of exchange across the capillary endothelium. Lipid-soluble substances like oxygen and carbon dioxide readily exchange across capillary endothelial cells by diffusion. Water and electrolytes move across the endothelium primarily by bulk flow through intercellular clefts ("pores"). Vesicular transport mechanisms move large molecules across the endothelium. Active transport mechanisms move ions and other small molecules across the endothelium.

are primarily transported by one mechanism, whereas other substances are able to use more than one mechanism. This is determined by the physical and chemical characteristics of the substance as well as the type of capillary endothelium, which differs among organs.

## Diffusion

*Diffusion is the movement of a molecule from a high concentration to a low concentration.* This mechanism of exchange is particularly important for gases ($O_2$ and $CO_2$) and other lipid-soluble substances (e.g., steroid hormones, anesthetics). Fluid and electrolytes also are exchanged across the endothelium, in part, by diffusion.

The movement of a substance by diffusion is described by **Fick's first law** of diffusion (Equation 8-1), in which the movement of a molecule per unit time (flux $J_S$; moles/s) equals the diffusion constant (D) of the barrier (e.g., capillary wall) multiplied by the surface area (A) available for diffusion and the concentration gradient ($\Delta C/\Delta X$), which is the concentration difference across the barrier ($\Delta C$) divided by the diffusion distance ($\Delta X$).

**Eq. 8-1**
$$J_S = DA \frac{\Delta C}{\Delta X}$$

*The **diffusion constant** is a value that represents the ease with which a specific substance can cross the capillary wall (or other barrier) by diffusion.* The higher the diffusion constant for a specific substance, the greater its flux across the barrier at a given concentration gradient. The diffusion constant is determined by the physical and chemical structure of the barrier as well as the physical and chemical characteristics (e.g., size, electrical charge) of the diffusing molecule. For example, the diffusion constant for oxygen (small and highly lipophilic) across cell membranes (which are lipid bilayers) is very high compared to glucose (large and hydrophilic).

Equation 8-1 indicates that *the rate of diffusion is directly related to the concentration difference, the diffusion constant, and the area available for diffusion, and it is inversely related to the diffusion distance.* The diffusion distance ($\Delta X$) in Equation 8-1 is sometimes combined with the diffusion constant (D) and called the **permeability coefficient** (P). This simplifies Equation 8-1 to $J_S = PS(\Delta C)$ in which S is the surface area available for exchange. The combined value of the permeability coefficient times the surface area has been calculated for different substances in many organs and tissues; it is called the **PS product.**

## Bulk Flow

A second mechanism for exchange is **bulk flow**. This mechanism is important for the movement of water and small lipid-insoluble substances across capillaries. *Bulk flow of fluid and electrolytes, and of small molecules, occurs through intercellular clefts between endothelial cells* (see Fig. 8.1). These extracellular pathways are sometimes referred to as "pores."

The physical structure of capillaries varies considerably among organs; these differences greatly affect exchange by bulk flow. Some capillaries (e.g., skeletal muscle, skin, lung, and brain) have a very "tight" endothelium and continuous basement membrane (termed **continuous capillaries**), which reduces bulk flow across the capillary wall. In contrast, some vascular beds have **fenestrated capillaries** (e.g., in exocrine glands, renal glomeruli, and intestinal mucosa), which have perforations (fenestrae) in the endothelium, resulting in relatively high permeability and bulk flow. **Discontinuous capillaries** (found in the liver, spleen, and bone marrow) have large intercellular gaps, as well as gaps in the basement membrane, and therefore have the highest permeability.

Bulk flow follows Poiseuille's equation for hydrodynamic flow (see Chapter 5, Equation 5-7). Changes in pressure gradients (either hydrostatic or colloid osmotic) across a capillary alter fluid movement across the capillary. In addition, changes in the size and number of "pores" or intercellular clefts alter exchange. Pore size and path length are analogous to vessel radius and length in Poiseuille's equation; they are major factors in the resistance to bulk flow across capillaries. In some organs, the number of perfused capillaries can be regulated. As described in Chapter 7, the number of perfused capillaries in contracting skeletal muscle, for example, is greater than at rest. An increase in perfused capillaries increases the surface area available for fluid exchange and the net movement of fluid across capillaries by bulk flow.

## Vesicular and Active Transport

**Vesicular transport** is a third mechanism by which exchange occurs between blood and tissue. This mechanism is particularly important for the translocation of macromolecules (e.g. proteins) across capillary endothelium. Compared to diffusion and bulk flow, vesicular transport plays a relatively minor role in transcapillary exchange (except for macromolecules). Evidence exists, however, that vesicles can sometimes fuse together, creating a channel through a capillary endothelial cell, thereby permitting bulk flow to occur across the cell.

**Active transport** is a fourth mechanism of exchange. Some molecules (e.g., ions, glucose, amino acids) are actively transported across capillary endothelial cells; however, this is not normally thought of as a mechanism for exchange between plasma and interstitium, but rather as a mechanism for exchange between an individual cell and its surrounding milieu.

## EXCHANGE OF OXYGEN AND CARBON DIOXIDE

### Oxygen Diffusion

Oxygen diffuses from the blood to tissue cells to support mitochondrial respiration. The lipid solubility of oxygen enables it to readily diffuse through tissues; however, the distance that oxygen is able to diffuse within a tissue is limited by cellular utilization of oxygen. For example, as oxygen diffuses out of a capillary into surrounding skeletal muscle cells, oxygen is consumed by the mitochondria. Consequently, little oxygen diffuses all the way through one cell to reach another. Therefore, in tissues having a high demand for oxygen, it is essential that the capillary density is great enough to provide short diffusion distances.

Large amounts of oxygen diffuse across the capillaries not only because of their thin walls and high diffusion constant for oxygen, but more importantly, because of their large surface area available for diffusion. It has been observed that significant amounts of oxygen also diffuse out of arterioles. Some of this oxygen diffuses through arteriolar walls into the surrounding cells, and in some cases, it diffuses from arterioles into the venules that often are found adjacent to arterioles. Normally, systemic arterial blood is fully saturated with oxygen and has a $PO_2$

of about 95 mm Hg. Direct measurements of $PO_2$ in small arterioles (20 to 80 µm diameter) of some tissues reveal that the $PO_2$ is only 25 to 35 mm Hg, which corresponds to a 30% to 60% loss of oxygen content of the blood. Therefore, substantial amounts of oxygen can diffuse out of the blood before the blood reaches the capillaries; however, capillaries are still the most important site for tissue oxygenation because the relatively high capillary density ensures that diffusion distances between the blood and tissue cells are short.

Figure 8.2 illustrates the diffusion of oxygen from blood within a capillary, across the capillary endothelium, and then into a cell. The $PO_2$ is only slightly reduced just outside of the capillary (from 25 to 24 mm Hg) because little oxygen is consumed as it diffuses through the endothelial cell and into the interstitial fluid surrounding the capillary. The oxygen in the interstitium then diffuses down a concentration gradient into nearby cells. Because the mitochondria inside a cell are consuming oxygen, the $PO_2$ may be very low inside the cytoplasm of the cell. Although an intracellular $PO_2$ of 5 mm Hg is shown in Figure 8.2, the value depends on where the $PO_2$ is measured within the cell, the rate of mitochondrial oxygen consumption, and the capillary blood $PO_2$. Just inside the cell membrane, the $PO_2$ is much higher than at the center of the cell; the lowest $PO_2$ is found within the mitochondria. Therefore, significant oxygen gradients exist within cells.

In Figure 8.2, the overall concentration gradient driving oxygen diffusion into the cell is 20 mm Hg. According to Fick's first law (Equation 8-1), the rate of oxygen diffusion ($JO_2$) is proportionate to the concentration difference of oxygen (expressed as $PO_2$ difference) between the capillary blood and inside the cell, assuming a fixed diffusion constant, diffusion distance, and surface area. Therefore, increasing capillary blood $PO_2$ (as occurs when a person breathes pure oxygen) or decreasing tissue $PO_2$ (as occurs with increased tissue oxygen consumption) increases the rate of oxygen diffusion into the tissue. Capillary $PO_2$ is also increased by dilation of resistance vessels. This increases

microvascular blood flow, thereby delivering more oxygen to the capillaries per unit time, which results in higher $PO_2$ values in the capillary blood. If vasodilation is accompanied by an increase in the number of flowing capillaries (as occurs during skeletal muscle contraction), this increases the surface area available for oxygen diffusion and further enhances oxygen transport into the tissue. For example, if the cell shown in Figure 8.2 were surrounded by three capillaries instead of one, then there would be an increase in the rate of oxygen diffusion into the cell, which would be necessary if the mitochondrial oxygen consumption increased significantly.

## Oxygen Delivery and Extraction

The previous discussion described oxygen diffusion from blood into tissue cells, and how the $PO_2$ gradient from the blood to the tissue cell plays an important role in determining the rate of diffusion. While the $PO_2$ gradient

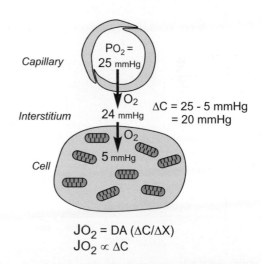

$$JO_2 = DA \, (\Delta C/\Delta X)$$
$$JO_2 \propto \Delta C$$

■ **FIGURE 8.2** Diffusion of oxygen ($JO_2$) from capillaries into the tissue follows Fick's first law of diffusion. Because the diffusion constant ($D$), the area for exchange ($A$), and the diffusion distance ($\Delta X$) remain relatively constant in a single capillary, the diffusion of oxygen is governed primarily by the difference in partial pressure of oxygen ($PO_2$) between the blood and cells ($\Delta C$), which is 20 mm Hg in this illustration. Most of this $PO_2$ gradient is between the interstitium and cell when mitochondria are actively consuming oxygen; there is only a small gradient across the capillary endothelium. Increasing the overall $PO_2$ gradient increases the rate of diffusion.

determines the rate of oxygen diffusion, the total amount of oxygen that is available per unit time for diffusion is determined by the amount of hemoglobin-bound oxygen in the blood and the rate of blood flow into the tissue.

The amount of oxygen in the blood (oxygen content) is determined by the $PO_2$ of the blood, along with the amount of hemoglobin in the red cells and the hemoglobin binding affinity for oxygen (Fig. 8.3). This relationship is called the **hemoglobin–oxygen dissociation curve**. At normal arterial $PO_2$ values (95 mm Hg), about 97% of the hemoglobin is bound to oxygen (97% hemoglobin saturation; $SaO_2$). If the blood contains 15 g of hemoglobin per 100 mL of blood (normal value), and a gram of hemoglobin can bind to 1.34 mL oxygen, then 20.1 mL oxygen (15 g/100 mL × 1.34 mL $O_2$/g) will be bound to hemoglobin in 100 mL of blood when 100% saturated, and 19.5 mL $O_2$/100 mL blood is bound at 97% saturation. A small amount of oxygen (~0.3 mL $O_2$/100 mL blood) is dissolved in the free water of the plasma and cells at normal arterial $PO_2$ values. Therefore, the total amount of hemoglobin-bound and dissolved oxygen

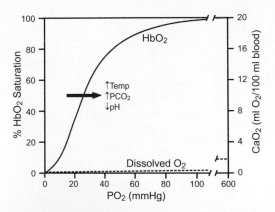

at normal arterial $PO_2$ values is approximately 20 mL $O_2$/100 mL blood (or, 20 vol %).

The hemoglobin–oxygen dissociation curve is sigmoidal in shape; therefore, small decreases in arterial $PO_2$ from normal values do not significantly reduce the oxygen content of the arterial blood. However, as the arterial $PO_2$ begins to fall below 80 mm Hg, and especially in the range of tissue $PO_2$ values (20 to 40 mm Hg), the curve becomes very steep and there is a large decrease in the amount of oxygen bound to hemoglobin as $PO_2$ decreases. At a $PO_2$ of about 25 mm Hg, hemoglobin is only 50% saturated ($P_{50}$ = 25 mm Hg). Therefore, as blood flows into tissues, the relatively low $PO_2$ in the tissue results in oxygen diffusing from the blood into the tissue. This lowers the blood $PO_2$ and causes oxygen to dissociate from the hemoglobin so that it can diffuse into the tissue. Unloading of oxygen from hemoglobin can also be enhanced by factors that cause a rightward shift in the oxygen dissociation curve. For example, increased temperature and $PCO_2$, and decreased pH shift the curve to the right, which shifts the $P_{50}$ to the right. Therefore, at any given tissue $PO_2$ value, a rightward shift causes more unloading of oxygen from the hemoglobin because of reduced binding affinity to oxygen. This is an important mechanism to increase tissue oxygenation when the metabolic activity of a tissue increases (e.g., contracting muscle), which increases tissue temperature and $CO_2$ production, and decreases pH.

The oxygen content of the arterial blood ($CaO_2$; mL $O_2$/100 mL blood) multiplied by the arterial blood flow (F; mL/min) represents the oxygen delivery ($DO_2$; mL $O_2$/min) to the tissue (Fig. 8.4).

$$DO_2 = F \cdot CaO_2$$

Therefore, the *oxygen delivery to a tissue is determined by the arterial blood flow and the arterial oxygen content*. Because arterial blood is normally near its maximal oxygen capacity (>95% saturated), oxygen delivery to a tissue can only be enhanced by increasing blood flow. On the other hand, oxygen delivery can be reduced by decreasing either flow

■ **FIGURE 8.3** Hemoglobin–oxygen dissociation curve. Percent oxygen saturation of hemoglobin (*% HbO₂*) has a sigmoidal relationship with the partial pressure of oxygen (*PO₂*). In this example, 100% saturation corresponds to an arterial blood oxygen content (*CaO₂*) of about 20 mL $O_2$/100 mL blood. This assumes that the hemoglobin concentration is 15 g/100 mL blood and that 1.34 mL $O_2$ bind to each gram of hemoglobin. Note that the amount of dissolved oxygen is very small relative to the amount of oxygen bound to hemoglobin. The dissociation curve shifts to the right (decreased hemoglobin affinity for oxygen) with increased temperature and $PCO_2$, and decreased pH.

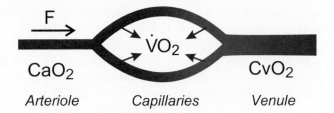

$$O_2 \text{ Delivery: } DO_2 = F \cdot CaO_2$$

$$O_2 \text{ Consumption: } \dot{V}O_2 = F \cdot (CaO_2 - CvO_2)$$

$$\text{Venous } O_2 \text{ Content: } CvO_2 = CaO_2 - \frac{\dot{V}O_2}{F}$$

■ **FIGURE 8.4** Model for oxygen delivery and balance in tissues. Oxygen delivery ($DO_2$) is the product of blood flow ($F$) and the arterial oxygen content ($CaO_2$). Oxygen consumption ($\dot{V}O_2$) is the product of flow and arterial–venous oxygen difference (oxygen extraction; $CaO_2 - CvO_2$) according to the Fick principle. Rearranging the equation shows that venous oxygen content ($CvO_2$) depends on $CaO_2$ minus the ratio of $\dot{V}O_2$ to F.

(e.g., ischemia) or arterial oxygen content (e.g., anemia, hypoxemia).

Oxygen delivery represents only what is available to the tissue, not what is utilized by the tissue. As arterial blood enters the microcirculation, and particularly the capillaries, oxygen diffuses from the blood into the tissues, and this reduces the oxygen content of the blood (see Fig. 8.4). The greater the oxygen consumption of the tissue, the greater the amount of oxygen that diffuses from the blood. Therefore, as the blood leaves the tissues, the venous blood has a lower oxygen content than the arterial blood. For example, if 5 mL $O_2$/100 mL blood were removed as the blood passes through a tissue (i.e., **oxygen extraction**), then the venous blood oxygen content ($CvO_2$) will be 15 mL $O_2$/100 mL blood if $CaO_2$ is 20 mL $O_2$/100 mL blood. Note, that as previously described in Chapter 7, oxygen extraction differs among organs and depends on their oxygen consumption and blood flow. When the oxygen extraction ($CaO_2 - CvO_2$; mL $O_2$/mL blood) is multiplied by the blood flow ($F$; mL/min), this represents the amount of oxygen consumed by the tissue ($\dot{V}O_2$; mL $O_2$/min), which is described by the Fick Principle (see Equation 4-3 and below). Note that oxygen content needs to be expressed as mL $O_2$/mL blood instead of mL $O_2$/100 mL blood when calculating values using the Fick Principle.

$$\dot{V}O_2 = F(CaO_2 - CvO_2)$$

If this equation is solved for the oxygen extraction, then we see that oxygen extraction is determined by the ratio of oxygen consumption to blood flow.

$$(CaO_2 - CvO_2) = \frac{\dot{V}O_2}{F}$$

Therefore, oxygen extraction is increased if oxygen consumption increases or blood flow decreases. Because the arterial oxygen content normally does not change significantly, then increased extraction reduces the venous oxygen content. This is more clearly seen by solving the previous equation for venous oxygen content:

$$CvO_2 = CaO_2 - \frac{\dot{V}O_2}{F}$$

Venous oxygen measurements are used for monitoring patients in intensive care settings, and therefore, the above relationship helps to explain what can cause venous oxygen levels (usually measured as venous oxygen saturation or $PO_2$) to fall. Venous oxygen saturation measured in the pulmonary artery ($SvO_2$) is normally about 75% and has a $PO_2$ of about 40 mm Hg. If it is abnormally low, this can be caused by elevated organ consumption by organs, reduced organ blood flow, or reduced arterial oxygen content. In intensive care settings, if arterial oxygen saturation is normal, reduced $SvO_2$ is usually caused by underperfusion of organs resulting from reduced cardiac output, which causes greater extraction of oxygen from the blood, thereby lowering venous oxygen saturation and content.

---

**PROBLEM 8-1**

An experiment is done on a human subject that measures the $PO_2$ of venous blood leaving the forearm during reactive hyperemia following a period of ischemia. During the initial phase of reactive hyperemia, venous $PO_2$ is transiently lower than normal and then becomes elevated. As blood flow returns toward normal near the end of the hyperemic response, the venous $PO_2$ also returns to its normal value. How would you explain these findings?

---

## Carbon Dioxide Diffusion

Carbon dioxide is a by-product of oxidative metabolism and must be removed from the tissue and transported to the lungs by the blood. Like oxygen, carbon dioxide is very lipid-soluble and readily diffuses from cells into the blood. In fact, its diffusion constant is about 20 times greater than oxygen in aqueous solutions. The removal of carbon dioxide from tissues is not diffusion-limited; its removal depends primarily on the blood flow. Therefore, reduced tissue perfusion leads to an increase in tissue and venous $PCO_2$. Increased oxidative metabolism of a tissue (e.g., contracting muscle) increases $CO_2$ production by cells, thereby increasing the concentration gradient for $CO_2$ diffusion from the tissue to the blood and increasing venous $PCO_2$. The magnitude of the increase in venous $PO_2$ depends on the relative increase in metabolism and blood flow.

## TRANSCAPILLARY FLUID EXCHANGE

The body is comprised of two basic fluid compartments: intravascular and extravascular. The intravascular compartment contains fluid (i.e., blood) within the cardiac chambers and blood vessels of the body. The extravascular system is everything outside of the intravascular compartment. The extravascular compartment is made up of many subcompartments such as the cellular, interstitial, and lymphatic subcompartments and a specialized system containing cerebrospinal fluid within the central nervous system.

Fluid readily exchanges between the intravascular and extravascular compartments. Fluid leaves blood vessels (primarily capillaries) and enters the tissue interstitium of the extravascular compartment. This is called **fluid filtration** (Fig. 8.5). It is estimated that about 1% of the plasma is filtered into the interstitium in a typical organ. The interstitial fluid is exchanged with the fluid found within the subcompartments of the extracellular compartment. It is crucial that a steady state is achieved in which the same volume of fluid that leaves the vasculature is returned to the vasculature; otherwise, the extravascular compartment would swell with fluid (i.e., become edematous).

There are two routes by which fluid is returned to the blood. First, **fluid reabsorption** returns most of the filtered fluid to the blood at the venular end of capillaries or at postcapillary venules (see Fig. 8.5). The rate of reabsorption is less than filtration; therefore, a second mechanism is required to maintain fluid balance. This second mechanism involves lymphatic vessels. These specialized vessels, similar in size to venules, comprise an endothelium with intercellular gaps surrounded by a highly permeable basement membrane. Terminal lymphatics end as blind sacs within the tissue. The terminal lymphatics take up the excess filtered fluid (including electrolytes and macromolecules) and transport it into larger lymphatics that leave the tissue. It is estimated that 5% to 10% of capillary filtration is transported out of tissues by the lymphatics. The larger lymphatics have smooth muscle cells that undergo spontaneous vasomotion that serves to "pump" the lymph. Vasomotion is spontaneous rhythmic contraction and relaxation of the lymphatic vessels. Evidence exists that as a lymphatic vessel fills with fluid,

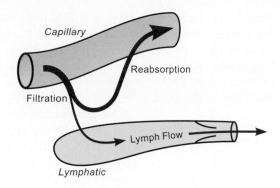

Filtration = Reabsorption + Lymph Flow

■ **FIGURE 8.5** Capillary filtration, reabsorption, and lymph flow. Fluid filters out of the arteriolar end of the capillary and into the interstitium. Most of this fluid is reabsorbed at the venular end of the capillary, with the rest of the fluid entering terminal lymphatics to be carried away from the tissue and eventually returned to the blood. Fluid exchange is in balance (i.e., at a steady state) when filtration equals reabsorption plus lymph flow.

the increased pressure stretches the vessel and induces a myogenic contraction. Sympathetic nerves can modulate this vasomotion. Lymphatic vessels contain one-way valves that direct lymph away from the tissue and eventually back into the systemic circulation via the thoracic duct and subclavian veins. Approximately 2 to 4 L/d of lymph are returned to the circulation by this manner.

In the steady state, the rate of fluid entering the tissue interstitium by filtration is the same as that of the fluid leaving the tissue by capillary reabsorption and lymph flow. That is, filtration equals reabsorption plus lymph flow. When this balance is altered, the volume and pressure of fluid within the interstitium change. For example, if net filtration transiently increases and lymph flow does not increase to the same extent, interstitial volume and pressure will increase, causing edema. Factors that cause edema are discussed in the last section of this chapter.

## Physical Mechanisms Governing Fluid Exchange

The movement of fluid across a capillary is determined by several physical factors: the hydrostatic pressure, oncotic pressure, and physical nature of the barrier (i.e., the permeability of the capillary wall) separating the

fluid in the blood from the fluid within the interstitium. As described earlier, the transcapillary movement of fluid can be described by Poiseuille equation for hydrodynamic flow (see Equation 5-7), or in more simplified terms, it can be described by the general hydrodynamic equation (Equation 5-5) that relates flow (F), driving pressure (ΔP), and resistance (R) (i.e., F = ΔP/R). In single capillaries, a more common way to express this hydrodynamic equation for transcapillary fluid movement (fluid flux, J) is to substitute hydraulic conductivity (Lp) for resistance, which are reciprocally related. Hydraulic conductivity is related to the ease by which fluid passes across the capillary wall. Fluid flux is the number of molecules of water (or volume) per unit time that moves across the exchange barrier; therefore, fluid flux can be expressed in similar units as flow. For a single capillary, fluid flux equals the product of capillary hydraulic conductivity and the net driving force (i.e., J = Lp · NDF). The NDF combines both those hydrostatic and oncotic pressures that drive fluid movement across the capillary wall.

In an organ, fluid is moving across many capillaries, and therefore the net fluid flux is related not only to the hydraulic conductivity of single capillaries and to the net driving force, but also to the surface area available for fluid exchange. When examining fluid flux across capillaries within an organ, filtration constant ($K_F$) and surface area (A) are substituted for hydraulic conductivity of a single capillary. With these substitutions, a new expression relating net fluid flux is obtained (Equation 8-2):

**Eq. 8-2**     $J = K_F \cdot A \ (NDF)$

Equation 8-2 and Figure 8.6 show that net fluid movement (net fluid flux, J) is directly related to the filtration constant ($K_F$), the surface area available for fluid exchange (A), and the net driving force (NDF). *At a given NDF (assuming that the NDF is not equal to zero), the amount of fluid filtered or reabsorbed per unit time is determined by the filtration constant and surface area available for exchange.* The filtration constant is determined by the physical properties of the barrier (i.e., size and number of "pores" and the thickness of the capillary barrier), and therefore, it represents the permeability of the capillaries to fluid. Fenestrated capillaries, for example,

have a much higher $K_F$ (i.e., permeability) than continuous capillaries. Furthermore, paracrine substances such as histamine, bradykinin, and leukotrienes can significantly increase $K_F$. The surface area (A) is primarily related to the length, diameter, and number of vessels (capillaries and postcapillary venules) available for exchange. The surface area is dynamic in vascular beds such as skeletal muscle. In that tissue, the number of perfused capillaries can increase severalfold during exercise. In experimental studies using whole organs, $K_F$ and A, which cannot be independently measured, are combined and called the **capillary filtration coefficient** (CFC).

The direction of fluid movement (filtration or reabsorption) in Equation 8-2 depends on whether the NDF is positive (filtration) or negative (reabsorption). If the NDF is zero, no net fluid movement occurs even if $K_F$ and A are very large.

As already mentioned, the NDF is determined by hydrostatic and oncotic forces. Two hydrostatic and two oncotic pressures affect transcapillary fluid exchange: capillary

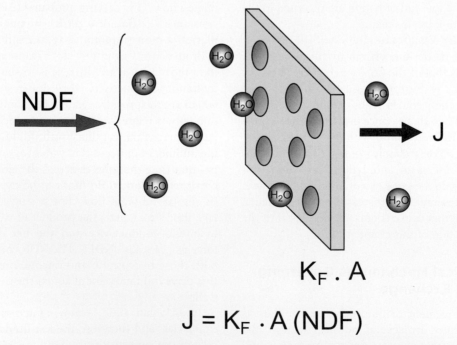

■ **FIGURE 8.6** Factors determining fluid movement. The rate of fluid movement (flux, *J*) across the capillary endothelium, designated as water molecules in this figure, is determined by the net driving force (*NDF*), the capillary filtration constant (*$K_F$*), and the capillary surface area (*A*) available for exchange.

hydrostatic pressure, tissue (interstitial) hydrostatic pressure, capillary (plasma) oncotic pressure, and tissue (interstitial) oncotic pressure (Fig. 8.7). These physical forces are sometimes referred to as **Starling forces** in honor of Ernest Starling who proposed in 1896 that these forces govern capillary fluid exchange. The net hydrostatic pressure driving fluid out of the capillary (filtration) is the hydrostatic pressure inside the capillary minus the interstitial hydrostatic pressure ($P_c - P_i$). The net oncotic pressure drawing fluid into the capillary (reabsorption) is the capillary plasma oncotic pressure minus the interstitial oncotic pressure ($\pi_c - \pi_i$).

## CAPILLARY HYDROSTATIC PRESSURE

Capillary hydrostatic pressure ($P_C$) drives fluid out of the capillary, and it is highest at the arteriolar end of the capillary and lowest at the venular end. Depending on the organ, the pressure may drop along the length of the capillary (axial or longitudinal pressure gradient) by 15 to 30 mm Hg owing to capillary resistance. Because of this pressure gradient along the capillary length, filtration is favored

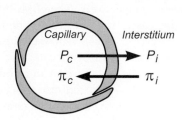

$$NDF = (P_c - P_i) - \sigma(\pi_c - \pi_i)$$

Filtration:          NDF > 0
Reabsorption:    NDF < 0

■ **FIGURE 8.7** Net driving force for fluid movement across capillaries. Hydrostatic and oncotic pressures within the capillary ($P_c$, $\pi_c$) and the tissue interstitium ($P_i$, $\pi_i$) determine the net driving force (*NDF*) for fluid movement out of the capillary (filtration) or into the capillary (reabsorption). The hydrostatic pressure difference favors filtration (*red arrow*) because $P_c$ is greater than $P_i$. The oncotic pressure difference favors reabsorption (*black arrow*) because $\pi_c$ is greater than $\pi_i$. The oncotic pressure difference is multiplied by the reflection coefficient ($\sigma$), a factor that represents the permeability of the capillary to the proteins responsible for generating the oncotic pressure.

at the arteriolar end of the capillary where capillary hydrostatic pressure is greatest.

The average capillary hydrostatic pressure is determined by arterial and venous pressures ($P_A$ and $P_V$), and by the ratio of post-to-precapillary resistances ($R_V/R_A$). An increase in either arterial or venous pressure increases capillary pressure; however, the effects of elevations in venous pressure are much greater than those of an equivalent elevation in arterial pressure. The reason for this is that postcapillary resistance is much lower than precapillary resistance. In most organs, the postcapillary resistance is only 10% to 20% of the precapillary resistance; therefore, $R_V/R_A$ ranges from 0.1 to 0.2. If we assume that $R_V/R_A = 0.2$, the following relationship (Equation 8-3) can be derived:

$$\text{Eq. 8-3} \quad P_C = \frac{\left(R_V/R_A\right)P_A + P_V}{1 + \left(R_V/R_A\right)} \Rightarrow P_C = \frac{0.2\,P_A + P_V}{1.2}$$

The above equation assumes that $P_C$ represents a point between two series resistances—an arterial or precapillary resistance ($R_A$) and a venous or postcapillary resistance ($R_V$). It also assumes that the flow that enters the capillary and exits the capillary is the same (i.e., there is conservation of flow). Therefore, on the precapillary side, flow into the capillary can be expressed as: $F_{in} = (P_A - P_c)/R_A$. On the postcapillary, the flow out of the capillary can be expressed as: $F_{out} = (P_c - P_V)/R_V$. Assuming that $F_{in}$ equals $F_{out}$, solving for $P_c$ results in Equation 8-3.

Equation 8-3 shows that increasing venous pressure by 20 mm Hg increases mean capillary pressure by 16.7 mm Hg when $R_V/R_A = 0.2$. In contrast, increasing arterial pressure by 20 mm Hg increases mean capillary pressure by only 3.3 mm Hg. The reason for this difference is that the high precapillary resistance blunts the effects of increased arterial pressure on the downstream capillaries. Therefore, *mean capillary hydrostatic pressure is more strongly influenced by changes in venous pressure than by changes in arterial pressure.* This has significant clinical implication. Conditions that increase venous pressure (e.g., right ventricular failure, cirrhosis of the liver, venous thrombosis) can lead to edema in peripheral organs and tissues by significantly increasing capillary hydrostatic pressure and capillary fluid filtration. This relationship also shows that arteriolar vasodilation or venous constriction increases capillary hydrostatic pressure, which increases filtration.

## TISSUE (INTERSTITIAL) HYDROSTATIC PRESSURE

Tissue (interstitial) hydrostatic pressure ($P_i$) is the pressure within the tissue interstitium that is exerted against the outside wall of the capillary and therefore opposes the capillary hydrostatic pressure. In many tissues under normal states of hydration, tissue hydrostatic pressure is subatmospheric by a few millimeters of mercury (mm Hg), whereas in others it is slightly positive by a few mm Hg. Increased tissue fluid volume, as occurs during states of enhanced capillary fluid filtration or lymphatic blockage, increases tissue hydrostatic pressure. In contrast, dehydration reduces tissue fluid volume and hydrostatic pressure.

The effect of changes in interstitial fluid volume on interstitial pressure is determined by interstitial compliance (C). This is defined as the change in interstitial fluid volume ($\Delta V_i$) divided by the change in interstitial fluid pressure ($\Delta P_i$). Rearranging this relationship gives the following:

$$\Delta P_i = \frac{\Delta V_i}{C}$$

Therefore, an increase in interstitial fluid volume increases interstitial fluid pressure, and the magnitude of the change varies inversely with the compliance of the interstitium.

Figure 8.8 is a graphical representation of the relationship between interstitial fluid volume and pressure, and interstitial compliance. The slope of the relationship between interstitial volume and pressure is interstitial compliance. Note that the compliance decreases at higher interstitial volumes, which causes the pressure to increase disproportionately as volume increases. Some tissues and

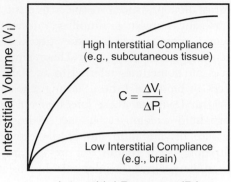

**■ FIGURE 8.8** Effects of interstitial compliance on interstitial fluid volumes and pressures. Compliance (*C*) is the change in interstitial volume ($\Delta V_i$) divided by the change in interstitial pressure ($\Delta P_i$), which is the slope of the relationship between volume and pressure. Low interstitial compliance (e.g., brain tissue) causes large increases in interstitial fluid pressure when interstitial fluid volume increases, which can occur during cerebral edema or hemorrhage within the brain. In contrast, tissue with high interstitial compliance (e.g., subcutaneous tissues), show relatively small increases in interstitial pressure as interstitial volume increases.

organs, such as the brain and kidney, have a low interstitial compliance. The reason is that the tissue is surrounded by a rigid boney skull or capsule, respectively. Therefore, relatively small increases in interstitial volume can lead to large increases in interstitial pressure. A large increase in pressure can be very damaging to the tissues and lead to cellular dysfunction and death. In contrast, subcutaneous tissues have a relatively high interstitial compliance so that large increases in interstitial volume can occur with relatively small increases in interstitial pressure. Despite a relatively high compliance at low interstitial fluid volumes, subcutaneous interstitial pressures can still increase to high values at very high interstitial volumes during severe limb edema.

## CAPILLARY PLASMA ONCOTIC PRESSURE

Capillary plasma oncotic pressure ($\pi_c$) is the osmotic pressure within the capillary that is determined by the presence of proteins. Because this is an osmotic force within the plasma, it opposes filtration and promotes reabsorption. Because the capillary barrier is readily permeable to ions, the ions have no significant effect on osmotic pressure within the capillary. Instead, the osmotic pressure is principally determined by plasma proteins that are relatively impermeable. Rather than being called "osmotic" pressure, this pressure is referred to as the "oncotic" pressure or "colloid osmotic" pressure because it is generated by macromolecular colloids. Albumin, the most abundant plasma protein, generates about 70% of the oncotic pressure; globulins and fibrinogen generate the remainder of the oncotic pressure. The plasma oncotic pressure typically is 25 to 30 mm Hg. When capillaries are filtering fluid, the oncotic pressure increases along the length of the capillary, particularly in capillaries having high filtration rates (e.g., renal glomerular capillaries). This occurs because the filtered fluid leaves behind proteins, increasing the plasma protein concentration.

When oncotic pressure is determined, it is measured across a semipermeable membrane, that is, a membrane that is permeable to fluid and electrolytes but not permeable to large protein molecules. In most capillaries, however, the endothelial barrier has a finite permeability to proteins. The actual permeability to proteins depends on the type of capillary and on the nature of the proteins (size, shape, and charge). Because of this finite permeability, the effective oncotic pressure generated across the capillary membrane is less than that calculated from the protein concentration. The **reflection coefficient** ($\sigma$) across a capillary wall represents the effective oncotic pressure divided by the oncotic pressure measured with a true semipermeable membrane. If the capillary is impermeable to protein, $\sigma = 1$. If the capillary is freely permeable to protein, $\sigma = 0$. Continuous capillaries have a high $\sigma$ (>0.9), whereas discontinuous capillaries (e.g., liver and spleen), which are very "leaky" to proteins, have a relatively low $\sigma$. In the latter case, plasma and tissue oncotic pressures may have a negligible influence on the NDF. If the capillary endothelium becomes damaged by physical injury or inflammation, the reflection coefficient may decrease significantly, which reduces the ability of plasma oncotic pressure to oppose filtration, thereby increasing net filtration.

## TISSUE (INTERSTITIAL) ONCOTIC PRESSURE

The tissue (or interstitial) oncotic pressure ($\pi_i$), a force that promotes filtration, is determined by the interstitial protein concentration and the reflection coefficient of the capillary wall for those proteins. The protein concentration is influenced, in part, by the amount of fluid filtration into the interstitium. For example, increased capillary filtration into the interstitium decreases interstitial protein concentration and reduces the oncotic pressure. This effect of filtration on protein concentration serves as a mechanism to limit excessive capillary filtration. The interstitial oncotic pressure, which is typically about 5 mm Hg, acts on the capillary fluid to enhance filtration and oppose reabsorption; therefore, when the interstitial proteins are diluted and this pressure falls, filtration is reduced. The interstitial protein concentration is also determined by the capillary permeability to protein. If this is increased, for example, by vascular damage or inflammation, then more proteins will be filtered with the fluid into the interstitium. An increase in interstitial protein concentration facilitates net filtration by reducing the net force for reabsorption.

## SUMMARY OF STARLING FORCES AND TRANSCAPILLARY FLUID MOVEMENT

Together, the hydrostatic and oncotic forces are related to the NDF as shown in Equation 8-4 and in Figure 8.7. The net hydrostatic pressure, which normally promotes filtration, is represented by ($P_c - P_i$). The net oncotic pressure, which promotes reabsorption, is represented by ($\pi_c - \pi_i$), multiplied by the reflection coefficient ($\sigma$). This equation shows that the NDF is increased by increases in $P_c$ and $\pi_i$ and decreased by increases in $P_i$ and $\pi_c$:

**Eq. 8-4**   $\text{NDF} = (P_c - P_i) - \sigma(\pi_c - \pi_i)$

If the above expression for NDF is incorporated into Equation 8-2, the following equation is derived, which is sometimes referred to as the **Starling equation**:

**Eq. 8-5**   $J = K_F \cdot A[(P_c - P_i) - \sigma(\pi_c - \pi_i)]$

The expression in brackets represents the NDF. If the NDF is positive, filtration occurs (J > 0), and if it is negative, reabsorption occurs (J < 0). For a given NDF, the rate of fluid movement (J) is determined by the product of $K_F$ and A.

## Capillary Exchange Model

Capillary fluid exchange can be modeled as shown in Figure 8.9. This model assumes that the following values remain constant along capillary length: $P_i$ = 1 mm Hg, $\pi_c$ = 25 mm Hg, $\pi_i$ = 6 mm Hg, and σ = 1. According to Equation 8-4, if $P_c$ is 30 mm Hg at the entrance to the capillary and falls linearly to 15 mm Hg at the end of the capillary, the NDF changes from +10 at the entrance of the capillary to –5 at the end of the capillary. Filtration occurs along most of the length of the capillary wherever NDF is greater than zero. Reabsorption occurs where NDF is less than zero, which is near the venular end of the capillary. Net fluid movement is zero at the point along the capillary where NDF = 0. Experimental studies have shown that the hydraulic conductivity in single capillaries increases severalfold from the arteriolar to the venular end of the capillary. Therefore, significant reabsorption can still occur at the distal end of a capillary when the NDF is only slightly negative.

This model is highly simplified because it assumes that $P_i$, $\pi_c$, and $\pi_i$ remain constant, which does not occur in vivo. As fluid leaves the arteriolar end of the capillary, $\pi_c$ increases, $P_i$ increases, and $\pi_i$ decreases. These changes oppose the filtration. For most capillaries, the fraction of fluid filtered from the capillary (filtration fraction) is <1%, so $P_i$, $\pi_c$, and $\pi_i$ do not change appreciably. Renal capillaries, however, are different because the filtration fraction in these capillaries is very high (~20%), which leads to significant increases in plasma oncotic pressure. In nonrenal capillaries, if capillary permeability is increased, or if capillary hydrostatic pressure is increased to high levels by venous occlusion or heart failure, the increase in filtration can lead to significant changes in $P_i$, $\pi_c$, and $\pi_i$ in a manner that opposes and therefore limits the net filtration of fluid.

Lymphatics (not shown in Fig. 8.9) pick up excess filtered fluid and transport it out of the tissue. When net filtration increases,

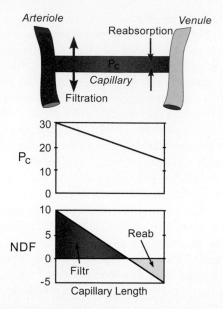

■ **FIGURE 8.9** Model of capillary fluid exchange. Assuming that $P_i$ = 1, $\pi_c$ = 25, $\pi_i$ = 6 mm Hg, and σ = 1, and assuming that capillary hydrostatic pressure ($P_c$) at the beginning and end of the capillary are 30 mm Hg and 15 mm Hg, respectively, the net driving force [NDF = ($P_c$ – $P_i$) – ($\pi_c$ – $\pi_i$)] is greater than zero along most of the length of the capillary, which causes filtration (*Filtr*) to occur. Near the venular end of the capillary, the *NDF* is less than zero and reabsorption (*Reab*) occurs.

lymphatic flow also increases. The lymphatics, therefore, along with the dynamic changes in $P_c$, $P_i$, $\pi_c$, and $\pi_i$ help to maintain a proper state of interstitial hydration and thereby prevent edema from occurring.

Finally, it is important to note that there is considerable heterogeneity among capillaries in terms of filtration and reabsorption. Some capillaries may filter along most or all of their length, whereas others may display reabsorption along most of their length. Furthermore, this can change depending on the balance of hydrostatic and oncotic forces, which can vary under different physiological and pathophysiological conditions. With arteriolar vasodilation or increased venous pressure, capillaries may filter along most or all of their length. Inflammation is accompanied by arteriolar vasodilation and increased capillary permeability, along with increased permeability of small postcapillary venules, which can become the major site of fluid filtration under inflammatory conditions.

<table>
<tr><td>

**PROBLEM 8-2**

Given that $P_c$ = 22 mm Hg, $P_i$ = −3 mm Hg, $\pi_c$ = 26 mm Hg, $\pi_i$ = 6 mm Hg, and σ = 0.9, answer the following questions:

a) What is the net driving force for transcapillary fluid exchange?

b) Is filtration or reabsorption occurring?

c) If the product of $K_F$ and A is doubled, what will happen to the net rate of fluid movement across the capillary, assuming that the net driving force does not change?

</td></tr>
</table>

## EDEMA FORMATION

When the fluid volume within the interstitial compartment increases because filtration exceeds the rate of capillary reabsorption plus lymphatic flow, the interstitial compartment increases in volume, leading to tissue swelling (i.e., edema). As already discussed, the change in interstitial pressure that results from an increase in interstitial volume depends on the compliance of the interstitial compartment.

Edema can damage organs and, in some cases, cause death. For example, cerebral edema following brain trauma can lead to cellular death because the increased interstitial pressure damages neurons and causes tissue ischemia by compressing blood vessels. Even in tissues that are relatively compliant, such as skin and skeletal muscle, severe edema can lead to tissue necrosis. Pulmonary edema can be life threatening because gas exchange is impaired.

Table 8-1 lists some of the many causes of edema. Every cause of edema can be related to one or more of the following:

• Increased capillary hydrostatic pressure
• Increased capillary permeability
• Decreased plasma oncotic pressure
• Lymphatic obstruction

The most common cause of edema is elevated capillary pressure, such as occurs during heart failure or venous obstruction. Both conditions increase venous pressure, which is transmitted back to the capillaries, causing an increase in fluid filtration. Localized edema in tissues is commonly caused by injury or inflammation

**TABLE 8-1  CAUSES OF EDEMA**

*Increased Capillary Pressure*
  Increased venous pressure
    - Heart failure
    - Increased blood volume
    - Venous obstruction (thrombosis or compression)
    - Incompetent venous valves
    - Gravity
  Increased arterial pressure
    - Hypertension
  Decreased arterial resistance
    - Vasodilation (physiologic or pharmacologic)
*Increased Capillary Permeability*
  Vascular damage (e.g., burns, trauma)
  Inflammation
*Decreased Plasma Oncotic Pressure*
  Reduced plasma proteins
  (e.g., malnutrition, burns, liver dysfunction)
*Lymphatic Blockage (Lymphedema)*
  Tissue injury
  Inflammation of lymphatics
  Lymphatic invasion by parasites
  (e.g., filariasis)

(e.g., sprained ankle, bee sting), which causes the release of local paracrine substances (e.g., histamine, bradykinin, and leukotrienes) that increase capillary and venular permeability. Some of these substances (e.g., histamine) also increase capillary pressure by dilating arterioles and constricting venules.

The treatment for edema involves modifying one or more of the physical factors that regulates fluid movement. For example, in pulmonary or systemic edema secondary to heart failure, diuretics are given to the patient to reduce blood volume and venous pressure, thereby reducing capillary hydrostatic pressure. A patient suffering from ankle edema following an injury will be instructed to keep that foot elevated whenever possible to diminish the effects of gravity on capillary pressure and to use a tight-fitting elastic stocking or bandage around the ankle to increase tissue hydrostatic pressure (which opposes filtration). Drugs (e.g., corticosteroids, antihistamines) are sometimes used to block the release or action of paracrine substances that increase capillary permeability following tissue injury or inflammation.

## SUMMARY OF IMPORTANT CONCEPTS

- Diffusion is the primary mechanism for the exchange of gases (e.g., oxygen) and lipid-soluble substances across the capillary barrier. The rate of diffusion is directly related to the concentration difference of the molecule across the capillary wall.

- Exchange of water and electrolytes across capillaries (and postcapillary venules) occurs primarily by bulk flow through intercellular clefts ("pores") between endothelial cells. Bulk flow is governed by the same factors that determine the blood flow through vessels.

- Movement of fluid across a capillary is determined by hydrostatic and osmotic driving forces, the permeability of the capillary to fluid movement, and the surface area for exchange of fluid.

- The net driving force that determines fluid movement is the net hydrostatic pressure difference across the capillary wall minus the opposing effective oncotic pressure difference across the capillary wall.

- Capillary hydrostatic pressure, which plays a major role in regulating transcapillary fluid exchange, is determined by arterial and venous pressures, and precapillary and postcapillary resistances.

- Changes in venous pressure have a much greater quantitative influence on capillary pressure than do similar changes in arterial pressure.

- Filtration occurs when the net driving force is greater than zero, which generally occurs at the arteriolar end of the capillary. Reabsorption occurs when the net driving force is less than zero, which generally occurs at the venular end of the capillary where capillary hydrostatic pressure is lower.

- An increase in tissue fluid volume (edema) occurs when the rate of fluid filtration exceeds the sum of the rate of fluid reabsorption and lymphatic flow.

- Edema can be caused by increased capillary hydrostatic pressure, increased capillary permeability, decreased plasma oncotic pressure, or lymphatic blockage.

## REVIEW QUESTIONS

For each question, choose the one best answer:

1. Which of the following mechanisms is most important quantitatively for the exchange of electrolytes across capillaries?

   a. Bulk flow
   b. Diffusion
   c. Osmosis
   d. Vesicular transport

2. Which of the following can increase the rate of oxygen diffusion from blood to tissue?

   a. Arteriolar vasodilation
   b. Decreased arteriolar $PO_2$
   c. Increased tissue $PO_2$
   d. Decreased number of flowing capillaries

3. A trauma patient in the hospital emergency department is found to have a venous oxygen saturation ($SvO_2$) of 50%; arterial oxygen saturation ($SaO_2$) is 95%. The $SvO_2$ value suggests that

 a. Cardiac output is low relative to the organ oxygen demand.
 b. Organ oxygen consumption is depressed.
 c. Tissue oxygen delivery is elevated.
 d. Tissue oxygen extraction is reduced.

4. Net capillary fluid filtration is enhanced by

 a. Decreased capillary plasma oncotic pressure.
 b. Decreased venous pressure.
 c. Increased precapillary resistance.
 d. Increased tissue hydrostatic pressure.

5. If capillary hydrostatic pressure = 15 mm Hg, capillary oncotic pressure = 28 mm Hg, tissue interstitial pressure = –5 mm Hg, and tissue oncotic pressure = 6 mm Hg (assume that $\sigma$ = 1), these Starling forces will result in

 a. Net filtration.
 b. Net reabsorption.
 c. No net fluid movement.

6. A malnourished, protein-deficient child presents with abdominal swelling, which is determined to be caused by increased fluid in the abdominal cavity (ascites). The ascites in this child is most likely caused by

 a. Decreased blood volume.
 b. Decreased interstitial oncotic pressure.
 c. Increased capillary reabsorption of fluid.
 d. Reduced plasma oncotic pressure.

7. A patient being treated for hypertension with an arterial vasodilator develops peripheral edema. The most likely cause of this edema is

 a. Decreased capillary hydrostatic pressure.
 b. Decreased capillary filtration constant.
 c. Increased postcapillary/precapillary resistance ratio.
 d. Reduced venous pressure.

## ANSWERS TO REVIEW QUESTIONS

1. The correct answer is "a" because this is the mechanism by which fluid and accompanying electrolytes move through capillary intercellular junctions. Choice "b" is incorrect because diffusion, although an important mechanism of exchange, is quantitatively less important than bulk flow. Furthermore, electrolytes are charged ions and therefore do not diffuse through membrane lipid bilayers. Choice "c" is incorrect because osmosis concerns the movement of water. Choice "d" is incorrect because vesicular transport is primarily for the transport of large macromolecules.

2. The correct answer is "a" because arteriolar vasodilation increases blood flow to the capillaries and increases capillary $PO_2$, which increases the concentration gradient for diffusion out of the blood. Choice "b" is incorrect because decreased arteriolar $PO_2$ decreases capillary $PO_2$ and therefore the oxygen gradient between the blood and tissue. Choice "c" is incorrect because increased tissue $PO_2$ decreases the concentration gradient for oxygen diffusion from the blood into the tissue. Choice "d" is incorrect because a decrease in the number of flowing capillaries decreases the surface area available for oxygen exchange.

3. The correct answer is "a" because when cardiac output is reduced, oxygen delivery to organs is reduced (choice "c" is therefore incorrect) because of reduced organ flow. If this flow reduction occurs under conditions of normal organ oxygen consumption, there will be an increase in oxygen extraction (choice "d" is therefore incorrect), which will reduce $SvO_2$. Choice "b" is incorrect because decreased oxygen consumption would increase $SvO_2$. Note that the reduced $SvO_2$ is not a consequence of reduced $SaO_2$ in this case because that value is within the normal range.

4. The correct answer is "a" because capillary plasma oncotic pressure opposes filtration; therefore, decreasing this pressure enhances filtration. Choices "b" and "c" are incorrect because decreasing venous pressure or increasing precapillary resistance reduces capillary hydrostatic pressure, thereby decreasing filtration. Choice "d" is incorrect because increased tissue hydrostatic pressure opposes filtration.

5. The correct answer is "b" because the net driving force, calculated from the given values, is –2 mm Hg, which causes reabsorption. Choices "a" and "c" are

incorrect because the net driving force is a negative value.

6. The correct answer is "d" because protein deficiency leads to hypoproteinemia, which reduces plasma oncotic pressure, thereby increasing net capillary fluid filtration. Choice "a" is incorrect because decreased blood volume caused by dehydration in this child would decrease capillary hydrostatic pressure and fluid filtration. Choice "b" is incorrect because decreased interstitial oncotic pressure opposes filtration. Choice "c" is incorrect because increased capillary fluid reabsorption would decrease edema and ascites.

7. The correct answer is "c" because increased postcapillary/precapillary resistance ratio caused by arterial (precapillary) vasodilation increases capillary hydrostatic pressure and fluid filtration. Choice "a" is incorrect because a decreased capillary hydrostatic pressure decreases fluid filtration. Choice "b" is incorrect because a decreased capillary filtration constant decreases net filtration. Choice "d" is incorrect because a reduced venous pressure decreases capillary pressure and filtration.

## ANSWERS TO PROBLEMS AND CASES

### PROBLEM 8-1

During the period of ischemia, the $PO_2$ and oxygen content of the static blood within the microcirculation fall as oxygen diffuses from the blood into the tissues. When blood flow is restored, this oxygen-depleted blood is washed out of the tissue; a sample of this blood will have reduced $PO_2$ and oxygen content. During the phase of reactive hyperemia, the increased blood flow and oxygen delivery to the tissue is greater than what is needed to supply the oxidative metabolism of the tissue. If the ratio of oxygen delivery to oxygen consumption is increased above normal, then the venous oxygen content and $PO_2$ will increase. As the balance is restored

toward the end of the hyperemic response, the $PO_2$ will normalize.

### PROBLEM 8-2

a) The net driving force, NDF = $[(P_c - P_i) - \sigma(\pi_c - \pi_i)]$. Substituting the given values, the NDF = 7 mm Hg.

$$NDF = \left[22 - (-3)\right] - 0.9\left[(26 - 6)\right]$$
$$= 7 \text{ mm Hg}$$

b) Because the NDF is greater than zero, filtration is occurring.

c) The net rate of fluid movement, J = $K_F \cdot A$ (NDF). Therefore, if the product of $K_F$ and A is doubled, then J (the filtration in this problem) is doubled because the NDF ≠ 0.

## SUGGESTED RESOURCES

Duling BR, Berne RM. Longitudinal gradients in periarteriolar oxygen tension. A possible mechanism for the participation of oxygen in local regulation of blood flow. Circ Res 1970;27:669–678.

Intaglietta M, Johnson PC. Principles of capillary exchange. In, Johnson PC, ed. Peripheral Circulation. New York: John Wiley & Sons, 1978.

Michel CC, Curry RE. Microvascular permeability. Physiol Rev 1999;79:703–761.

Takahashi E, Sato K, Endoh H, Xu Z, Doi K. Direct observation of radial intracellular $PO_2$ gradients in a single cardiomyocyte of the rat. Am J Physiol 1998;275:H225–H233.

# CARDIOVASCULAR INTEGRATION, ADAPTATION, AND PATHOPHYSIOLOGY

CHAPTER

# 9

**LEARNING OBJECTIVES**

Understanding the concepts presented in this chapter will enable the student to:

1. Describe the cardiac and vascular changes that occur during exercise, the mechanisms responsible for those changes, and factors that can alter the responses.

2. Describe how cardiovascular function is altered during pregnancy.

3. Describe the conditions that can lead to hypotension and the compensatory mechanisms that are activated to restore arterial pressure.

4. Explain how positive feedback mechanisms can lead to irreversible shock and death following severe hemorrhage.

5. Describe several different causes of hypertension and how it is treated.

6. Define systolic and diastolic ventricular failure and describe how these two types of failure alter cardiac and vascular function at rest and during physical exertion.

7. Describe the compensatory mechanisms that operate during heart failure.

8. Describe how heart valve stenosis and regurgitation affect cardiac function.

## INTRODUCTION

Previous chapters emphasized physiologic concepts concerning cardiac and vascular function at the cellular and organ level. In addition, they examined mechanisms, such as baroreceptors and circulating hormones, that regulate overall cardiovascular function. This chapter integrates all the components of the cardiovascular system and shows how they work together to maintain normal perfusion of organs under conditions of increased organ demand for blood flow (e.g., during exercise and pregnancy) or during abnormal stressful conditions such as hemorrhage. This chapter also examines changes that occur in cardiovascular function during pathologic conditions such as hypertension, heart failure, and valve disease.

## CARDIOVASCULAR RESPONSES TO EXERCISE

The cardiovascular system must be able to respond to a wide range of demands placed on it by the body. Previous chapters focused on cardiovascular function in normal resting states; however, physical activity is (or should be!) a normal, daily activity of humans. Physical movement is associated with increases in the metabolic activity of contracting muscles. This increased metabolic activity is largely oxidative; therefore, the cardiovascular system needs to increase blood flow and oxygen delivery to the contracting muscles.

The cardiovascular responses to physical activity are summarized in Table 9-1. If large muscle groups are involved in the physical

| TABLE 9-1 | SUMMARY OF CARDIOVASCULAR CHANGES DURING EXERCISE |
|---|---|

↑ **Cardiac output**
- ↑ heart rate (↑ sympathetic adrenergic and ↓ parasympathetic activity)
- ↑ stroke volume (↑ CVP; ↑ inotropy; ↑ lusitropy)

↑ **Mean arterial pressure and pulse pressure**
- CO increases more than SVR decreases
- ↑ stroke volume increases pulse pressure

↑ **Central venous pressure**
- Venous constriction (↑ sympathetic adrenergic activity)
- Muscle pump activity
- Abdominothoracic pump

↓ **Systemic vascular resistance**
- Metabolic vasodilation in active muscle and heart
- Cutaneous vasodilation (↓ sympathetic adrenergic activity)
- Vasoconstriction in splanchnic, nonactive muscle, and renal circulation (↑ sympathetic adrenergic activity)

*CVP*, central venous pressure; *CO*, cardiac output; *SVR*, systemic vascular resistance.

activity (e.g., running, bicycling), metabolic vasodilation (see Chapter 7) in these muscles causes a large fall in systemic vascular resistance. Ordinarily, this would cause arterial pressure to fall; however, during physical activity, arterial pressure normally increases because cardiac output increases at the same time that systemic vascular resistance begins to fall. Furthermore, increased sympathetic activity (see Chapter 6) leads to vasoconstriction in the gastrointestinal tract, nonactive muscles, and kidneys, which helps to limit the fall in systemic vascular resistance as well as shift blood flow to the active muscles. Venous return to the heart is augmented by venous constriction and by the skeletal muscle and abdominothoracic pumps (see Chapter 5). Enhanced venous return enables the cardiac output to increase by preventing a fall in cardiac preload that would otherwise

occur as heart rate and inotropy increase (see Chapter 4). Therefore, all the cardiovascular changes occurring during physical activity ensure that active muscles are supplied with increased blood flow and oxygen while maintaining normal, or even elevated, arterial pressures.

## Mechanisms Involved in Cardiovascular Response to Exercise

Four fundamental mechanisms are responsible for cardiovascular changes during physical activity: mechanical, metabolic, autonomic, and hormonal. When a person suddenly begins to run, cardiac output increases before metabolic and neurohumoral mechanisms are activated. This initial increase in cardiac output results primarily from the skeletal muscle pump system, which enhances venous return and increases cardiac output by the Frank-Starling mechanism. Within a few seconds of the initiation of muscle contraction, metabolic mechanisms in the contracting muscle dilate resistance vessels and increase blood flow. At about the same time, changes begin to occur in the autonomic nervous system (Fig. 9.1). Hypothalamic centers coordinate a pattern of increased sympathetic and decreased parasympathetic (vagal) outflow from the medulla (see Chapter 6). This leads to an increase in heart rate, inotropy, and lusitropy, which increases cardiac output. Increased sympathetic efferent activity constricts resistance and capacitance vessels in the splanchnic circulation and nonactive muscles to help maintain arterial pressure and central venous pressure. In addition, during strenuous activity, sympathetic nerves constrict the renal vasculature.

Exercise activates several different hormonal systems that affect cardiovascular function. Many of the hormonal systems are activated by the enhanced sympathetic activity. Because hormonal changes take longer to occur, cardiovascular responses to these changes lag behind the direct effects of autonomic activation on the heart and circulation.

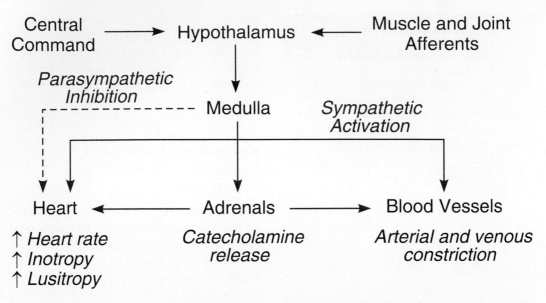

**■ FIGURE 9.1** Summary of adrenergic and cholinergic control mechanisms during exercise. The hypothalamus functions as an integrative center that receives information from the brain and muscle and joint receptors, then modulates sympathetic and parasympathetic (vagal) outflow from the medulla. Sympathetic nerves are activated leading to cardiac stimulation, arterial and venous constriction (not in active muscles), and adrenal release of catecholamines; parasympathetic inhibition removes vagal tone on the heart.

Sympathetic nerves innervating the adrenal medulla cause the secretion of epinephrine and lesser amounts of norepinephrine into the blood (see Chapter 6). Plasma norepinephrine concentrations increase more than 10-fold during exercise. A large fraction of this norepinephrine comes from sympathetic nerves. Normally, most of the norepinephrine released by sympathetic nerves is taken back up by the nerves (neuronal reuptake); however, some of the norepinephrine can diffuse ("spillover") into the capillary blood and enter the systemic circulation. This spillover is greatly enhanced when the level of sympathetic activity is high in the body. The blood transports the epinephrine and norepinephrine to the heart and other organs, where these hormones act upon $\alpha$- and $\beta$-adrenoceptors to enhance cardiac function and either constrict or dilate blood vessels. In Chapter 6, we learned that epinephrine (at low concentrations) binds to $\beta_2$-adrenoceptors in skeletal muscle, which causes vasodilation. At high concentrations, epinephrine also binds to postjunctional $\alpha_1$- and $\alpha_2$-adrenoceptors on blood vessels to cause vasoconstriction.

Circulating norepinephrine constricts blood vessels by binding preferentially to $\alpha_1$-adrenoceptors in most organs. During exercise, circulating levels of norepinephrine and epinephrine can become very high so that the net effect on the vasculature is $\alpha$-adrenoceptor-mediated vasoconstriction, except in those organs (e.g., heart and active skeletal muscle) in which metabolic mechanisms produce vasodilation. It is important to note that vasoconstriction produced by sympathetic nerves and circulating catecholamines does not occur in the active skeletal muscle, coronary circulation, or brain because blood flow in these organs is primarily controlled by local metabolic vasodilator mechanisms.

Increased sympathetic activity stimulates renal release of renin, which leads to the formation of angiotensin II. Increased angiotensin II increases renal sodium and water reabsorption by directly affecting renal function and by stimulating aldosterone secretion; in addition, angiotensin II augments sympathetic activity (see Chapter 6). Circulating arginine vasopressin (antidiuretic hormone) also increases during exercise, most likely resulting from increased plasma osmolarity. Although these hormonal changes promote renal retention of sodium and water, especially after prolonged periods of exercise, blood volume often decreases during exercise (particularly in hot environments) because of water loss through sweating and increased respiratory exchange.

Two mechanisms operate to activate the autonomic nervous system during exercise. One mechanism is referred to as "**central command.**" When physical activity is anticipated or already under way, higher brain centers (e.g., the cortex) relay information to hypothalamic centers to coordinate autonomic outflow to the cardiovascular system. By this central command mechanism, anticipation of exercise can lead to autonomic changes that increase cardiac output and arterial pressure before exercise begins. This serves to prime the cardiovascular system for exercise. A second mechanism involves muscle mechanoreceptors and chemoreceptors. Once physical activity is underway, these muscle receptors respond to changes in muscle mechanical activity and tissue chemical environment (e.g., increased lactic acid), and then relay that information to the central nervous system via afferent fibers. This information is processed by the hypothalamus and medullary autonomic control regions to enhance the sympathetic outflow to the heart and systemic vasculature.

Arterial baroreceptor function is altered during physical activity. Exercise normally is associated with a rise in both arterial pressure and heart rate. If arterial baroreceptor function were not modified, the increase in arterial pressure would result in a reflex bradycardia. Instead, the baroreceptor reflex is modified (reset to a higher control point) by the central nervous system (see Chapter 6).

## Steady-State Changes in Cardiovascular Function during Exercise

Changes in cardiovascular function during physical activity depend upon the level of physical exertion. If the level of physical exertion is expressed as workload, heart rate, cardiac output, and arterial pressure increase in nearly direct proportion to the increase in workload (Fig. 9.2, panel A). In contrast, systemic vascular resistance falls as workload increases because of vasodilation in the active muscles. Ventricular stroke volume increases at low-to-moderate workloads and then plateaus. Although not shown in Figure 9.2, the increase in stroke volume is responsible for an

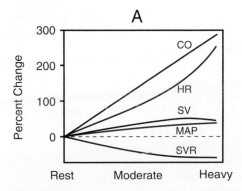
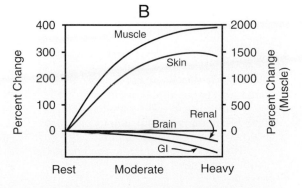

■ **FIGURE 9.2** Systemic hemodynamic and organ blood flow responses at different levels of exercise intensity. **Panel A** shows systemic hemodynamic changes. Systemic vascular resistance (*SVR*) decreases because of vasodilation in active muscles; mean arterial pressure (*MAP*) increases because cardiac output (*CO*) increases more than SVR decreases. CO and heart rate (*HR*) increase almost proportionately to the increase in workload. Stroke volume (*SV*) plateaus at high heart rates. **Panel B** shows organ blood flow changes. Muscle blood flow increases to very high levels because of active hyperemia; skin blood flow increases because of the need to remove excess heat from the body. Sympathetic-mediated vasoconstriction decreases gastrointestinal (*GI*) blood flow and renal blood flow. Brain blood flow changes very little.

increase in arterial pulse pressure that accompanies the increase in mean arterial pressure.

Stroke volume may decline at very high workloads because ventricular filling time is reduced as heart rate increases. Decreased filling time decreases ventricular filling (decreases preload), which decreases stroke volume by the Frank-Starling mechanism. This would prevent the heart from increasing cardiac output during physical activity if not for several mechanisms that work together to ensure that stroke volume is maintained and even increased as heart rate increases (Table 9-2). For example, during a physical activity such as running, enhanced venous return by the muscle pump and abdominothoracic pump systems helps to maintain preload despite the increase in heart rate (see Chapter 5). Furthermore, increased atrial and ventricular inotropy enhances ventricular stroke volume and ejection fraction, and increased lusitropy helps to augment ventricular filling. When the heart rate approaches its maximal rate, the effects of reduced filling time can predominate over these compensatory mechanisms, thereby compromising ventricular filling and reducing stroke volume. The point at which increased heart rate begins to decrease stroke volume varies considerably among individuals because of age, health, and physical conditioning. Furthermore, this point can vary

within an individual, depending on the type of exercise and the environmental conditions.

Blood flow to major organs depends upon the level of physical activity (Fig. 9.2, panel B). During whole-body exercise (e.g., running), the blood flow to the working muscles may increase more than 20-fold (see Chapter 7). At rest, muscle blood flow is about 20% of cardiac output; this value may increase to 90% during strenuous exercise. Coronary blood flow can increase severalfold as the metabolic demands of the myocardium increase and local regulatory mechanisms cause coronary vasodilation. The need for increased blood flow to active muscles and the coronary circulation would exceed the reserve capacity of the heart to increase its output if not for blood flow being reduced to other organs. During exercise, blood flow decreases to the splanchnic circulation (gastrointestinal, splenic, and hepatic circulations) and nonactive skeletal muscle as workload increases. This is brought about primarily by increased sympathetic nerve activity to these organs. With very strenuous exercise, renal blood flow is also decreased by sympathetic-mediated vasoconstriction.

Skin blood flow increases with increasing workloads, but it can then decrease at very high workloads, especially in hot environments. Increases in cutaneous blood flow are controlled by hypothalamic thermoregulatory centers (see Chapter 7). During physical activity, increased blood temperature is sensed by thermoreceptors in the hypothalamus. To enhance heat loss through the skin, the hypothalamus decreases sympathetic nerve activity to cutaneous blood vessels, which increases skin blood flow. At the same time, activation of sympathetic cholinergic nerves to the skin causes sweating.

While cutaneous vasodilation is essential for thermoregulation during physical activity, this requirement must be balanced by the need to maintain arterial pressure. Cutaneous vasodilation contributes to the fall in systemic vascular resistance primarily brought about by vasodilation in active muscles. If increased cardiac output is unable to maintain arterial pressure at very high workloads, baroreceptor

| TABLE 9-2 | **MECHANISMS MAINTAINING STROKE VOLUME AT HIGH HEART RATES DURING EXERCISE** |
|---|---|

- Increased venous return promoted by the abdominothoracic and skeletal muscle pumps maintains central venous pressure and therefore ventricular preload.
- Venous constriction (decreased venous compliance) maintains central venous pressure.
- Increased atrial inotropy augments atrial filling of the ventricles.
- Increased ventricular inotropy decreases end-systolic volume, which increases stroke volume and ejection fraction.
- Enhanced rate of ventricular relaxation (lusitropy) aids in filling.

mechanisms restore sympathetic tone to the skin and decrease its blood flow. Although this may help to preserve arterial pressure temporarily, reduced heat exchange through the skin can lead to dangerous elevations in core temperature, resulting in organ damage and loss of autonomic control. **Heat stroke** is a potentially lethal condition that occurs when core temperatures rise above 105°F.

---

### CASE 9-1

A 45-year-old male patient with type 2 diabetes is diagnosed with autonomic neuropathy, which impairs autonomic function. He complains of becoming weak and "light headed" when he performs physical work such as mowing the lawn. Explain how this patient's autonomic dysfunction may account for his inability to be engaged in normal physical activities.

---

## Factors Influencing Cardiovascular Response to Exercise

The cardiovascular changes associated with physical activity are modified by many different factors. The level of activity, which is commonly expressed as work performed or whole-body oxygen consumption, affects the cardiac and vascular responses. Several other important factors influence cardiovascular responses at a given workload.

The **type of exercise** significantly affects cardiovascular responses. The previous section described the cardiovascular responses to dynamic exercise such as running, walking, bicycling, or swimming. Dynamic exercise results in joint movement as muscles contract rhythmically. In contrast, muscle contraction without joint movement (isometric or static contraction) elicits a different cardiovascular response. An example of this activity would be trying to lift a very heavy weight at maximal effort (e.g., bench or leg press). This type of activity does not incorporate rhythmic contraction of synergistic and antagonistic muscle groups; therefore, the muscle pump

system cannot operate to promote venous return, and so, cardiac output increases relatively little. Furthermore, the abdominothoracic pump does not contribute to enhancing venous return, particularly if the subject holds his or her breath during the forceful contraction, effectively performing a Valsalva maneuver. Unlike dynamic exercise, static exercise leads to a large increase in systemic vascular resistance, particularly if a large muscle mass is being contracted at maximal effort. The increased systemic vascular resistance results from enhanced sympathetic adrenergic activity to the peripheral vasculature and from mechanical compression of the vasculature in the contracting muscles. As a result, systolic arterial pressure may increase to over 250 mm Hg during forceful isometric contractions, particularly those involving large muscle groups. This acute hypertensive state can produce vascular damage (e.g., hemorrhagic stroke) in susceptible individuals. In contrast, dynamic exercise leads to only modest increases in arterial pressure.

**Body posture** also influences how the cardiovascular system responds to exercise because of the effects of gravity on venous return and central venous pressure (see Chapter 5). When a person exercises in the supine position (e.g., swimming), central venous pressure is higher than when the person is exercising in the upright position (e.g., running). In the resting state before the physical activity begins, ventricular stroke volume is higher in the supine position than in the upright position owing to increased right ventricular preload. Furthermore, the resting heart rate is lower in the supine position. When exercise commences in the supine position, the stroke volume cannot be increased appreciably by the Frank-Starling mechanism because the high resting preload reduces the reserve capacity of the ventricle to increase its end-diastolic volume. Stroke volume still increases during exercise although not as much as when exercising while standing because, in the supine position, the increased stroke volume is resulting primarily from increases in inotropy and ejection fraction with minimal contribution from the Frank-Starling mechanism. Because heart rate is initially lower in the supine position, the percent increase in heart rate is greater in the supine position, which compensates for the reduced ability to increase stroke volume. Overall, the change in cardiac output during exercise, which depends upon the fractional increases in both stroke volume and heart rate, is not appreciably different in the supine versus standing position.

**Physical conditioning** permits a person to achieve a higher cardiac output, whole-body oxygen consumption, and workload than a person who has a sedentary lifestyle. The increased cardiac output capacity is a consequence, in part, of increased ventricular and atrial responsiveness to inotropic stimulation by sympathetic nerves. Conditioned individuals also have stronger, hypertrophied hearts, much like what happens to skeletal muscle in response to weight training. Coupled with enhanced capacity for promoting venous return by the muscle pump system, these cardiac changes permit highly conditioned individuals to achieve ventricular ejection fractions that can exceed 90% during exercise. In comparison, a sedentary individual may not be able to increase ejection fraction above 75%.

In a conditioned individual, resting heart rate is lower and resting stroke volume is higher than in a sedentary person—resting cardiac output is not necessarily different. Because the maximal heart rate of a conditioned individual is similar to that of a sedentary individual of the same age, the lower resting heart rates of a conditioned person allow for a greater percent increase in heart rate during exercise. This greater capacity to increase heart rate, coupled with a greater capacity to enhance stroke volume, permits a conditioned individual to achieve maximal cardiac outputs that can be 50% higher than those found in sedentary people. Another important distinction between a sedentary and conditioned person is that for a given workload, the conditioned person has a lower heart rate. Furthermore, a conditioned person is able to sustain higher workloads for a longer duration and recover from the exercise much more rapidly.

**Environmental conditions** can significantly alter cardiovascular responses to exercise. High altitudes, for example, decrease maximal stroke volume and cardiac output. The reason for this is that arterial $PO_2$ and oxygen content are reduced at higher elevations because of decreased atmospheric pressure. This decreases oxygen delivery to tissues, particularly to contracting muscle (both skeletal and cardiac), thereby resulting in insufficient oxygenation at lower workloads. Myocardial hypoxia decreases maximal inotropy, which results in reduced stroke volume. Reduced oxygen delivery to exercising muscle reduces exercise capacity in the muscle and results in increased production of lactic acid as the muscle switches over to anaerobic metabolism in the absence of adequate oxygen; that is, the anaerobic threshold is reached at a lower workload.

Increased temperature and humidity affect cardiovascular responses during exercise by diverting a greater fraction of cardiac output to the skin to enhance heat removal from the body. This decreases the availability of blood flow for the contracting muscles. With elevated temperature and humidity, maximal cardiac output and oxygen consumption are reached at lower workloads, thereby reducing exercise capacity as well as endurance. Furthermore, dehydration can accompany high temperatures. Dehydration reduces blood volume and central venous pressure, which attenuates the normal increase in cardiac output associated with exercise. This can lead to a fall in arterial pressure and heat exhaustion. Signs of **heat exhaustion** include general fatigue, muscle weakness, nausea, and mental confusion; it usually results from dehydration and loss of sodium chloride associated with physical activity in a hot environment—core temperature is not necessarily elevated.

**Increased age** reduces maximal exercise capacity. Maximal oxygen consumption decreases about 40% between 20 and 70 years of age. There are many reasons for this decline. With increasing age, maximal heart rate decreases. Maximal heart rate is approximately 220 beats/min minus the age of a person. Therefore, the maximal heart rate of a 70-year-old person is about 25% lower than the maximal heart rate of a 20-year-old person. Increasing age also reduces maximal stroke volume because of impaired ventricular filling (decreased ventricular compliance) and reduced inotropic responsiveness to sympathetic stimulation. Together, these changes reduce maximal cardiac output substantially. Older individuals have reduced skeletal muscle mass as well as decreased maximal muscle blood flow per unit weight of muscle. A reduction in vasodilatory capacity of resistance vessels in skeletal muscle in older persons may be related to reduced endothelial production or bioavailability of nitric oxide and altered vascular smooth muscle responsiveness to metabolic vasodilators. Although increasing age inevitably limits exercise capacity, exercise habits and general health can significantly influence the decline in maximal cardiac output with age.

**Gender** influences cardiovascular responses to exercise. Generally, males can reach and sustain significantly higher workloads and maximal oxygen consumptions than can females. Maximal cardiac outputs are about 25% less in females, although the maximal heart rates are similar. This difference is partly owing to increased skeletal muscle mass and to increased cardiac mass in males.

Finally, **cardiac disease** can significantly limit exercise capacity. As described later in this chapter, diseases that impair cardiac function (e.g., heart failure) can limit the ability of the heart to increase cardiac output during physical activity. Arrhythmias, such as atrial fibrillation or AV nodal block, can reduce exercise capacity by decreasing maximal cardiac output.

## MATERNAL CHANGES IN CARDIOVASCULAR FUNCTION DURING PREGNANCY

Pregnancy causes significant changes in the cardiovascular system (Fig. 9.3). Increased uterine mass and the developing fetus require large amounts of blood flow. To supply this flow, cardiac output increases by 30% to 50% during the first and second trimesters and then plateaus during the third trimester. In the first half of the pregnancy, the cardiac output is primarily increased through

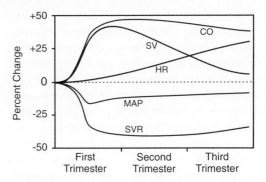

■ **FIGURE 9.3** Changes in maternal hemodynamics during pregnancy. Early in the course of pregnancy, cardiac output (*CO*) increases because stroke volume (*SV*) increases owing to an increase in blood volume; systemic vascular resistance (*SVR*) and mean arterial pressure (*MAP*) decrease. Heart rate (*HR*) gradually increases throughout pregnancy; SV declines as HR increases.

increases in stroke volume. By the third trimester, however, stroke volume may be only slightly elevated. At this stage of pregnancy, the increased cardiac output is sustained by an elevated heart rate, which may increase by 10 to 20 beats/min.

Cardiac output increases because blood volume (and therefore ventricular preload) increases dramatically during pregnancy. By week 6, blood volume may be increased by 10%. By the end of the third trimester, blood volume may be increased by 50%. The increase in blood volume is brought about by estrogen-mediated activation of the renin-angiotensin-aldosterone system, which increases sodium and water retention by the kidneys.

Although cardiac output is elevated, mean arterial pressure generally falls owing to a disproportionate decrease in systemic vascular resistance. The fall in systemic vascular resistance may be caused in part by hormonal changes that dilate resistance vessels; however, the major factor contributing to the reduced resistance is the development of low-resistance uterine circulation, particularly in the later stages of pregnancy. Diastolic pressure falls more than systolic pressure because of reduced systemic vascular resistance, so there is an increase in pulse pressure. Increased pulse pressure results from the increase in stroke volume during the first and second trimesters.

Pregnancy significantly alters the cardiovascular responses to exercise. Because cardiac output at rest is substantially elevated, there is less capacity for it to increase during exercise. In addition, compression of the inferior vena cava caused by an elevated intra-abdominal pressure, particularly during the third trimester, limits venous return and thereby prevents stroke volume from increasing as it normally would during exercise. Compression of the inferior vena cava, especially in the supine position, can also diminish venous return at rest, thereby reducing cardiac output and arterial pressure (supine hypotensive syndrome).

## HYPOTENSION

### Causes of Hypotension

Hypotension is often defined clinically as a systolic arterial pressure <90 mm Hg, or a diastolic pressure <60 mm Hg. There are many causes of hypotension as summarized in Figure 9.4. Because arterial pressure is the product of cardiac output and systemic

vascular resistance, a decrease in either will reduce arterial pressure (see Chapter 5).

A reduction in systemic vascular tone or impaired vasoconstrictor responsiveness to baroreceptor reflexes can lead to hypotension. For example, **septic shock** (or Systemic Inflammatory Response Syndrome, SIRS), which usually results from a bacterial infection in the blood, causes a loss of vascular tone and hypotension. Septic shock is caused by the release of bacterial endotoxins (e.g., lipopolysaccharide) that activate the inflammatory cascade. This leads to the production of cytokines (e.g., tumor necrosis factor, interleukins) and excessive amounts of nitric oxide, causing systemic vasodilation. Severe allergic reactions can lead to **anaphylactic shock**. Another cause of vasodilatory circulatory shock is damage to the spinal cord sympathetic tracts (**neurogenic shock**) resulting in loss of vascular sympathetic tone. Systemic vascular resistance can also be decreased if **autonomic dysfunction** occurs. For example, in diabetic individuals having autonomic neuropathy, baroreceptor-mediated reflex

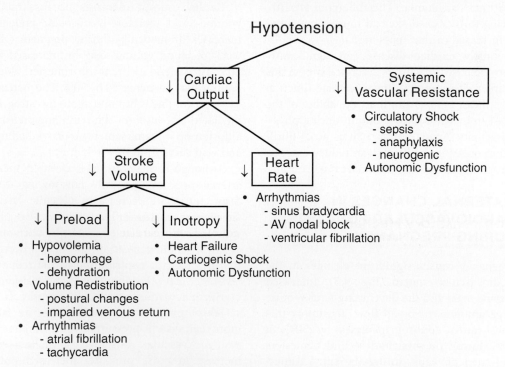

**■ FIGURE 9.4** Mechanisms and causes of hypotension. Ultimately, hypotension occurs because there is a reduction in cardiac output, systemic vascular resistance, or both.

vasoconstriction may be impaired, which can result in a fall in arterial pressure when the person stands up (**orthostatic hypotension**) and when the person exercises.

Hypotension can also occur when cardiac output is reduced by a decrease in either heart rate or stroke volume. Ventricular rate can be reduced by **sinus bradycardia**, which may be caused by excessive vagal activation of the SA node. A **vasovagal reflex** can lower heart rate and arterial pressure sufficiently to cause syncope (see Chapter 6). Second- and third-degree **AV nodal blockade** (see Chapter 2) reduce ventricular rate. **Ventricular fibrillation** prevents coordinated ventricular beats so the effective ventricular rate is zero.

Stroke volume can be reduced by decreases in either inotropy or ventricular filling (preload) (see Chapter 4). Reduced inotropy occurs during **heart failure** (systolic failure) or when autonomic dysfunction decreases sympathetic outflow to the heart. A sudden loss of mechanical efficacy by the heart, as occurs following acute ischemic damage (e.g., myocardial infarction), is a frequent cause of **cardiogenic shock**. Decreased preload can be caused by several conditions: (1) **hypovolemia**, which results from blood loss (hemorrhage) or dehydration; (2) a redistribution of blood volume, as occurs when a person stands up (**orthostatic hypotension**; see Chapter 5); (3) reduced venous return, which can result from compression of the vena cava (e.g., **supine hypotensive syndrome** during pregnancy); and (4) **tachyarrhythmias**, such as atrial fibrillation and ventricular tachycardia, which reduce ventricular filling.

## Compensatory Mechanisms during Hypotension

When hypotension occurs, the body attempts to restore arterial pressure by activating neurohumoral compensatory mechanisms (see Chapter 6). Initial, short-term mechanisms involve baroreceptor reflex activation of sympathetic nerves, which constrict systemic vascular beds and stimulate the heart. More slowly activated, long-term compensatory mechanisms include the renin-angiotensin-aldosterone system and

vasopressin. These hormone systems serve to increase blood volume and reinforce the vasoconstriction caused by increased sympathetic activity. Neurohumoral compensatory mechanisms increase arterial pressure and thereby help to maintain normal cerebral and coronary perfusion at the expense of reduced blood flow to less essential organs. The following discussion specifically addresses compensatory mechanisms in hypotension caused by hemorrhage-induced hypovolemia.

The fall in blood volume during hemorrhage reduces central venous pressure, which reduces cardiac filling and stroke volume through the Frank-Starling mechanism. The fall in cardiac output causes the arterial pressure fall. The baroreceptor reflex is the first compensatory mechanism to become activated in response to blood loss (Fig. 9.5). This reflex occurs within seconds of a fall in arterial pressure. As described in Chapter 6, a reduction in mean arterial pressure and arterial pulse pressure decreases the firing of arterial baroreceptors. This activates the sympathetic nervous system and inhibits vagal influences to the heart, thereby increasing heart rate and inotropy. It is important to note that cardiac stimulation alone does not lead to a significant increase in cardiac output. For cardiac output to increase, some mechanism must increase central venous pressure and therefore filling pressure for the ventricles. This is accomplished, at least initially following hemorrhage, by an increase in venous tone produced by sympathetic stimulation of the venous capacitance vessels. The partially restored central venous pressure increases stroke volume through the Frank-Starling mechanism. The increased preload, coupled with cardiac stimulation, attenuates the decline in cardiac output. The partially compensated cardiac output along with systemic vasoconstriction causes the arterial pressure to increase toward its normal value.

Although the baroreceptor reflex can respond quickly to a fall in arterial pressure and provide initial compensation, the long-term recovery of cardiovascular homeostasis requires activation of hormonal compensatory mechanisms to restore blood volume through

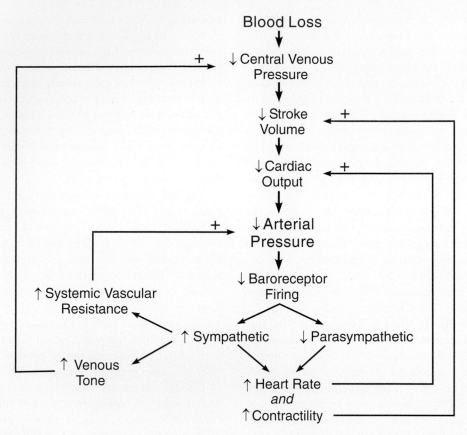

■ **FIGURE 9.5** Activation of baroreceptor mechanisms following acute blood loss (hemorrhage). Blood loss reduces central venous pressure (cardiac preload), which decreases cardiac output and arterial pressure. Reduced firing of arterial baroreceptors activates the sympathetic nervous system, which stimulates cardiac function, and constricts resistance and capacitance vessels. These actions help to elevate (+) the reduced central venous pressure, stroke volume, cardiac output, and arterial pressure, and thereby help to restore arterial pressure.

renal mechanisms (Fig. 9.6). Some of these humoral systems also reinforce the baroreceptor reflex by causing cardiac stimulation and vasoconstriction.

The renin-angiotensin-aldosterone system is activated by increased renal sympathetic nerve activity and renal artery hypotension via decreased sodium delivery to the macula densa, which releases renin leading to the formation of angiotensin II (see Chapter 6). Increased circulating angiotensin II constricts the systemic vasculature directly by binding to $AT_1$ receptors and indirectly by enhancing sympathetic effects. Angiotensin II stimulates aldosterone secretion. Vasopressin secretion is stimulated by reduced atrial stretch, sympathetic stimulation, and angiotensin II.

Working together, angiotensin II, aldosterone, and vasopressin cause the kidneys to retain sodium and water, thereby increasing blood volume, cardiac preload and cardiac output. Increased vasopressin also stimulates thirst so that more fluid is ingested. The renal and vascular responses to these hormones are further enhanced by decreased secretion of atrial natriuretic peptide by the atria, resulting from decreased atrial stretch associated with the hypovolemic state.

The vascular responses to angiotensin II and vasopressin occur rapidly in response to increased plasma concentrations of these vasoconstrictors. The renal effects of angiotensin II, aldosterone, and vasopressin, in contrast, occur more slowly as decreased sodium and

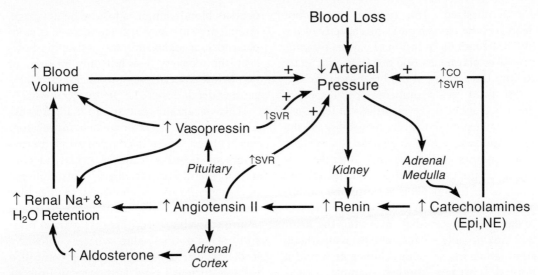

**■ FIGURE 9.6** Activation of humoral mechanisms following acute blood loss (hemorrhage). Decreased arterial pressure activates the sympathetic nervous system (baroreceptor reflex), which stimulates catecholamine release (*Epi*, epinephrine; *NE*, norepinephrine) from the adrenal medulla. This increases cardiac output (*CO*) and systemic vascular resistance (*SVR*), which elevates (+) arterial pressure. Renin release is stimulated by the enhanced sympathetic activity, increased circulating catecholamines, and hypotension; this leads to the formation of angiotensin II and aldosterone. Vasopressin release from the posterior pituitary is stimulated by angiotensin II, reduced atrial pressure (not shown), and increased sympathetic activity (not shown). These hormones act together to increase blood volume through their renal actions (sodium and water retention), which elevates arterial pressure. Angiotensin II and vasopressin also elevate arterial pressure by increasing SVR. These changes in systemic vascular resistance, blood volume, and cardiac output thereby help to restore the arterial pressure.

water excretion gradually increases blood volume over several hours and days.

Enhanced sympathetic activity stimulates the adrenal medulla to release catecholamines (epinephrine and norepinephrine). This causes cardiac stimulation ($\beta_1$-adrenoceptor mediated) and peripheral vasoconstriction ($\alpha$-adrenoceptor mediated), and contributes to the release of renin by the kidneys through renal $\beta$-adrenoceptors.

Other mechanisms besides the baroreceptor reflex and hormones have a compensatory role in hemorrhagic hypotension. Severe hypotension can lead to activation of chemoreceptors (see Chapter 6). Low perfusion pressures and reduced organ blood flow cause increased production of lactic acid as organs are required to switch over to anaerobic glycolysis for the production of ATP. Acidosis stimulates peripheral and central chemoreceptors, leading to increased sympathetic activity to the systemic vasculature. Stagnant hypoxia

in the carotid body chemoreceptors, which results from reduced carotid body blood flow, stimulates chemoreceptor firing. If cerebral perfusion becomes impaired and the brain becomes ischemic, intense sympathetic-mediated vasoconstriction of the systemic vasculature will result.

Reduced arterial and venous pressures, coupled with a decrease in the post-to-precapillary resistance ratio, decreases capillary hydrostatic pressures (see Chapter 8). This leads to enhanced capillary fluid reabsorption. This mechanism can result in up to 1 L/h of fluid being reabsorbed back into the intravascular compartment, which can lead to a significant increase in blood volume and arterial pressure after a few hours. Although capillary fluid reabsorption increases intravascular volume and serves to increase arterial pressure, it also leads to a reduction in hematocrit and dilution of plasma proteins until new blood cells and plasma proteins are synthesized. The reduced hematocrit decreases the oxygen-carrying capacity of the blood. Eventually, dilution of plasma proteins decreases plasma oncotic pressure sufficiently to limit the amount of fluid reabsorption.

Most of the compensatory responses described above occur regardless of the cause of hypotension; however, the ability of the heart and vasculature to respond to a specific compensatory mechanism may differ depending upon the cause of the hypotension. For example, if hypotension is caused by cardiogenic shock (a form of acute heart failure) secondary to a myocardial infarction, the heart will not be able to respond to sympathetic stimulation in the same manner as would a normal heart. As another example, vascular responsiveness to sympathetic-mediated vasoconstriction is significantly impaired in a person in septic shock. Finally, drugs that a person is taking for hypertension (e.g., beta-blockers, alpha-blockers, ACE inhibitors) can interfere with neurohumoral compensatory responses to hypotension.

---

**CASE 9-2**

A patient who is being aggressively treated for severe hypertension with a diuretic, an angiotensin-converting enzyme (ACE) inhibitor, and a calcium channel blocker is in a serious automobile accident that causes significant intra-abdominal bleeding. How might these drugs affect the compensatory mechanisms that are activated following hemorrhage? How might this alter the course of this patient's recovery?

---

## Decompensatory Mechanisms Following Severe and Prolonged Hypotension

Severe, prolonged hypotension can lead to irreversible shock and death. This occurs when normal compensatory mechanisms (and additional medical resuscitation) are unable to restore arterial pressure to adequate levels in a timely manner. For example, if 40% of a person's blood volume is lost by hemorrhage, arterial pressure may begin to recover as compensatory mechanisms are activated; however, the recovery may last only an hour or two before arterial pressure once again falls, causing death despite heroic interventions.

This secondary fall in arterial pressure results from the activation of decompensatory mechanisms. These decompensatory mechanisms are **positive feedback** cycles, in contrast to the negative feedback control offered by compensatory mechanisms. A negative feedback mechanism attempts to restore a controlled variable (in this case arterial pressure) to its normal value, whereas a positive feedback mechanism causes the controlled variable to move even farther away from its control point.

In the case of severe hemorrhagic shock and some other forms of hypotensive shock (e.g., cardiogenic and septic shock), several potential positive feedback mechanisms can lead to irreversible shock and death. These mechanisms include cardiac depression, sympathetic escape, metabolic acidosis, cerebral ischemia, rheological factors, and systemic inflammatory responses.

Figure 9.7 illustrates how cardiac depression and sympathetic escape can lead to decompensation in severe hemorrhage. If mean arterial pressure falls below 60 mm Hg, coronary blood flow is insufficient to support the metabolic demands of the heart because this pressure is below the coronary autoregulatory range (see Chapter 7). Reduced coronary blood flow causes myocardial hypoxia, which impairs cardiac contractions (reduces inotropy). When this occurs, stroke volume and cardiac output decrease, causing additional decreases in arterial pressure and coronary perfusion—a positive feedback cycle. Also shown in Figure 9.7 is the effect of hypotension on organ blood flow. Hypotension decreases organ blood flow by decreasing perfusion pressure and through baroreceptor-mediated sympathetic activation that constricts resistance vessels. This reduced flow causes tissue hypoxia. The more hypoxic a tissue becomes and the longer it remains hypoxic (especially under low flow

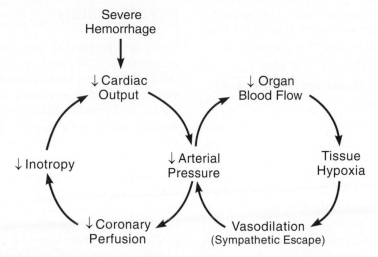

■ **FIGURE 9.7** Positive feedback decompensatory mechanisms triggered by severe hypotension. Impairment of coronary perfusion leads to a loss in cardiac inotropy and an additional decrease in cardiac output and pressure. Prolonged tissue ischemia (reduced blood flow) and hypoxia caused by hypotension and sympathetic vasoconstriction lead to vasodilation (sympathetic escape), which reduces systemic vascular resistance and arterial pressure.

conditions), the greater the buildup of vasodilator metabolites. These metabolites eventually override the sympathetic-mediated vasoconstriction (sympathetic escape), and blood flow begins to increase within the organ. When this sympathetic escape occurs within major organs of the body (e.g., skeletal muscle and gastrointestinal tract), systemic vascular resistance falls. This reduces arterial pressure and further reduces organ perfusion, which leads to further vasodilation and hypotension—a positive feedback cycle.

Several other positive feedback cycles can contribute to irreversible shock:

- Prolonged hypotension with accompanying tissue hypoxia results in metabolic acidosis as organs begin to generate ATP by anaerobic pathways. Acidosis impairs cardiac contraction and vascular smooth muscle contraction, which decreases cardiac output and systemic vascular resistance, thereby lowering arterial pressure even more.
- Cerebral ischemia and hypoxia during severe hypotension, although initially causing strong sympathetic activation, eventually results in depression of all autonomic outflow as the cardiovascular

regulatory centers cease to function because of the lack of oxygen. This withdrawal of sympathetic tone causes arterial pressure to fall, which further reduces cerebral perfusion.

- Reduced organ perfusion during hypotension and intense sympathetic vasoconstriction causes increased blood viscosity within the microcirculation, microvascular plugging by leukocytes and platelets, and disseminated intravascular coagulation. Low-flow states within the microcirculation cause red blood cells to adhere to each other, which increases the viscosity of the blood. Furthermore, low-flow states enhance leukocyte–endothelial adhesion and platelet–platelet adhesion. This reduces organ perfusion even more and can lead to ischemic damage and stimulation of inflammatory processes, which can further enhance metabolic acidosis and impair cardiac and vascular function.

In summary, the body responds to hypotension by activating neurohumoral mechanisms that serve as negative feedback, compensatory mechanisms to restore arterial pressure. With severe hypotension, positive feedback control mechanisms may become operative. These mechanisms counteract the compensatory mechanisms and eventually lead to an additional reduction in arterial pressure.

## Physiologic Basis for Therapeutic Intervention

Treatment for hypotension depends upon the underlying cause of the hypotension. If hypotension is caused by hypovolemia owing to hemorrhage or excessive fluid loss (e.g., dehydration), increasing blood volume by administration of blood or fluids becomes a treatment priority. Restoring blood volume increases preload on the heart and thereby increases cardiac output, which is reduced in hypovolemic states. Administration of fluids is occasionally accompanied by the administration of pressor agents. These drugs increase arterial pressure by increasing systemic vascular resistance (e.g., α-adrenoceptor agonists such as norepinephrine and phenylephrine; or vasopressin) or by stimulating cardiac function (e.g., β-adrenoceptor agonists such as dobutamine). Treatment of hypotension caused by cardiogenic shock can include drugs that stimulate the heart (e.g., β-adrenoceptor agonists such as dobutamine or dopamine, or cAMP-dependent phosphodiesterase inhibitors such as milrinone that inhibit the degradation of cAMP); however, depending upon the magnitude of the hypotension, either pressor or depressor agents may be used. Because the primary cause of hypotension in cardiogenic shock is impaired cardiac function, drugs such as phosphodiesterase inhibitors that stimulate the heart and dilate arterial vessels can improve cardiac function by enhancing inotropy and decreasing afterload on the heart. Systemic vasodilators, however, cannot be used alone if the hypotension is severe, because arterial pressure may fall further. Hypotension associated with septic shock results from systemic vasodilation and, in its later stages, cardiac depression. Therefore, pressor agents are commonly used with this form of shock in addition to administration of fluid and antibiotics.

## HYPERTENSION

High blood pressure (hypertension) is a condition that afflicts about one-third of American adults and is a leading cause of morbidity and mortality. Hypertension is much more than a "cardiovascular disease" because it can damage other organs such as kidney, brain, and eye. One-third of hypertensive people are not aware of being hypertensive because it is usually asymptomatic until the damaging effects of hypertension (such as stroke, myocardial infarction, renal dysfunction, visual disturbances, etc.) are observed.

The term "hypertension" is applied to elevations in diastolic or systolic pressures above normal values. Normal arterial pressure is defined as a systolic pressure <120 mm Hg (but >90 mm Hg) and diastolic pressure <80 mm Hg (but >60 mm Hg). Diastolic pressures of 80 to 89 mm Hg and systolic pressures of 120 to 139 mm Hg are considered prehypertension. Hypertension is defined as diastolic or systolic pressures ≥90 or 140 mm Hg, respectively. Both diastolic and systolic hypertension have been shown to be significant risk factors for causing other cardiovascular disorders such as stroke and myocardial infarction. Mean arterial pressure is usually not discussed in the context of hypertension because it is not normally measured in a patient.

Chronic hypertension is caused by increases in systemic vascular resistance and cardiac output. The elevation in cardiac output is normally caused by an increase in blood volume, which increases ventricular preload and stroke volume. It is important to note that to sustain a hypertensive state it is necessary to increase blood volume through renal retention of sodium and water. Evidence for this comes from studies showing that elevations in arterial pressure produced by infusing a vasoconstrictor drug for several days are not sustained because of **pressure natriuresis** in the kidneys. When renal artery pressure is elevated by increasing systemic vascular resistance, the kidneys respond by increasing glomerular filtration and excretion of sodium and water. The loss of sodium and water decreases blood volume and restores pressure after a day to two despite continued infusion of the vasoconstrictor. Therefore, with normal renal function, an acute elevation in arterial pressure caused by increasing systemic vascular resistance (or by stimulating the heart) is compensated by a reduction in blood volume, which restores the arterial pressure to normal.

Considerable evidence shows that in chronic hypertension, the renal pressure natriuresis curve is shifted to the right so that a higher arterial pressure is required to maintain sodium balance. The elevated pressure is sustained by an increase in blood volume. These changes in renal handling of sodium and water can be brought about by changes in sympathetic activity and hormones that affect renal function (e.g., angiotensin II, aldosterone, vasopressin). In addition, altered kidney filtration and sodium balance in renal disease can shift the pressure natriuresis curve to the right, leading to an increase in blood volume and sustained hypertension.

## Essential (Primary) Hypertension

Essential (or primary) hypertension accounts for approximately 90% to 95% of patients

| TABLE 9-3 **CAUSES OF HYPERTENSION** |
|---|
| **Essential hypertension** (90%–95%) |
| • Unknown causes |
| • Involves: |
|   - increased blood volume |
|   - increased systemic vascular resistance (vascular disease) |
| • Associated with: |
|   - heredity |
|   - abnormal response to stress |
|   - diabetes and obesity |
|   - age, race, and socioeconomic status |
| **Secondary hypertension** (5%–10%) |
| • Renal artery stenosis |
| • Renal disease |
| • Hyperaldosteronism (primary) |
| • Pheochromocytoma (catecholamine-secreting tumor) |
| • Aortic coarctation |
| • Pregnancy (preeclampsia) |
| • Hyperthyroidism/hypothyroidism |
| • Cushing syndrome (excessive glucocorticoid secretion) |
| • Sleep apnea |

diagnosed with hypertension (Table 9-3). This diagnosis is made after known causes of hypertension (i.e., secondary hypertension) are eliminated. Therefore, essential hypertension is a diagnosis by exclusion. Despite many years of research, no unifying hypothesis accounts for the pathogenesis of essential hypertension. However, a natural progression of this disease suggests that early elevations in blood volume and cardiac output might precede and then initiate subsequent increases in systemic vascular resistance. This has led some investigators to suggest that the basic underlying defect in hypertensive patients is an inability of the kidneys to adequately handle sodium. Increased sodium retention could account for the increase in blood volume. Indeed, many excellent experimental studies as well as clinical observations have shown that impaired renal natriuresis (sodium excretion) can lead to chronic hypertension.

Besides the renal involvement in hypertension, it is well known that vascular changes can contribute to hypertensive states, especially in the presence of impaired renal function. For example, essential hypertension is usually associated with increased systemic vascular resistance caused by a thickening of the walls of resistance vessels and by a reduction in lumen diameters. In some forms of hypertension, this is mediated by enhanced sympathetic activity or by increased circulating levels of angiotensin II, causing smooth muscle contraction and vascular hypertrophy. Experimental studies have suggested that changes in vascular endothelial function may cause these vascular changes. For example, in hypertensive patients, the vascular endothelium produces less nitric oxide. Nitric oxide, besides being a powerful vasodilator, inhibits vascular hypertrophy. Increased endothelin-1 production may enhance vascular tone and induce hypertrophy. Evidence suggests that hyperinsulinemia and hyperglycemia in type 2 diabetes (non–insulin-dependent diabetes) cause endothelial dysfunction through increased formation of reactive oxygen species and decreased nitric oxide bioavailability, both of which may contribute to the abnormal vascular function and hypertension often associated with diabetes.

Essential hypertension is related to heredity, age, race, and socioeconomic status. The strong hereditary correlation may be related to genetic abnormalities in renal function and neurohumoral control mechanisms. The incidence of essential hypertension increases with age, and people of African descent are more likely to develop hypertension than are Caucasians. Hypertension is more prevalent among lower socioeconomic groups.

Some patients with essential hypertension are more strongly influenced by stressful conditions than are normotensive individuals. Stress not only leads to acute elevations in arterial pressure, but it can also lead to chronic elevations in pressure. Stress activates the sympathetic nervous system, which increases cardiac output and systemic vascular resistance. Furthermore, stress causes the adrenal medulla to secrete more catecholamines (epinephrine and norepinephrine) than normal. Sympathetic activation increases circulating angiotensin II, aldosterone, and vasopressin, which together can increase systemic vascular resistance and, through their renal effects, increase sodium and water retention. In addition, prolonged elevation of angiotensin II and catecholamines leads to vascular and cardiac hypertrophy.

## Secondary Hypertension

Secondary hypertension accounts for 5% to 10% of hypertensive cases. This form of hypertension has identifiable causes that often can be remedied. Regardless of the underlying cause, arterial pressure becomes elevated through an increase in cardiac output, an increase in systemic vascular resistance, or both. When cardiac output is elevated, it is often related to increased blood volume and neurohumoral activation of the heart. Several causes of secondary hypertension are summarized in Table 9-3 and discussed below.

**Renal artery stenosis** occurs when the renal artery becomes narrowed (stenotic) owing to atherosclerotic or fibromuscular lesions. This reduces the pressure at the afferent arteriole, which stimulates the release of renin by the kidney (see Chapter 6). Increased plasma renin activity increases circulating angiotensin II and aldosterone. Angiotensin II causes vasoconstriction by binding to vascular $AT_1$ receptors and by augmenting sympathetic influences. Furthermore, angiotensin II along with aldosterone increases renal sodium and water reabsorption. The net effect of the renal actions is an increase in blood volume that augments cardiac output by the Frank-Starling mechanism. In addition, chronic elevation of angiotensin II promotes cardiac and vascular hypertrophy. Therefore, hypertension caused by renal artery stenosis is associated with increases in cardiac output and systemic vascular resistance.

**Renal disease** (e.g., diabetic nephropathy, glomerulonephritis) damages nephrons in the kidney. When this occurs, the kidney cannot excrete normal amounts of sodium, and the pressure natriuresis curve shifts to the right, which leads to sodium and water retention, increased blood volume, and increased cardiac output. Renal disease may increase the release of renin, leading to a renin-dependent form of hypertension. The elevation in arterial pressure secondary to renal disease can be viewed as an attempt by the kidney to increase renal perfusion, thereby restoring normal glomerular filtration and sodium excretion.

**Primary hyperaldosteronism** is increased secretion of aldosterone by an adrenal adenoma or adrenal hyperplasia. This condition causes renal retention of sodium and water, thereby increasing blood volume and arterial pressure. Aldosterone acts upon the distal convoluted tubule and cortical collecting duct of the kidney to increase sodium reabsorption in exchange for potassium and hydrogen ion, which are excreted in the urine. Plasma renin levels generally are decreased as the body attempts to suppress the renin-angiotensin system. In addition, hypokalemia is associated with the high levels of aldosterone.

A **pheochromocytoma** (a catecholamine-secreting tumor, usually in the adrenal medulla) can cause high levels of circulating catecholamines (both epinephrine and norepinephrine). A pheochromocytoma is diagnosed by measuring plasma or urine catecholamine levels and their metabolites (vanillylmandelic acid and metanephrine). This condition leads to α-adrenoceptor-mediated systemic vasoconstriction and $\beta_1$-adrenoceptor-mediated cardiac stimulation that can cause substantial elevations in arterial pressure. Although arterial pressure rises to very high levels, tachycardia still occurs because of the direct effects of the catecholamines on the heart and vasculature. Excessive $\beta_1$-adrenoceptor stimulation in the heart often leads to arrhythmias in addition to the hypertension.

Aortic coarctation is a narrowing of the aortic arch usually just distal to the left subclavian artery. It is a congenital defect that obstructs aortic outflow, leading to elevated pressures proximal to the coarctation (i.e., elevated arterial pressures in the head and arms). Distal pressures, however, are not necessarily reduced as would be expected from the hemodynamics associated with a stenosis. The reason for this is that reduced systemic blood flow, and in particular reduced renal blood flow, leads to an increase in the release of renin and an activation of the renin-angiotensin-aldosterone system. This in turn elevates blood volume and arterial pressure. Although the aortic arch and carotid sinus baroreceptors are exposed to higher-than-normal pressures, the baroreceptor reflex is blunted owing to structural changes in the walls of vessels where the baroreceptors are located. Furthermore, baroreceptors become desensitized to chronic elevation in pressure and become "reset" to the higher pressure.

Preeclampsia is a type of hypertension that occurs in about 5% of pregnancies during late second and third trimesters. Preeclampsia differs from less severe forms of pregnancy-induced hypertension (gestational hypertension) in that preeclampsia is associated with a loss of albumin in the urine because of renal damage, and pulmonary and systemic edema. Preeclampsia is also associated with increased vascular responsiveness to vasoconstrictors, which can lead to vasospasm. It is unclear why some women develop this condition during pregnancy; however, it usually disappears after parturition unless an underlying hypertensive condition exists.

Hyperthyroidism induces systemic vasoconstriction, an increase in blood volume, and increased cardiac activity, all of which can lead to hypertension. It is less clear why some patients with hypothyroidism also develop hypertension, but it may be related to decreased tissue metabolism reducing the release of vasodilator metabolites, thereby producing vasoconstriction and increased systemic vascular resistance.

Cushing syndrome, which results from excessive glucocorticoid secretion, can lead to hypertension. Glucocorticoids such as cortisol, which are secreted by the adrenal cortex, share some of the same physiologic properties as aldosterone, a mineralocorticoid also secreted by the adrenal cortex. Therefore, excessive glucocorticoids can lead to volume expansion and hypertension.

Sleep apnea is a disorder in which people repeatedly stop breathing for short periods of time (10 to 30 seconds) during their sleep; this can occur dozens of times per hour. Breathing is most commonly interrupted by airway obstruction, and less commonly by disorders of the central nervous system. This condition is often associated with obesity. Individuals suffering from sleep apnea have a higher incidence of hypertension. The mechanism of hypertension may be related to sympathetic activation and hormonal changes associated with repeated periods of apnea-induced hypoxia and hypercapnia, and from stress associated with the loss of sleep.

## Physiologic Basis for Therapeutic Intervention

If a person has secondary hypertension, it is sometimes possible to correct the underlying cause. For example, renal artery stenosis can be corrected by placing a wire stent within the renal artery to maintain vessel patency; aortic coarctation can be surgically corrected; a pheochromocytoma can be removed. However, for the majority of people who have essential hypertension, the cause is unknown, so it cannot be targeted for correction. Therefore, the therapeutic approach for these patients involves modifying the factors that determine arterial pressure by using drugs.

Because hypertension results from an increase in cardiac output and increased systemic vascular resistance, these are the two physiologic mechanisms that are targeted in drug therapy. In most hypertensive patients, altered renal function causes sodium and water retention. This increases blood volume, cardiac output, and arterial pressure. Therefore, the most common treatment for hypertension is the use of a diuretic to stimulate renal excretion of sodium and water. This reduces blood volume and arterial pressure very effectively in many patients. In addition to a diuretic, most hypertensive patients are given at least one other drug. This is because decreasing blood volume with a diuretic leads to activation of the renin-angiotensin-aldosterone system, which counteracts the effects of the diuretic. Therefore, these patients may be given an ACE inhibitor or angiotensin receptor blocker (ARB) as well.

In addition to using diuretics, cardiac output can be reduced using beta-blockers and the more cardioselective calcium channel blockers (e.g., verapamil). Beta-blockers are particularly useful in patients who may have excessive sympathetic stimulation caused by emotional stress, and these drugs also inhibit sympathetic-mediated release of renin.

In combination with a diuretic, some hypertensive patients can be effectively treated with an α-adrenoceptor antagonist, which dilates resistance vessels and reduces systemic vascular resistance. Other drugs that reduce systemic vascular resistance include ACE inhibitors, ARBs, calcium channel blockers (especially dihydropyridines), and direct-acting arterial dilators such as hydralazine.

Although pharmacologic intervention is an important therapeutic modality in treating hypertension, improved diet and exercise have been shown to be effective in reducing arterial pressure in many patients. A proper, balanced diet that includes sodium restriction can prevent the progression of, and in some cases reverse, cardiovascular changes associated with hypertension. Regular exercise, especially aerobic exercise, reduces arterial pressure and has beneficial effects on vascular function.

## HEART FAILURE

Heart failure occurs when the heart is unable to supply adequate blood flow and therefore oxygen delivery to peripheral tissues and organs, or to do so only at elevated filling pressures. Heart failure most commonly involves the left ventricle. Right ventricular failure, although sometimes found alone or in association with pulmonary disease, more often occurs secondary to left ventricular failure. Mild heart failure is manifested as reduced exercise capacity and the development of shortness of breath during physical activity (**exertional dyspnea**). In more severe forms of heart failure, a patient may have virtually no capacity for physical exertion and will experience dyspnea even while at rest. Furthermore, the patient will likely have significant pulmonary or systemic edema.

### Causes of Heart Failure

Heart failure can be caused by factors originating from the heart (i.e., intrinsic disease or pathology) or from external factors that place excessive demands upon the heart. The number-one cause of heart failure is coronary artery disease, which reduces coronary blood flow and oxygen delivery to the myocardium, thereby causing myocardial hypoxia and impaired function. A related common cause of heart failure is myocardial infarction. Infarcted tissue does not contribute to the generation of mechanical activity, and noninfarcted regions must compensate for the loss of function. Over time, the additional demands placed upon the noninfarcted tissue can cause functional changes leading to failure. Other heart conditions that can lead to failure include:

- Valvular disease and congenital defects, which place increased demands upon the heart
- Cardiomyopathies (intrinsic diseases of the myocardium) of known origin (e.g., bacterial

or viral; alcohol-induced) or unknown origin (idiopathic)

- Infective or noninfective myocarditis (inflammation of the myocardium)
- Chronic arrhythmias

External factors precipitating heart failure include increased afterload (pressure load; e.g., uncontrolled hypertension), increased stroke volume (volume load; e.g., arterial–venous shunts), and increased body demands (high output failure; e.g., thyrotoxicosis, pregnancy).

## Systolic versus Diastolic Dysfunction

Heart failure can result from impaired ability of the heart muscle to contract (**systolic failure**) or impaired filling of the heart (**diastolic failure**). Systolic failure is caused by changes in cellular signal transduction mechanisms and excitation–contraction coupling that impair inotropy (see Chapter 3). Functionally, this causes a downward shift in the Frank-Starling curve (Fig. 9.8). This decreases stroke volume and causes a compensatory rise in preload (clinically assessed as increased ventricular end-diastolic pressure or volume, or increased pulmonary capillary wedge pressure). Increased preload is an important compensatory mechanism because it activates the

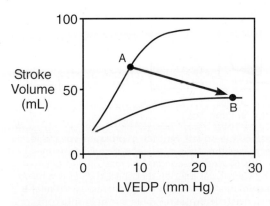

■ **FIGURE 9.8** Effects of systolic failure on left ventricular Frank-Starling curves. Systolic failure depresses the Frank-Starling curve, which decreases stroke volume and leads to an increase in ventricular preload (*LVEDP*, left ventricular end-diastolic pressure). Point *A*, control point; point *B*, systolic failure.

Frank-Starling mechanism to help maintain stroke volume despite the loss of inotropy. If preload did not undergo a compensatory increase, the decline in stroke volume would be even greater for a given loss of inotropy. As systolic failure progresses, the ability of the heart to compensate by the Frank-Starling mechanism becomes exhausted as sarcomeres stretch to their maximal length. Furthermore, with chronic systolic failure, the ventricle anatomically remodels by dilating. This is achieved by new sarcomeres being added in series to existing sarcomeres. Increased wall circumference with the addition of new sarcomere units prevents the individual sarcomeres from overstretching in the presence of elevated filling pressures and volumes. The dilated ventricle has increased compliance so that it can accommodate large end-diastolic volumes without excessive increases in end-diastolic pressure (see Fig. 4.5).

The effects of a loss of inotropy on stroke volume, end-diastolic volume, and end-systolic volume can be depicted using ventricular pressure–volume loops (Fig. 9.9, panel A) (the concept of pressure–volume loops was developed in Chapter 4; see Fig. 4.4). Systolic failure decreases the slope of the end-systolic pressure–volume relationship, which occurs because of reduced inotropy. Because of this change, at any given ventricular volume, less pressure can be generated during systole, and therefore, less volume can be ejected. This leads to an increase in end-systolic volume. The pressure–volume loop also shows that the end-diastolic volume increases (compensatory increase in preload). Ventricular preload increases because as the heart loses its ability to eject blood, more blood remains in the ventricle at the end of ejection. This results in the ventricle filling to a larger end-diastolic volume as venous return enters the ventricle. Increased ventricular filling is enhanced by ventricular remodeling that enlarges the chamber size (ventricular dilation) and increases compliance. This permits larger end-diastolic volumes with smaller increases in end-diastolic pressure, although this pressure can still rise to levels that lead to blood backing up into the left atrium and

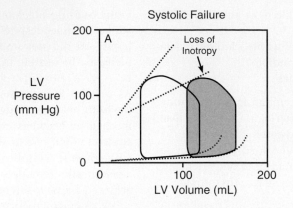

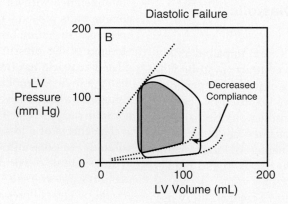

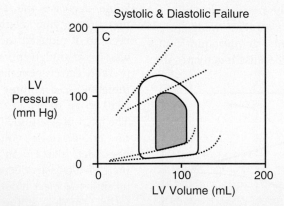

■ **FIGURE 9.9** Effects of systolic, diastolic, and combined failure on left ventricular pressure–volume loops. **Panel A** shows that systolic failure (loss of inotropy) decreases the slope of the end-systolic pressure–volume relationship and increases end-systolic volume. This causes a secondary increase in end-diastolic volume, which is augmented under chronic conditions by ventricular dilation that shifts the passive filling curve down and to the right. The net effect is that stroke volume and ejection fraction decrease. **Panel B** shows that diastolic failure increases the slope of the end-diastolic pressure–volume relationship (passive filling curve) because of reduced ventricular compliance caused by either hypertrophy or decreased lusitropy. This reduces the end-diastolic volume and increases end-diastolic pressure. End-systolic volume may decrease slightly as a result of reduced afterload. The net effect is reduced stroke volume; ejection fraction may or may not change. **Panel C** shows that combined systolic and diastolic failure reduces end-diastolic volume and increases end-systolic volume so that stroke volume is greatly reduced; end-diastolic pressure may become very high.

pulmonary vasculature, leading to pulmonary edema. The increase in end-diastolic volume, however, is not as great as the increase in end-systolic volume. Therefore, the net effect is a decrease in stroke volume (decreased width of the pressure–volume loop). Because stroke volume decreases and end-diastolic volume increases, a substantial reduction in ejection fraction occurs. Ejection fraction (stroke volume divided by end-diastolic volume) is normally >55%, but it can fall below 20% in severe systolic failure.

The second type of heart failure is diastolic failure, which is caused by impaired ventricular filling. Diastolic failure can be caused by either decreased ventricular compliance (e.g., as occurs with ventricular hypertrophy; see Chapter 4) or impaired relaxation (decreased lusitropy; see Chapter 3). Ventricular hypertrophy most commonly is caused by chronic, uncontrolled hypertension, which results in a thickening of the ventricular wall as new sarcomeres are added in parallel to existing sarcomeres. The hypertrophy enables the heart to contract more forcefully against the higher pressure in the aorta and helps to normalize wall stress (see Equation 4-2). Therefore, a hypertrophied heart may exhibit a leftward shift in the end-systolic pressure-volume relationship (not shown in Fig. 9.9, panel B). Other causes of diastolic failure include hypertrophic cardiomyopathy, a disease resulting from a genetic defect that alters myocardial structure. Normal age-related changes to cardiac structure can make the ventricle less compliant, leading to impaired ventricular filling in the elderly population.

Reduced ventricular compliance, whether of anatomic or physiologic origin, shifts the ventricular end-diastolic pressure–volume relationship (i.e., passive filling curve) up and to the left (Fig. 9.9, panel B). This results in less ventricular filling (decreased end-diastolic volume) and a greater end-diastolic pressure. Stroke volume, therefore, decreases. Depending upon the relative change in stroke volume and end-diastolic volume, ejection fraction may or may not change. For this reason, reduced ejection fraction is useful only as an indicator of systolic failure.

Increased ventricular end-diastolic pressure, which can exceed 30 mm Hg in left ventricular failure, can have serious clinical consequences because left atrial and pulmonary capillary pressures rise. Pulmonary edema can occur when the left ventricular end-diastolic pressure exceeds 20 mm Hg. If the right ventricle is in diastolic failure, the increase in end-diastolic pressure is reflected back into the right atrium and systemic venous vasculature. This can lead to peripheral edema and abdominal ascites.

It is not uncommon in chronic heart failure to have a combination of both systolic and diastolic dysfunction to varying degrees (Fig. 9.9, panel C). With both systolic and diastolic dysfunction, the slope of the end-systolic pressure–volume relationship is decreased, and the slope of the passive filling curve is increased. This causes a dramatic reduction in stroke volume because end-systolic volume is increased and end-diastolic volume is decreased. This combination of systolic and diastolic dysfunction can lead to high end-diastolic pressures that can cause pulmonary congestion and edema.

## Systemic Compensatory Mechanisms in Heart Failure

Heart failure, whether systolic or diastolic in nature, leads to a reduction in stroke volume and cardiac output. In the absence of compensatory mechanisms, a fall in cardiac output has two effects on pressure: decreased arterial pressure and increased central venous pressure (see Fig. 5.18). These changes activate neurohumoral mechanisms that attempt to restore cardiac output and arterial pressure (Fig. 9.10).

In response to an acute reduction in cardiac output and arterial pressure, decreased firing of arterial baroreceptors activates the sympathetic adrenergic nerves to the heart and vasculature. The baroreceptor reflex responds mainly to acute changes in arterial pressure and therefore cannot be responsible for maintaining the increased sympathetic drive when hypotension accompanies chronic heart failure. In addition, not all patients in chronic heart failure are hypotensive. It is not

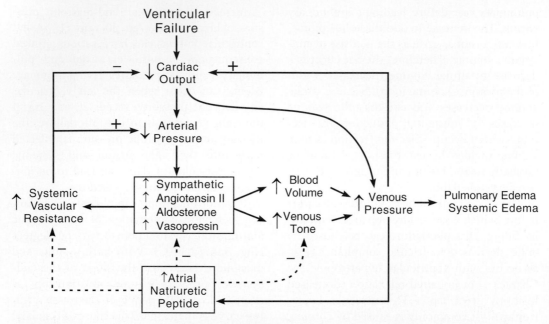

■ **FIGURE 9.10** Summary of neurohumoral changes associated with heart failure. Activation of the sympathetic nervous system, the renin-angiotensin-aldosterone system, and vasopressin cause an increase in systemic vascular resistance, blood volume, and central venous pressure. Although increased central venous pressure helps to elevate (+) cardiac output by the Frank-Starling mechanism, it can also lead to pulmonary and systemic edema. The increased systemic vascular resistance, although helping to elevate arterial pressure, can depress (−) cardiac output further because of increased afterload. Increased atrial natriuretic peptide counterregulates the other hormonal systems.

clear what drives the characteristic increase in sympathetic activity in chronic heart failure, although humoral changes and cardiac stretch receptors may be involved, along with baroreceptor resetting.

Important humoral changes occur during heart failure to help compensate for the reduction in cardiac output. Arterial hypotension, along with sympathetic activation, stimulates renin release, leading to the formation of angiotensin II and aldosterone. Vasopressin (antidiuretic hormone) release from the posterior pituitary is also stimulated. Increased vasopressin release seems paradoxical because right atrial pressure is often elevated in heart failure, which should inhibit the release of vasopressin (see Chapter 6). It may be that vasopressin release is stimulated in heart failure by sympathetic activation and increased angiotensin II. Circulating catecholamines (norepinephrine and epinephrine) are also elevated in heart failure because of sympathetic stimulation of the adrenals and

spillover of norepinephrine into the circulation from highly activated sympathetic nerves.

These changes in neurohumoral status constrict resistance vessels, which causes an increase in systemic vascular resistance to help maintain arterial pressure. Venous capacitance vessels constrict as well. This increased venous tone contributes to the increase in venous pressure. Angiotensin II and aldosterone, along with vasopressin, increase blood volume by increasing renal reabsorption of sodium and water, which further increases venous pressure. The increased venous pressure increases cardiac preload and helps to maintain stroke volume through the Frank-Starling mechanism. Increased right atrial pressure stimulates the synthesis and release of atrial natriuretic peptide to counterregulate the renin-angiotensin-aldosterone system. These neurohumoral responses function as compensatory mechanisms, but they can aggravate heart failure by increasing ventricular afterload (which depresses stroke volume) and increasing venous pressures and cardiac preload to the point at which pulmonary or systemic congestion and edema occur. The volume and afterload increases also increase oxygen demand by the heart, which can further exacerbate ventricular failure over time.

## Exercise Limitations Imposed by Heart Failure

Heart failure can severely limit exercise capacity. In early or mild stages of heart failure, cardiac output and arterial pressure may be normal at rest because of compensatory mechanisms. When the person in heart failure begins to perform physical work, however, the maximal workload is reduced, and he or she experiences fatigue and dyspnea at less than normal maximal workloads.

A comparison of exercise responses in a normal person and in a heart failure patient is shown in Table 9-4. In this example, the degree of heart failure is moderate to severe. At rest, the person with congestive heart failure (CHF) has reduced cardiac output (decreased 29%) caused by a 38% decrease in stroke volume. Mean arterial pressure is slightly decreased, and resting heart rate is elevated. Whole-body oxygen consumption is normal at rest, but the reduced cardiac output results in an increase in the arterial–venous oxygen difference as more oxygen is extracted from the blood because organ blood flow is reduced. At a maximally tolerated exercise workload, the CHF patient

can increase cardiac output by only 50%, compared to a 221% increase in the normal person. The reduced cardiac output is a consequence of the inability of the left ventricle to augment stroke volume as well as a lower maximal heart rate (exercise intolerance limits the heart rate increase). The CHF patient has a significant reduction in arterial pressure during exercise in contrast to the normal person's increase in arterial pressure. Arterial pressure falls because the increase in cardiac output is not sufficient to maintain arterial pressure as the systemic vascular resistance falls during exercise. The maximal whole-body oxygen consumption is greatly reduced in the CHF patient because reduced perfusion of the active muscles limits oxygen delivery and therefore the oxygen consumption of the muscles. The CHF patient experiences substantial fatigue and dyspnea during exertion, which limits the patient's ability to sustain the physical activity.

Some of the neurohumoral compensatory mechanisms that operate to maintain resting cardiac output in heart failure contribute to limiting exercise capacity. The chronic increase in sympathetic activity to the heart down-regulates $\beta_1$-adrenoceptors, which reduces the heart's chronotropic and inotropic responses to acute sympathetic activation during exercise. Increased sympathetic activity (and possibly circulating vasoconstrictors) to the skeletal muscle vasculature limits the degree of vasodilation during muscle contraction. This limits oxygen delivery to the working

| TABLE 9-4 | COMPARISON OF CARDIOVASCULAR FUNCTION IN A NORMAL PERSON AND A PATIENT WITH MODERATE-TO-SEVERE CHF AT REST AND AT MAXIMAL (MAX) EXERCISE | | | | | |
|---|---|---|---|---|---|---|
| | Co (L/Min) | Hr (Beats/Min) | Sv (Ml) | Map (Mm Hg) | Vo$_2$ (Ml O$_2$/Min) | CaO$_2$–CvO$_2$ (Ml O$_2$/100 Ml) |
| Normal (Rest) | 5.6 | 70 | 80 | 95 | 220 | 4.0 |
| Normal (Max) | 18.0 | 170 | 106 | 120 | 2500 | 13.9 |
| CHF (Rest) | 4.0 | 80 | 50 | 90 | 220 | 5.5 |
| CHF (Max) | 6.0 | 120 | 50 | 85 | 780 | 13.0 |

CO, cardiac output; HR, heart rate; SV, stroke volume; MAP, mean arterial pressure; VO$_2$, whole-body oxygen consumption; CaO$_2$–CvO$_2$, arterial–venous oxygen difference. VO$_2$ is calculated from the product of CO and CaO$_2$–CvO$_2$, after the units for CO are converted to mL/min and the units for CaO$_2$–CvO$_2$ are converted to mL O$_2$/mL blood.

muscle and leads to increased oxygen extraction (increased arterial–venous oxygen difference), enhanced lactic acid production (and a lower anaerobic threshold), and muscle fatigue at lower workloads. The increase in blood volume, although helping to maintain stroke volume at rest through the Frank-Starling mechanism, decreases the reserve capacity of the heart to increase preload during exercise.

## Physiologic Basis for Therapeutic Intervention

Therapeutic goals in the pharmacologic treatment of heart failure include (1) reducing the clinical symptoms of edema and dyspnea; (2) improving cardiovascular function to enhance organ perfusion and increase exercise capacity; and (3) reducing mortality.

Four pharmacologic approaches are taken to achieve these goals. The first approach is to reduce venous pressure to decrease edema and help relieve the patient of dyspnea. Diuretics are routinely used to reduce blood volume by increasing renal excretion of sodium and water. Drugs that dilate the venous vasculature (e.g., ACE inhibitors) also can reduce venous pressure. Judicious use of these drugs to decrease blood volume and venous pressure does not significantly reduce stroke volume because the Frank-Starling curve associated with systolic failure is relatively flat at left ventricular end-diastolic pressures above 15 mm Hg (see Fig. 9.8).

The second approach is to use drugs that reduce afterload on the ventricle by dilating the systemic vasculature. Drugs such as ACE inhibitors and ARBs have proven to be useful in this regard for patients with chronic heart failure. Decreasing the afterload on the ventricle can significantly enhance stroke volume and ejection fraction, which secondarily reduces ventricular end-diastolic volume (preload). Because arterial vasodilators enhance cardiac output in heart failure patients, the reduction in systemic vascular resistance does not usually lead to an unacceptable fall in arterial pressure. Vasodilators also have the benefit of decreasing myocardial oxygen demand.

The third approach is to use drugs that stimulate ventricular inotropy. A commonly used drug is digoxin, which inhibits the $Na^+/K^+$-ATPase and thereby increases intracellular calcium (see Chapter 2). This drug, however, has not been shown to reduce mortality associated with heart failure. Drugs that stimulate $\beta_1$-adrenoceptors (e.g., dobutamine) or inhibit cAMP-dependent phosphodiesterase (e.g., milrinone) are sometimes used as inotropic agents (see Chapter 3). With the exception of digoxin, inotropic drugs are used only in acute heart failure and end-stage failure because their long-term use has been shown to be deleterious to the heart.

The fourth therapeutic approach involves using beta-blockers. Although this might seem counterintuitive, many clinical trials have clearly demonstrated the efficacy of some beta-blockers (e.g., carvedilol and metoprolol). The mechanism of their efficacy is not clear, but it is known that long-term sympathetic activation of the heart is deleterious. Therefore, beta-blockers probably work by reducing the deleterious actions of long-term sympathetic activation. Beta-blockers (as well as ACE inhibitors) provide long-term benefit through ventricular remodeling (e.g., reducing ventricular hypertrophy or dilation). Furthermore, $\beta$-blockers significantly reduce mortality in heart failure.

It should be noted that vasodilators, inotropic drugs, and $\beta$-blockers are nearly always used in combination with a diuretic.

---

**CASE 9-3**

A patient is diagnosed with dilated cardiomyopathy. The echocardiogram shows substantial left ventricular dilation (end-diastolic volume is 240 mL) and an ejection fraction of 20%; the arterial pressure is 115/70 mm Hg. Calculate the stroke volume and end-systolic volume. How would combined therapy with an ACE inhibitor and diuretic alter ventricular volumes, ejection fraction, and arterial pressure?

## VALVE DISEASE

Normal valve function as described in Chapter 4 is characterized as having (1) low pressure gradients across the valve as blood flows through the orifice and (2) unidirectional flow. These normal features are altered when heart valves function abnormally. When this occurs, net ventricular outflow can decrease, leading to a fall in cardiac output and clinical signs of heart failure.

There are two general categories of valve defects: stenosis and insufficiency. **Valve stenosis** results from a narrowing of the valve orifice. Fibrosis, often accompanied by calcification, causes the valve leaflets to thicken so that they cannot open fully, which decreases cross-sectional area of the open orifice. Furthermore, the valve cusps can fuse together, which prevents them from fully opening. Congenital valve defects can also produce stenosis. **Valve regurgitation** (insufficiency) occurs when the valve leaflets do not completely seal when the valve is closed; this causes blood to flow backward (regurgitate) into the proximal chamber. Both of these valve defects alter intracardiac pressures and volumes during the cardiac cycle.

Valve defects produce murmurs that can be heard with a stethoscope. A murmur is a rumbling or rasping sound caused by vibrations generated by the abnormal movement of blood within or between cardiac chambers, or by turbulent flow within the pulmonary artery or aorta just distal to the outflow valve. If a murmur is heard during systole between the first ($S_1$) and second ($S_2$) heart sounds, it is termed a **systolic murmur**. If it is heard during diastole (between $S_2$ and $S_1$), it is termed a **diastolic murmur**. The sound intensifies with increasing flow and turbulence across the valve.

The following sections describe pressure and volume changes that occur during valve stenosis and regurgitation. Because valve disease is generally a chronic problem, neurohumoral activation and cardiac remodeling occur in an attempt to maintain normal cardiac output and arterial pressure. These compensatory responses include systemic vasoconstriction, increased blood volume, and increased heart rate and inotropy. Cardiac remodeling involves hypertrophy or dilation, depending on the valve defect. When these compensatory mechanisms fail to maintain cardiac output and arterial pressure within normal limits (termed "decompensation"), the patient develops symptoms of heart failure as described in the previous section.

The following discussion examines cardiac changes during valve disease in the absence of significant heart failure at rest, therefore representing compensated conditions.

### Valve Stenosis

Stenosis can occur at either an outflow valve (aortic or pulmonic valve) or inflow valve (mitral or tricuspid valve). Stenosis increases the resistance to flow across the valve, which causes a high pressure gradient across the valve. The pressure gradient across a valve is the pressure difference on either side of the leaflets as blood is flowing through the valve. For the aortic valve, the pressure gradient is the left ventricular pressure minus the aortic pressure; for the mitral valve, the pressure gradient is the left atrial pressure minus the left ventricular pressure. In normal valves, the pressure gradient is only a few mm Hg when blood is flowing across the open valve.

The following equation is the general hemodynamic expression that relates pressure gradient ($\Delta P$), flow (F), and resistance (R) under laminar, nonturbulent flow conditions:

$$\Delta P = F \cdot R$$

A reduced valve orifice increases the resistance to flow across the valve because resistance is inversely related to the radius (r) of the valve orifice to fourth power (equivalent to valve orifice area [A] to the second power because $A = \pi r^2$) (see Chapter 5). Therefore, the above equation can also be expressed as:

$$\Delta P \propto \frac{F}{A^2}$$

Using the above relationship, if the valve orifice area is reduced by 75%, the valve resistance is increased 16-fold, which increases the pressure gradient 16-fold if flow through the valve remains unchanged. In reality, the formation of turbulence increases the pressure gradient across the valve even further. Turbulence occurs because a reduced orifice area leads to an increase in the velocity of blood flow across the valve. Because flow (F) equals the product of velocity (V) and area (A), the velocity equals flow divided by area (V = F/A). Therefore, if flow remains unchanged, a 75% reduction in area causes a fourfold increase in velocity, which increases turbulence and produces a murmur. In summary, at a given flow across a valve, a reduction in valve orifice area increases the pressure gradient across the valve that is required to drive the flow, increases the velocity of flow, and increases the turbulence.

## AORTIC VALVE STENOSIS

In aortic valve stenosis, left ventricular pressure is increased above normal during systole to eject blood across the narrowed valve (Fig. 9.11, left panel). This leads to a large pressure gradient across the valve during ejection, the magnitude of which depends on the degree of stenosis and the flow across the valve. Increased flow velocity through the stenotic valve causes turbulence and a systolic murmur. In moderate-to-severe aortic stenosis, the aortic pressure may be reduced because ventricular stroke volume (and cardiac output) is reduced. The degree of hypotension depends on the ability of neurohumoral mechanisms to increase blood volume and systemic vascular resistance. Because ejection is impeded by the increase in ventricular afterload, more blood remains in the heart after ejection, which leads to an increase in left atrial volume and pressure.

Changes in left ventricular pressure–volume loops with moderate aortic stenosis are shown in Figure 9.11 (right panel). Because left ventricular emptying is impaired by the increased afterload (see Chapter 4), the stroke volume is reduced, which leads to an increase in end-systolic volume. With chronic aortic stenosis, the left ventricle hypertrophies. This decreases ventricular compliance, elevates end-diastolic pressure,

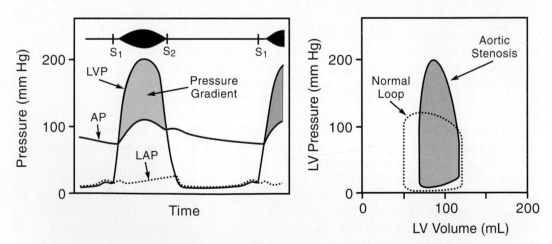

■ **FIGURE 9.11** Changes in cardiac pressures and volumes associated with chronic aortic valve stenosis in the absence of systolic failure. The **left panel** shows that during ventricular ejection, left ventricular pressure (*LVP*) exceeds aortic pressure (*AP*) (the gray area represents the pressure gradient generated by the stenosis); a systolic murmur is present between S$_1$ and S$_2$, and left atrial pressure (*LAP*) is elevated. Aortic pressure may be reduced because of decreased stroke volume. The **right panel** shows the effects of aortic valve stenosis (*red loop*) on the left ventricular (*LV*) pressure–volume loop. The end-systolic volume is increased, with little or no change in end-diastolic volume; therefore, stroke volume is decreased. Ventricular hypertrophy reduces ventricular compliance, which elevates end-diastolic pressure at any given end-diastolic volume.

and may impair filling (i.e., produces diastolic dysfunction). This is shown in the pressure–volume loop as an elevated and steeper filling curve (see Figs. 4.5 and 9.9). Whether end-diastolic volume is increased or decreased depends on the changes in compliance and filling pressure. Recall from Chapter 4 that an acute increase in afterload, which initially leads to an increase in end-systolic volume, usually causes a secondary increase in end-diastolic volume that helps to preserve stroke volume. But in chronic aortic stenosis, this secondary increase in preload often will not occur because of the reduced ventricular compliance.

In summary, aortic valve stenosis is characterized by a large pressure gradient across the aortic valve during systole, a systolic ejection murmur, reduced stroke volume, ventricular hypertrophy (reduced compliance), increased left ventricular filling pressure, and increased left atrial and pulmonary vascular pressures.

## MITRAL VALVE STENOSIS

Mitral valve stenosis increases the pressure gradient across the mitral valve during ventricular filling, which leads to an increase in left atrial pressure and a reduction in left ventricular filling pressure (Fig. 9.12, left panel). During ventricular filling, turbulence caused by the narrowed mitral valve causes a diastolic murmur. In moderate-to-severe mitral stenosis, reduced ventricular filling causes a reduction in ventricular preload (both end-diastolic volume and pressure decrease) (Fig. 9.12, right panel). This leads to a decrease in stroke volume (width of pressure–volume loop) through the Frank-Starling mechanism, and a fall in cardiac output and aortic pressure. Reduced afterload (particularly if aortic pressure falls) enables the end-systolic volume to decrease slightly, but not enough to overcome the decline in end-diastolic volume. These changes will be influenced by neurohumoral activation, which increases blood volume, systemic vascular resistance, cardiac inotropy, and heart rate.

In summary, mitral valve stenosis impairs ventricular filling, which reduces preload and therefore stroke volume. A diastolic murmur is present, and left atrial and pulmonary vascular pressures are elevated.

## PULMONIC AND TRICUSPID VALVE STENOSIS

Pulmonic stenosis produces changes to the right side of the heart that are analogous to

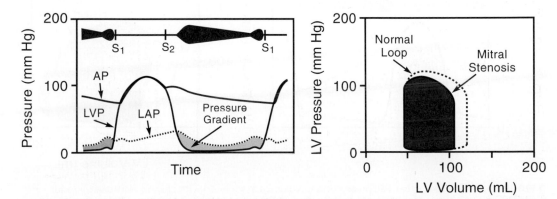

■ **FIGURE 9.12** Changes in cardiac pressures and volumes associated with chronic mitral valve stenosis in the absence of systolic failure. The **left panel** shows that during ventricular filling, left atrial pressure (*LAP*) exceeds left ventricular pressure (*LVP*) (the gray area represents the pressure gradient generated by the stenosis); a diastolic murmur is present between $S_2$ and $S_1$. Aortic pressure (*AP*) is reduced by severe mitral stenosis because of decreased cardiac output. The **right panel** shows the effects of mitral valve stenosis (*red loop*) on the left ventricular (*LV*) pressure–volume loop. End-diastolic volume is reduced because of impaired ventricular filling, and end-systolic volume may be slightly reduced because of reduced afterload; therefore, stroke volume is reduced.

those produced on the left side of the heart by aortic stenosis. Stenosis of the pulmonic valve results in a pressure gradient across that valve during right ventricular ejection, as well as a systolic murmur. Reduced right ventricular stroke volume decreases left ventricular filling and stroke volume, which leads to activation of neurohumoral compensatory mechanisms. The right ventricle hypertrophies, which contributes to elevated filling pressures that are transmitted back into the right atrium and systemic venous circulation.

Tricuspid stenosis impairs right ventricular filling and stroke volume, and elevates right atrial and systemic venous pressures. Because right ventricular output is reduced, left ventricular stroke volume is also diminished, which can trigger compensatory neurohumoral mechanisms. As with mitral stenosis, there is a diastolic murmur.

## Valve Regurgitation

Valvular insufficiency can occur with outflow valves (aortic or pulmonic) or inflow valves (mitral or tricuspid). In this condition, the valve does not close completely, which permits blood to flow backward (regurgitate) across the valve. Aortic or pulmonary insufficiency most commonly occurs through disease processes that alter valve structure. Mitral and tricuspid valve regurgitation can occur following rupture of the chordae tendineae, following ischemic damage to the papillary muscles, in response to infective or degenerative disease of the valve tissue, or when the ventricles are pathologically dilated (e.g., as occurs in dilated cardiomyopathy).

### AORTIC VALVE REGURGITATION

Aortic valve regurgitation causes blood to enter the left ventricle from the aorta (backward flow) during the time that the valve would normally be closed. Because blood leaves the aorta by two pathways (back into the ventricle as well as down the aorta), the aortic pressure falls more rapidly than usual during diastole, thereby reducing aortic diastolic pressure (Fig. 9.13, left panel). Ventricular (and aortic) peak systolic pressures are increased because there is an increase in stroke volume into the aorta because of increased ventricular filling. The increased systolic pressure and decreased

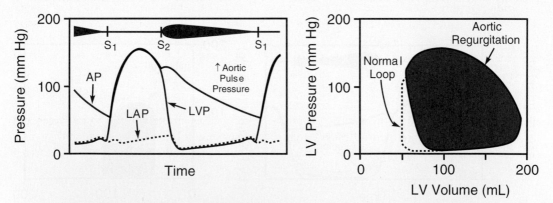

■ **FIGURE 9.13** Changes in cardiac pressures and volumes associated with chronic aortic valve regurgitation in the absence of systolic failure. The **left panel** shows that during ventricular relaxation, blood flows backwards from the aorta into the ventricle, causing a more rapid fall in aortic pressure (*AP*), which decreases diastolic pressure and increases aortic pulse pressure; left atrial pressure (*LAP*) increases because of blood backing up into the atrium as left ventricular end-diastolic volume and pressure increase. An increase in ventricular stroke volume (because of increased filling) leads to an increase in peak ventricular and aortic pressures; a diastolic murmur is present between $S_2$ and $S_1$. The **right panel** shows the effects of aortic valve regurgitation (*red loop*) on the left ventricular (*LV*) pressure–volume loop. End-diastolic volume and stroke volume are greatly increased, and there are no true isovolumetric phases because blood flows across the valve whenever there is a pressure difference across the valve.

diastolic pressure increase the aortic pulse pressure. The regurgitation, which takes place as the ventricle relaxes and fills, causes a diastolic murmur, which is louder early in diastole (decrescendo murmur).

Because of the backward flow of blood from the aorta into the left ventricle, there is no true phase of isovolumetric relaxation (see Fig. 9.13, right panel). Instead, the left ventricle begins to fill with blood from the aorta before the mitral valve opens. Once the mitral valve opens, ventricular filling occurs from the left atrium; however, blood continues to flow from the aorta into the ventricle throughout diastole because aortic pressure is higher than ventricular pressure during diastole. This greatly enhances ventricular filling (end-diastolic volume), which activates the Frank-Starling mechanism to increase the force of contraction and stroke volume as shown by the increased width of the pressure–volume loop. With chronic aortic regurgitation, the ventricle remodels by dilating, which increases compliance. This helps the ventricle to accommodate the large increase in volume without excessive increases in end-diastolic pressure. As long as the ventricle is not in failure, normal end-systolic volumes can be sustained; however, the end-systolic volume increases when the ventricle goes into systolic failure. Because the aortic valve never completely closes, blood will always be moving across the valve depending on the aortic and left ventricular pressure difference. Consequently, there is no true isovolumetric phase at the beginning of diastole or systole. When the ventricle first begins to contract, blood continues to enter the ventricle from the aorta until the ventricular pressure exceeds the aortic pressure. It is important to note that the stroke volume, calculated from the difference between the end-diastolic and end-systolic volumes, is increased. However, the net stroke volume into the aorta (net forward flow in the aorta) is lower than normal. For example, assume that stroke volume is normally 70 mL. During aortic regurgitation, the stroke volume calculated from the end-diastolic and end-systolic

volumes may be 120 mL. If half of that stroke volume flows backward into the ventricle (regurgitant fraction = 0.5), then the net outward stroke volume will be 60 mL, which is smaller than normal.

In summary, aortic valve insufficiency is characterized by an increase in aortic pulse pressure, a diastolic murmur, increased stroke volume but reduced net aortic flow, ventricular dilation, no true isovolumetric phases, increased ventricular filling pressure, and increased left atrial and pulmonary vascular pressures.

## MITRAL VALVE REGURGITATION

In mitral valve regurgitation, blood flows backward into the left atrium as the left ventricle contracts. This leads to a large increase in the v wave of the left atrial pressure tracing (Fig. 9.14, left panel) and the generation of a systolic murmur that spans briefly beyond $S_2$. Ventricular systolic and aortic pressures decrease if the net ejection of blood into the aorta is significantly reduced.

There are several important changes in the left ventricular pressure–volume loop in the presence of mitral insufficiency (Fig. 9.14, right panel). First, there is no true isovolumetric phase at the beginning of systole. As soon as the ventricle begins to contract and develop pressure, blood begins to flow across the mitral valve and back into the left atrium. Mitral regurgitation reduces the afterload on the left ventricle (total outflow resistance is reduced), which causes stroke volume to be larger and end-systolic volume to be smaller than normal; however, end-systolic volume increases if the heart goes into systolic failure in response to chronic mitral regurgitation. Because the mitral valve is never completely closed, blood flows back into the left atrium as long as intraventricular pressure is greater than left atrial pressure; therefore, there is no true phase of isovolumetric relaxation. During diastole, the elevated pressure within the left atrium is transmitted to the left ventricle during filling so that left ventricular end-diastolic pressure

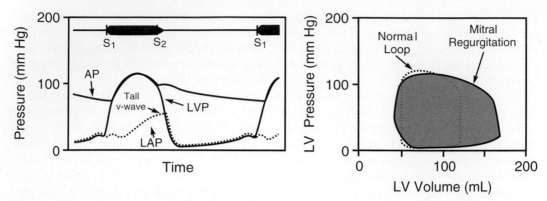

■ **FIGURE 9.14** Changes in cardiac pressures and volumes associated with chronic mitral valve regurgitation in the absence of systolic failure. The **left panel** shows that during ventricular contraction, the left ventricle ejects blood back into the left atrium as well as into the aorta, thereby increasing left atrial pressure (*LAP*), particularly the *v* wave. The aortic pressure (*AP*) and left ventricular pressure (*LAP*) may fall in response to a reduction in the net volume of blood ejected into the aorta; a systolic murmur is present between S$_1$ and just beyond S$_2$. The **right panel** shows the effects of mitral valve regurgitation (*red loop*) on the left ventricular (*LV*) pressure–volume loop. End-systolic volume is reduced because of decreased outflow resistance (afterload); end-diastolic volume is increased because increased left atrial pressure increases ventricular filling; stroke volume is greatly enhanced. There are no true isovolumetric phases because blood flows across the valve whenever there is a pressure difference across the valve.

and volume increase. In chronic mitral regurgitation, volume overload causes the ventricle to undergo dilation, thereby increasing its compliance. This dilation would cause wall stress (afterload) to increase if it were not for the reduced outflow resistance that tends to decrease afterload during ejection. The net effect of these changes is that the width of the pressure–volume loop (stroke volume) is increased; however, ejection into the aorta is reduced by the regurgitant fraction.

In summary, mitral regurgitation is characterized by a tall *v* wave, a systolic murmur, increased stroke volume but reduced net ventricular outflow into the aorta, ventricular dilation, no true isovolumetric phases, increased ventricular filling pressures, and increased left atrial and pulmonary vascular pressures.

### PULMONIC AND TRICUSPID VALVE REGURGITATION

Pulmonic regurgitation produces changes to the right side of the heart that are analogous to those produced on the left side of the heart by aortic regurgitation. Regurgitation across the pulmonic valve leads to increased pulmonary artery pulse pressure, increased right ventricular end-diastolic volume and pressure, and a diastolic murmur. There is no true isovolumetric phase during right ventricular systole and diastole. Because the right ventricle becomes volume overloaded, it responds by dilating, and right atrial and systemic venous pressures increase.

Tricuspid regurgitation causes a tall *v* wave in the right atrial pressure tracing, an overall increase in right atrial volume and systemic venous pressures, and a systolic murmur. Right ventricular stroke volume is increased, but ejection into the pulmonary artery may be reduced because of the large volume of blood ejected into the right atrium during ventricular systole. Reduced ejection into the pulmonary artery decreases left ventricular filling and stroke volume, leading to activation of neurohumoral compensatory mechanisms.

## SUMMARY OF IMPORTANT CONCEPTS

- Dynamic exercise such as running is associated with a large fall in systemic vascular resistance as active muscles dilate. To maintain (and elevate) arterial pressure, sympathetic activation and circulating hormones increase cardiac output and constrict blood vessels in other major organs of the body; the abdominothoracic and skeletal muscle pumps promote venous return to maintain adequate cardiac preload conditions.

- Cardiovascular responses to exercise are significantly influenced by the type of exercise (dynamic versus static), body posture, physical conditioning, environmental factors, age, gender, and the presence of heart disease.

- Pregnancy is associated with an increase in blood volume and cardiac output, and a decrease in systemic vascular resistance and mean arterial pressure; heart rate gradually increases during pregnancy.

- Arterial hypotension can result from mechanisms that reduce cardiac output or cause systemic vasodilation.

- Compensatory negative feedback mechanisms, triggered by hypotension, help to restore arterial pressure. Baroreceptor and renal mechanisms play a prominent role. Failure of these mechanisms and the expression of positive feedback mechanism lead to irreversible shock and death.

- Hypertension results from increased cardiac output, usually caused by increased blood volume, and from increased systemic vascular resistance. Essential hypertension is of unknown origin, whereas secondary hypertension results from identifiable causes such as renal disease, excessive sympathetic activation, or abnormal levels of hormones.

- Heart failure occurs when the heart is unable to supply adequate blood flow to organs, or when it is able to do so only at elevated filling pressures. It may involve systolic dysfunction (depressed ventricular inotropy) or diastolic dysfunction (impaired filling).

- The body compensates for heart failure by activating the sympathetic nervous system, renin-angiotensin-aldosterone system, and other circulating hormones. These compensatory mechanisms increase systemic vascular resistance, stimulate the heart, and increase blood volume.

- Structural defects in heart valves result in valve stenosis and/or regurgitation, which affect pressure and volume relationships within the heart during systole and diastole, and lead to reduced cardiac output and elevated venous pressures.

## REVIEW QUESTIONS

For each question, choose the one best answer:

1. During a moderate level of whole-body exercise (e.g., running),
   a. Arterial pulse pressure decreases owing to the elevated heart rate.
   b. Sympathetic-mediated vasoconstriction occurs in the skin.
   c. Systemic vascular resistance increases owing to sympathetic activation.
   d. Vagal influences on the sinoatrial node are inhibited.

2. One important reason why stroke volume is able to increase during running exercise is that

   a. Central venous pressure decreases.
   b. Heart rate increases.
   c. The rate of ventricular relaxation decreases.
   d. Venous return is enhanced by the muscle pump system.

3. In an exercise study, the subject's resting heart rate and left ventricular stroke volume were 70 beats/min and 80 mL/beat, respectively. While the subject was walking rapidly on a treadmill, the heart rate and stroke volume increased to 140 beats/min and 100 mL/beat, respectively; ejection fraction increased from 60% to 75%. The subject's mean arterial pressure increased from 90 mm Hg at rest to 110 mm Hg during exercise. One can conclude that

   a. Cardiac output doubled.
   b. Compared to rest, the cardiac output increased proportionately more during exercise than systemic vascular resistance decreased.
   c. Ventricular end-diastolic volume increased.
   d. The increase in mean arterial pressure during exercise indicates that systemic vascular resistance increased.

4. During the second trimester of pregnancy,

   a. Systemic vascular resistance is increased.
   b. Heart rate is decreased.
   c. Cardiac output is decreased.
   d. Blood volume is increased.

5. The baroreceptor reflex in hemorrhagic shock

   a. Decreases venous compliance.
   b. Decreases systemic vascular resistance.
   c. Increases vagal tone on the SA node.
   d. Stimulates angiotensin II release from the kidneys.

6. Long-term recovery of cardiovascular homeostasis following moderate hemorrhage involves

   a. Aldosterone inhibition of renin release.
   b. Enhanced renal loss (excretion) of sodium.
   c. Increased capillary fluid filtration.
   d. Vasopressin-mediated water reabsorption by the kidneys.

7. A trauma patient is admitted the Emergency Department following massive blood loss. The bleeding is controlled, and resuscitation with fluids and pressor agents elevates the mean arterial pressure to 60 mm Hg. Despite additional efforts to raise arterial pressure, the pressure begins to fall after 2 hours, and the patient dies. Which of the following most likely contributed to the cardiovascular collapse in this patient?

   a. Excessive fluid sodium and water retention by the kidneys
   b. Increased capillary fluid reabsorption
   c. Myocardial depression by metabolic acidosis
   d. Sympathetic-mediated vasoconstriction

8. A 43-year-old female patient consistently has arterial pressure values of about 150/105 mm Hg. This patient's hypertension could be the result of

   a. Diminished secretion of aldosterone.
   b. Excessive renal excretion of sodium.
   c. Suppressed release of renin.
   d. Thyroid disorder.

9. The echocardiogram report that you receive for your patient indicates that he has left ventricular diastolic dysfunction. Which of the following is usually associated with this condition?

   a. Increased ventricular compliance
   b. Elevated end-diastolic pressure
   c. Decreased end-systolic volume
   d. Large decrease in ejection fraction

10. Compared to the maximal exercise responses of a normal subject, a patient with moderate-to-severe heart failure during maximal exercise will have a
    a. Lower arterial pressure.
    b. Lower arterial–venous oxygen extraction.
    c. Higher ejection fraction.
    d. Similar maximal oxygen consumption.

11. A patient with a history of mild hypertension has recently been diagnosed with left ventricular systolic dysfunction associated with dilated cardiomyopathy. In addition to a diuretic, the patient is also prescribed a mixed arterial–venous dilator (e.g., an ACE inhibitor). The rationale for adding the vasodilator is that it will increase
    a. Stroke volume by increasing preload.
    b. Ventricular afterload by reducing preload.
    c. Ventricular ejection fraction by increasing stroke volume.
    d. Ventricular end-systolic volume by increasing stroke volume.

12. A patient is diagnosed with moderately severe aortic valve regurgitation. In the absence of ventricular failure, which of the following changes is associated with this valve defect?
    a. Aortic diastolic pressure is increased.
    b. Aortic systolic pressure is decreased.
    c. Left ventricular stroke volume into the aorta is increased.
    d. Left ventricular preload is decreased.

13. A patient is diagnosed with mitral valve stenosis with no evidence of systolic dysfunction. This patient will likely have
    a. A systolic murmur.
    b. Elevated left atrial pressure.
    c. Increased left ventricular end-diastolic pressure.
    d. Reduced left ventricular ejection fraction.

## ANSWERS TO REVIEW QUESTIONS

1. The correct answer is "d" because heart rate is increased during exercise through activation of sympathetic adrenergic nerves and inhibition of vagal (parasympathetic) nerves on the sinoatrial node. Choice "a" is incorrect because arterial pulse pressure increases during moderate exercise because of the increase in stroke volume. Choice "b" is incorrect because cutaneous vasodilation occurs during exercise to facilitate heat loss from the body. Choice "c" is incorrect because systemic vascular resistance falls owing to vasodilation in the active skeletal muscle.

2. The correct answer is "d" because the muscle pump system facilitates venous return, which maintains or elevates ventricular filling pressures. Choice "a" is incorrect because a decrease in central venous pressure would decrease stroke volume. Choice "b" is incorrect because an increase in heart rate, with no other compensatory changes, decreases stroke volume. Choice "c" is incorrect because the rate of ventricular relaxation (lusitropy) increases during exercise owing to sympathetic influences, which aids ventricular filling and enhances stroke volume.

3. The correct answer is "b" because arterial pressure increased; therefore, cardiac output must have increased more than systemic vascular resistance decreased because mean arterial pressure is approximately the product of cardiac output and systemic vascular resistance. Choice "a" is incorrect because cardiac output (the product of heart rate and stroke volume) increased from 5.6 to

14.0 L/min (i.e., it more than doubled). Choice "c" is incorrect because stroke volume increased by 25% (from 80 to 100 mL/beat), and the ejection fraction increased by 25% (from 60% to 75%). Therefore, end-diastolic volume could not have changed because ejection fraction equals stroke volume divided by end-diastolic volume. Choice "d" is incorrect because the percent change in cardiac output is much greater than the percent change in arterial pressure; the systemic vascular resistance can be approximated from the arterial pressure divided by the cardiac output.

4. The correct answer is "d" because activation of the renin-angiotensin-aldosterone system during pregnancy increases blood volume. Choice "a" is incorrect because systemic vascular resistance decreases during pregnancy owing to the developing uterine circulation. Choices "b" and "c" are incorrect because heart rate and cardiac output increase during pregnancy.

5. The correct answer is "a" because the baroreceptor reflex activates sympathetic adrenergic nerves that constrict arterial and venous vessels. Choice "b" is incorrect because sympathetic activation increases systemic vascular resistance. Choice "c" is incorrect because sympathetic activation is accompanied by withdrawal of vagal tone on the heart. Choice "d" is incorrect because renin, not angiotensin II, is released from the kidneys.

6. The correct answer is "d" because long-term recovery from hypovolemia requires renal retention of water, which is partially regulated by vasopressin. Choice "a" is incorrect because increased renin release and subsequent formation of angiotensin II and aldosterone contribute to renal reabsorption of sodium and water. Choice "b" is incorrect because sodium reabsorption, not loss, is enhanced following hemorrhage. Choice "c" is incorrect because increased capillary fluid filtration would decrease blood volume and not serve as a compensatory mechanism following hemorrhage.

7. The correct answer is "c" because reduced oxygen delivery to the peripheral organs stimulates anaerobic metabolism, leading to metabolic acidosis, which impairs cardiac contraction. Choices "a," "b," and "d" are incorrect because these are normal compensatory mechanisms that help to maintain arterial pressure following hemorrhage.

8. The correct answer is "d" because either hypothyroidism or hyperthyroidism can cause hypertension. Choices "a," "b," and "c" are incorrect because each of these can decrease blood volume, which would decrease arterial pressure.

9. The correct answer is "b" because diastolic dysfunction caused by decreased ventricular compliance (choice "a" is therefore incorrect) leads to an elevated end-diastolic pressure at any given end-diastolic volume. Choice "c" is incorrect because changes in end-systolic volume are normally associated with changes in systolic function. Choice "d" is incorrect because ejection fraction does not necessarily change much with diastolic dysfunction because reduced stroke volume is usually associated with reduced end-diastolic volume.

10. The correct answer is "a" because cardiac output is unable to increase sufficiently to maintain arterial pressure as systemic vascular resistance falls during exercise. Choice "b" is incorrect because reduced organ perfusion increases oxygen extraction from the arterial blood. Choice "c" is incorrect because impaired inotropic responses during exercise reduce ejection fraction. Choice "d" is incorrect because the heart failure patient achieves lower maximal oxygen consumption because maximal cardiac output is reduced.

11. The correct answer is "c" because reducing afterload increases stroke volume and reduces ventricular end-diastolic volume; these changes enhance ejection fraction. Choice "a" is incorrect because

the mixed vasodilator decreases preload as well as afterload. Choice "b" is incorrect because afterload is decreased. Choice "d" is incorrect because reducing afterload leads to a decrease in end-systolic volume, which increases in stroke volume.

12. The correct answer is "c" because ventricular filling (preload) is increased (choice "d" is therefore incorrect) because blood flows from the aorta back into the ventricle during diastole in aortic regurgitation; this increases the volume of blood ejected into the aorta, which increases aortic systolic pressure (choice "b" is therefore incorrect). Choice "a" is incorrect because the retrograde flow causes aortic pressure to fall more rapidly during diastole, which decreases the diastolic pressure.

13. The correct answer is "b" because with mitral stenosis, blood has difficulty flowing from the left atrium into the left ventricle. This leads to blood backing up into the left atrium and increasing its pressure. Choice "a" is incorrect because turbulence occurs as blood flows across the narrowed valve during diastole, thereby producing a diastolic murmur. Choice "c" is incorrect because left ventricular filling can be impaired, which decreases its end-diastolic volume and pressure. Choice "d" is incorrect because reduced ventricular filling is accompanied by a reduced stroke volume; therefore, ejection fraction does not change much.

ANSWERS TO CASES

## CASE 9-1

Autonomic neuropathy affects the function of most organ systems of the body because autonomic nerves play a vital role in regulating normal function. In the cardiovascular system, autonomic nerves, particularly sympathetic adrenergic nerves, regulate arterial pressure through their actions on the heart and vasculature. Patients with type 2 diabetes who have impaired autonomic control of the cardiovascular system may have abnormal responses to exercise because heart rate and inotropy may not increase normally, and sympathetic stimulation of the arterial and venous system may be impaired. This loss of sympathetic control may result in a fall in arterial pressure during exercise owing to a greater-than-normal reduction in systemic vascular resistance, a decrease in central venous pressure owing to loss of venous tone, and a reduction in cardiac output caused by smaller-than-normal increases in heart rate and stroke volume. Hypotension during exercise impairs muscle perfusion, causing fatigue. Decreased cerebral perfusion caused by hypotension can lead to dizziness, visual disturbances, and syncope.

## CASE 9-2

Recovery from hemorrhage partly involves arterial and venous constriction, cardiac stimulation, and renal retention of sodium and water. The diuretic would counter the normal renal compensatory mechanisms of sodium and water retention. The ACE inhibitor would reduce the formation of circulating angiotensin II that normally plays an important compensatory role through constricting blood vessels and increasing blood volume by enhancing renal reabsorption of sodium and water. The calcium channel blocker, depending upon its class, would depress cardiac function and cause systemic vasodilation, both of which would counteract normal compensatory responses to hemorrhage. These drugs, therefore, would impair and prolong the recovery process following hemorrhage.

Fortunately, many of these drugs have relatively short half-lives so that their effects diminish within several hours.

## CASE 9-3

Given that the ejection fraction is 20% and the end-diastolic volume is 240 mL, the stroke volume is 48 mL/beat using the following relationship: stroke volume = ejection fraction × end-diastolic volume. The end-systolic volume is the end-diastolic volume minus the stroke volume, which equals 192 mL. The administration of a diuretic would decrease the end-diastolic volume by decreasing blood volume. The ACE inhibitor, by reducing circulating angiotensin II and aldosterone, would reinforce the effects of the diuretic on the kidney and also cause dilation of resistance and capacitance vessels. These actions would further decrease end-diastolic pressure by decreasing venous pressure, and would reduce the afterload. This latter effect enhances stroke volume by decreasing the end-systolic volume and increasing the cardiac output. The increased stroke volume and decreased end-diastolic volume would cause the ejection fraction to increase. Although the ACE inhibitor would decrease systemic vascular resistance, the increased cardiac output might prevent arterial pressure from falling, or at least partially offset the pressure-lowering effect of systemic vasodilation.

## SUGGESTED RESOURCES

Chapman AB, Abraham WT, Zamudio S, et al. Temporal relationships between hormonal and hemodynamic changes in early human pregnancy. Kidney Int 1998;54:2056–2063.

Chobanian AV, Bakris GL, Black HR, et al. Joint National Committee on prevention, detection, evaluation, and treatment of high blood pressure: the JNC 7 report. JAMA 2003;289:2560–2572.

Hall JE. The kidney, hypertension, and obesity. Hypertension 2003;41:625–633.

Janicki JS, Sheriff DD, Robotham JL, Wise RA. Cardiac output during exercise: contributions of the cardiac, circulatory, and respiratory systems. In: Rowell LB, Shepherd JT, eds. Handbook of Physiology; Exercise: Regulation and Integration of Multiple Systems. New York: Oxford University Press, 1996.

Laughlin MH, Korthius RJ, Duncker DJ, Bache RJ. Control of blood flow to cardiac and skeletal muscle during exercise. In: Rowell LB, Shepherd JT, eds. Handbook of Physiology; Exercise: Regulation and Integration of Multiple Systems. New York: Oxford University Press, 1996.

Lilly LS. Pathophysiology of Heart Disease. 5th Ed. Philadelphia: Lippincott Williams & Wilkins, 2011.

Rowell LB, O'Leary DS, Kellogg DL: Integration of cardiovascular control systems in dynamic exercise In: Rowell LB, Shepherd JT, eds. Handbook of Physiology; Exercise: Regulation and Integration of Multiple Systems. New York: Oxford University Press, 1996.

Wei JY. Age and the cardiovascular system. N Engl J Med 1992;327:1735–1739.

# INDEX

Page numbers in *italics* denote figures; those followed by a t denote tables.